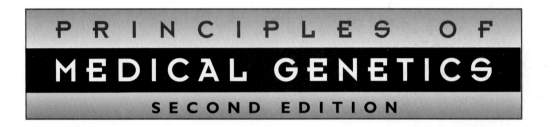

PRINCIPLES OF
MEDICAL GENETICS
SECOND EDITION

PRINCIPLES OF

MEDICAL GENETICS

SECOND EDITION

Thomas D. Gelehrter, M.D.

Professor and Chairman

Department of Human Genetics

Professor of Internal Medicine

University of Michigan Medical School

Ann Arbor, Michigan

Francis S. Collins, M.D., Ph.D.

Director

National Human Genome Research Institute

National Institutes of Health

Bethesda, Maryland

David Ginsburg, M.D.

Professor

Departments of Internal Medicine and Human Genetics

Investigator, Howard Hughes Medical Institute

The University of Michigan Medical School

Ann Arbor, Michigan

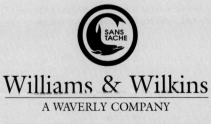

Williams & Wilkins

A WAVERLY COMPANY

BALTIMORE • PHILADELPHIA • LONDON • PARIS • BANGKOK
BUENOS AIRES • HONG KONG • MUNICH • SYDNEY • TOKYO • WROCLAW

Editor: Paul J. Kelly
Managing Editor: Crystal Taylor
Marketing Manager: Rebecca Himmelheber
Production Coordinator: Carol Eckhart
Project Editor: Jeffrey S. Myers
Designer: Dan Pfisterer
Illustration Planner: Ray Lowman
Illustrators: Mollie Dunker and Jacqueline A. Schaffer
Cover Designer: Karen Klinedinst
Typesetter: Peirce Graphic Services, Inc.
Printer and Binder: World Color

Copyright © 1998 Williams & Wilkins

351 West Camden Street
Baltimore, Maryland 21201-2436 USA

Rose Tree Corporate Center
1400 North Providence Road
Building II, Suite 5025
Media, Pennsylvania 19063-2043 USA

Accurate indications, adverse reactions and dosage schedules for drugs are provided in this book, but it is possible that they may change. The reader is urged to review the package information data of the manufacturers of the medications mentioned.

Printed in the United States of America
First Edition,1990

Library of Congress Cataloging-in-Publication Data

Gelehrter, Thomas D.
 Principles of medical genetics / Thomas D. Gelehrter, Francis S. Collins, David Ginsburg. —
2nd ed.
  p.   cm.
 Includes bibliographical references and index.
 ISBN (invalid) 0-683-03445-6
 1. Medical genetics. I. Collins, Francis S. II. Ginsburg, David, 1920– . III. Title.
 [DNLM: 1. Genetics, Medical. QZ 50 G316p 1997]
RB155.G358 1997
6169.042—dc21
DNLM/DLC
for Library of Congress   97-21931
                                                                      CIP

The publishers have made every effort to trace the copyright holders for borrowed material. If they have inadvertently overlooked any, they will be pleased to make the necessary arrangements at the first opportunity.

To purchase additional copies of this book, call our customer service department at (800) 638-0672 or fax orders to (800) 447-8438. For other book services, including chapter reprints and large quantity sales, ask for the Special Sales department.

Canadian customers should call (800) 665-1148, or fax (800) 665-0103. For all other calls originating outside of the United States, please call (410) 528-4223 or fax us at (410) 528-8550.

Visit Williams & Wilkins on the Internet: http://www.wwilkins.com or contact our customer service department at custserv@wwilkins.com. Williams & Wilkins customer service representatives are available from 8:30 am to 6:00 pm, EST, Monday through Friday, for telephone access.

                                              97 98 99 00 01
                                          1 2 3 4 5 6 7 8 9 10

To our students

Preface

In the preface to the first edition of this text, we wrote, perhaps ambitiously, "The intent of *Principles of Medical Genetics* is to allow students and physicians to understand ongoing developments in genetics and to apply them to patient care." We hope we have been at least partially successful, because during the past seven years, our understanding of the genetic basis of disease has grown explosively. The impact of genetics on clinical practice has also dramatically increased. Understanding the basic principles of medical genetics is now more important than ever—for medical students and practicing physicians.

Virtually every chapter in this new edition reflects the stunning developments in human molecular genetics. Improved techniques for the detection and characterization of mutations, the development of automated sequencing techniques, and the generation of mice in which specific genes have been precisely inactivated are but a few examples. The discovery of triplet-repeat expansions as a mechanism of disease has opened up our understanding of the fragile X syndrome, myotonic dystrophy, and Huntington disease and related neurodegenerative disorders. Molecular cytogenetics has advanced particularly with the application of fluorescence in situ hybridization (FISH) techniques, which have had a major impact on gene mapping and molecular cytogenetic diagnoses. Advances in cancer genetics have now been applied to identifying individuals at risk for common cancers, such as colon and breast.

Perhaps most striking of all have been the advances in the genetic and physical mapping of the human genome. The positional cloning of a disease gene, a major feat in 1990, has become almost routine today. The Human Genome Project has fostered an exponential increase in our knowledge of genetic anatomy and the identification of disease-causing genes, and is the subject of a separate chapter in this new edition. These advances have expanded the range of genetic screening programs for identifying presymptomatic individuals and those at risk for transmitting genetic diseases, amplified the number of diseases for which there is now prenatal diagnosis available to couples at risk, and facilitated approaches to understanding the genetic bases of common complex diseases. Finally, all of these advances have raised a number of difficult ethical issues, giving rise to a new chapter on ethical issues in genetics.

The growth of medical genetics has necessarily resulted in some expansion in the size of this book. However, it remains an exposition of the *principles* of medical genetics and is not intended to be a compendium of human or medical genetics. Excellent, up-to-date references, both published and electronic, are available for this purpose, and are listed in the text area at the end of relevant chapters.

Genetics, like other branches of medicine, has its own special language. Key terms, when first introduced, appear in bold face and are defined in the Glossary. A special, tabbed section at the end of the book contains study questions, and their answers, relevant to each chapter. The questions are of two types. First, there are questions that can be answered, either directly by studying the material contained in that chapter, or indirectly by applying the principles learned to areas not specifically covered in the text. A second class of questions, indicated by an asterisk, may not necessarily have any simple, straightforward, or correct answers. Rather, these questions are designed to stimulate thought and discussion, to encourage the reader to extend his or her analysis beyond that presented in the text, and hopefully, to apply the principles included herein to new situations with uncertain outcomes.

We would like to acknowledge the help of many colleagues who contributed to the preparation of this book. First, we thank Drs. Thomas Glover, Elizabeth Petty, and Eric Fearon, and Genetic Counselors Wendy Uhlmann and Diane Baker, all of the University of Michigan, for critical reading of sections of the text. We also thank several colleagues, both at our institutions and elsewhere, for providing photographs and other materials. Mollie Dunker again provided expert medical illustrations, and Crystal Taylor tried hard to keep us on some sort of schedule. We very much appreciate Karen Grahl, June Balog, Suzann Labun, Pam Fitzgerald, and Patti Fakunding for their critical secretarial help. Finally, we thank our families for continuing encouragement and, above all, patience with us during this task.

Preface to the First Edition

Increasing awareness of the role of genetic factors in the causation of human disease has made clinical genetics one of the fastest growing fields in medicine during the past two decades. Our objective here is to present the basic principles of medical genetics and their application to clinical medicine; our emphasis is on molecular genetics because we believe that advances in this area have provided the major impetus to the rapid development of medical genetics, especially in the areas of diagnosis and prevention of disease. The intent of *Principles of Medical Genetics* is to allow students and physicians to understand ongoing developments in genetics and to apply them to patient care. This book is aimed primarily at first- or second-year medical students taking a course in medical genetics. We anticipate that the book will also prove useful to house officers who wish to review basic principles of medical genetics, to physicians whose training preceded current advances in medical genetics, to genetic counselors, and to nurses and other allied health professionals.

Although this is not a book about clinical medicine, human diseases are used to illustrate basic genetic principles. Furthermore, we have used certain diseases repeatedly because they illustrate several aspects of medical genetics and serve as useful paradigms. Our choice of examples reflects more than 25 years combined experience as clinical geneticists.

Principles of Medical Genetics covers basic principles of chromosome structure and function, Mendelian patterns of inheritance, mitochondrial diseases, and multifactorial inheritance and its role in human variation and human disease. We have included a detailed discussion of the molecular structure of the gene, regulation of its expression, and techniques for manipulation of genetic material. A detailed discussion of the hemoglobinopathies serves as a model for the molecular genetics of human disease. Other single gene disorders, however, are also discussed from the clinical to the molecular level as paradigms of molecular diseases. Human biochemical genetics, including pharmacogenetics, and cytogenetic disorders are also covered. Gene mapping is considered from the perspective of a background in molecular genetics, cytogenetics, and population genetics to provide a modern approach to this important area. There is a chapter devoted to the genetics of cancer due to the significant advances in cytogenetic and molecular genetic understanding of this group of disorders. Important aspects of the practice of clinical genetics, such as obtaining and interpreting a family history, genetic counseling, and genetic screening, are discussed as are current and future approaches to prenatal diagnosis and treatment. The final chapter points to further areas in which major advances can be expected and to which the basic principles learned can be applied.

In a field that changes and progresses so rapidly, the role of a textbook might be questioned. The intent of this book is not simply to present a body of facts, but rather to present the principles that allow one to keep up with rapid progress in the laboratory and its applications at the bedside.

Each chapter is followed by a group of study questions. These are of two types: First, there are questions that can be answered, either directly by studying the material contained in that chapter, or indirectly by applying the principles learned to areas not specifically covered in the text. A second class of questions, indicated by an asterisk, may not necessarily have any simple, straightforward, or correct answers. Rather, these questions are designed to stimulate thought and discussion, to encourage the reader to extend his or her analysis beyond that presented in the text, and hopefully, to apply the principles included herein to new situations with uncertain outcomes.

We wish to acknowledge the help of many colleagues who have made major contributions to the preparation of this book. First, we thank Drs. Richard King (University of Minnesota), Margretta Seashore (Yale University), and Claire Leonard (University of Utah) for reviewing the text and providing constructive criticisms. We thank Professor Peter Smouse (Rutgers University), formerly of the University of Michigan, for his help with the chapter on population genetics and multifactorial inheritance, and Dr. Thomas Glover of the University of Michigan, for his review of the cytogenetics chapter. We thank Drs. Glover and Constance Stein and Beth Cox of the University of Michigan Clinical Cytogenetics Service for the excellent chromosome photomicrographs. We owe special thanks to Dr. Robert Nussbaum (University of Pennsylvania) for preparing the study questions, to Mollie Dunker and Jacqueline A. Schaffer for preparing the illustrations, to Dr. Pamela Talalay for help in preparing the glossary, and Lee Marks, Danielle Paille, June McGee, and Bernice Sandri for secretarial help. We especially thank our editor, John Gardner, and managing editor, Linda Napora, for their support, encouragement, threats, and other interactions that kept this project going during the years of its creation. A textbook is a teaching device, and teaching has no meaning without students. The first-year medical students at the University of Michigan were our laboratory, our critics, and ultimately, our reason for writing this book. Finally, we thank our families: our parents for providing the support and nurture to bring us to our professional calling, and, most of all, our spouses and children whose forbearance, patience, and support throughout this project were essential for its completion.

Contents

The Role of Genetics in Medicine

"Nature is nowhere accustomed more openly to display her secret mysteries than in cases where she shows traces of her workings apart from the beaten path; nor is there any better way to advance the proper practice of medicine than to give our minds to the discovery of the usual law of Nature by careful investigation of cases of rare forms of diseases. For it has been found in almost all things, that what they contain of useful or applicable nature is hardly perceived unless we are deprived of them, or they become deranged in some way."

—WILLIAM HARVEY, 1657

The recognition of the role of genetic factors in the causation of human disease has made clinical genetics one of the most rapidly developing fields in medicine. With the marked reduction in nutritional and infectious diseases in the developed countries, there has been an increasing awareness of the role of genetic determinants of human disease. Important genetic contributions to the etiology of major diseases, such as coronary artery disease, diabetes mellitus, hypertension, and the major psychoses, have been identified. At the same time, there has been a veritable explosion of knowledge in basic genetics. Much of this progress has been propelled by recent advances in the area of molecular genetics and gene mapping. Almost 600 chromosomal loci have been identified at which one or more specific disease-causing mutations have been defined. Much of this new information has been applied directly to a better understanding of the pathogenesis of disease and to improved diagnosis and management of patients. Appropriately, a major contribution of these new developments in genetics has been in the area of *prevention and/or avoidance of disease*, the aspect of medicine that must become the focus of modern medicine. Genetic screening programs to detect individuals at risk, improved genetic diagnosis, genetic counseling, and prenatal diagnosis are some of these current applications of new genetic knowledge to medical practice. Gene therapy trials have already begun to treat specific diseases and will have a major impact on medical practice of the future. Medical Genetics has recently become the 24th member of the American Board of Medical Specialties, the first new specialty so recognized in 12 years. Given the rapidly growing contribution of genetics to the prevention and avoidance of clinical disease, genetic services must become an integral part of any new health care plan.

Impact of Genetic Diseases

Contrary to common belief, many genetic diseases are far from rare and, in fact, are a significant cause of illness and death. Even those individually rare conditions are, in aggregate, a major cause of morbidity and mortality. Approximately 3% of all pregnancies result in the birth of a child with a significant genetic disease or birth defect that can cause crippling, mental retardation, or early death. A survey of more than 1 million consecutive births in British Columbia indicated that at least 1 in 20 individuals younger than 25 years of age developed a serious disease with an important genetic component. The chronic nature of many genetic diseases imposes a heavy medical, financial, and emotional burden on affected patients and their families, as well as on society at large.

Two studies of the causes of death of more than 1200 children admitted to hospitals in the United Kingdom identified genetically determined diseases as contributing 38 and 42% of the total mortality (Table 1.1). In two North American studies of nearly 17,000 pediatric hospital admissions, clearly genetic disorders accounted for 5–10% of the admissions. When diseases in which genetic factors are thought to play a role were included, a third to more than half of the admissions were the result of genetic disorders (Table 1.2). Furthermore, patients with genetic diseases were hospitalized more frequently and for longer periods. Although the frequency of genetically caused diseases in the adult population is less clear, it is estimated that at least 10% of adult hospital admissions are as a result of genetic diseases. Thus, the financial and medical burdens of genetic diseases are indeed significant.

Aside from trauma, the term "nongenetic" may be a misnomer, for it is hard to conceive of any disease as being wholly nongenetic. The development of any individual depends on the interplay of genetic and environmental influences. Genetic factors are present from conception although their expression varies throughout development, whereas environmental influences are constantly changing. Since all human variation in both health and disease is to some extent genetic, all diseases are therefore genetic. Infectious diseases were once thought to represent clear examples of nongenetic diseases because specific exogenous agents of disease could be identified. However, it is now appreciated that host defense factors, many of them genetically determined, play an important role in susceptibility to infection and in the nature of the immune response to infectious agents. Thus, even in diseases with well-defined exogenous causes, genetic factors may play a critical role. More subtle examples of this same principle may be involved in the causation of such common problems as alcoholism.

The nature and extent of the genetic contribution to human variation and disease is the substance of the fields of human and medical genetics. Identification of genetic factors predisposing to disease and identification of genetically predisposed individuals are powerful keys for discovering the critical environmental agents of disease.

Paradoxically, one of the most important benefits of identifying the genetic factors in disease susceptibility may not be the potential for gene therapy, as exciting a prospect as that is, but rather the opportunity for treatment and prevention of clinical disease by manipulating the environment of individuals identified to be genetically at risk.

Table 1.1.   Genetic Components of Childhood Mortality in the United Kingdom[a]

Cause of Death	Newcastle	London
Chromosomal	2.5%	} 12.0%
Single gene	8.5%	
Polygenic	31.0%	25.5%
Nongenetic/unknown	58.0%	62.5%
Total deaths	1041	200

[a] Adapted from Roberts DF, Chavez J, Court SDM: The genetic component in child mortality. Arch Dis Child 45:33–38, 1970 and Carter CO: Changing patterns in the causes of death at the Hospital for Sick Children. Great Ormond St J 11:65–68, 1956.

Table 1.2. Frequency of Genetic Disorders among Pediatric Hospital Admissions in North America[a]

Cause	Seattle	Montreal
Chromosomal	0.6%	0.4%
Single gene	3.9%	6.9%
Polygenic	48.9%	29.0%
Nongenetic	46.6%	63.7%
No. of Admissions	4,115	12,801

[a] Adapted from Hall JG, Powers EK, McIlvaine RT, Ean VH: The frequency and financial burden of genetic disease in a pediatric hospital. Am J Med Genet 1:417–436, 1978 and Scriver CR, Neal JL, Saginur R, Clow A: The frequency of genetic disease and congenital malformation among patients in a pediatric hospital. Can Med Assoc J 108:1111–1115, 1973.

Genetically determined diseases are often classified into three major categories: chromosomal, single gene defects, and polygenic, or multifactorial, diseases. Recent studies on the molecular basis of human cancer require the addition of a fourth category, somatic cell genetic defects. Each of these will be discussed briefly below and more extensively in subsequent chapters.

Major Types of Genetic Disease

CHROMOSOMAL DISORDERS

These diseases are the result of the addition or deletion of entire chromosomes or parts of chromosomes and will be discussed in detail in chapter 8. Because each chromosome contains tens of thousands of genes, physical manifestations of chromosome disorders are often quite striking. Most major chromosome disorders are characterized by growth retardation, mental retardation, and a variety of somatic abnormalities. Clinically significant chromosome abnormalities occur in nearly 1% of liveborn babies and account for about 1% of pediatric hospital admissions and 2.5% of childhood deaths. The loss or gain of whole chromosomes is often incompatible with survival, and such abnormalities are a major cause of spontaneous abortions or miscarriages. Major chromosomal anomalies are found in almost half of spontaneous abortuses. Since approximately 15% of recognized pregnancies end in a miscarriage and it is estimated that 50% of conceptions do so, it appears that a quarter of conceptions may suffer from major chromosome problems. Thus, the major impact of chromosomal disorders occurs before birth (Fig. 1.1).

A typical example of a major chromosomal disease is Down syndrome, which is caused by trisomy 21, or three copies of chromosome 21 instead of the usual two copies. This abnormality occurs in approximately 1 in 800 liveborn infants and increases in frequency with advancing maternal age. It is characterized by growth retardation, variable but often severe mental retardation, and characteristic physical abnormalities including the upward-slanting eyes that have in the past given the condition the unfortunate name "mongolism." Most significant among the congenital abnormalities associated with this condition are congenital heart defects, which are the major cause of death in children with Down syndrome. Trisomy 21 also significantly decreases intrauterine viability and the majority of affected fetuses are spontaneously aborted. Down syndrome was the first chromosomal disease defined in humans and demonstrated for the first time that alterations in chromosomal material could cause mental retardation and severe congenital anomalies. Down syndrome was also one of the first diseases amenable to prenatal diagnosis by amniocentesis.

Figure 1.1. The age of expression of the major types of genetic disease. This schematic diagram shows the relative numbers of individuals affected with chromosomal, single gene, and multifactorial genetic disorders at different prenatal and postnatal ages. (Redrawn from a diagram provided by Dr. Barton Childs, The Johns Hopkins Hospital.)

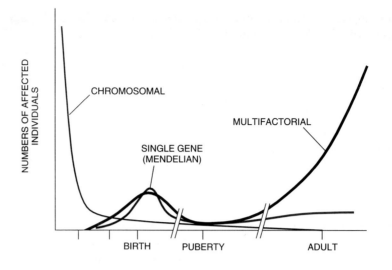

SINGLE GENE DISORDERS

These disorders are caused by single mutant genes with a large effect on the patient's health. As might be expected, single gene disorders are inherited in a simple Mendelian fashion (discussed in chapter 3) and are also referred to as Mendelian diseases. Some 4000 distinct disorders are now known to be single gene diseases inherited in autosomal dominant, autosomal recessive, or X-linked fashion. Some of these disorders will be discussed in greater detail in subsequent chapters. Single gene disorders account for approximately 5–10% of pediatric hospital admissions and childhood mortality. The major impact of single gene disorders occurs in the newborn period and early childhood (Fig. 1.1), although their importance in adult life is increasingly being appreciated. Although many single gene disorders are rare, others are common and pose major health problems. Familial hypercholesterolemia with its attendant high risk of premature coronary artery disease occurs in 1 in 500 individuals. Familial breast cancer and hereditary colon cancer each affect approximately 1 in 300. Sickle cell anemia affects 1 in 400 blacks in the United States, and cystic fibrosis affects 1 in 2000 whites. Sickle cell anemia was the first genetic disease to be defined at the molecular level, and its study serves as a model for the application of modern molecular genetic analysis to clinical disease. Single gene disorders have thus far proven to be the area in which advances in molecular genetics have made the major contribution to understanding and managing disease.

Mutations can also occur in genes on the mitochondrial chromosome, as well as in those on nuclear chromosomes. Mitochondrial diseases often affect energy production in nerve and muscle, and may play a role in cellular aging. These disorders are inherited in a uniquely maternal fashion, and are discussed in chapter 3.

POLYGENIC OR MULTIFACTORIAL DISEASES

These diseases result from the interaction of multiple genes, some of which may have a major effect, but many of which may have a relatively minor effect. This group of diseases is both the most common and the least understood of human genetic diseases; understanding the genetic basis of common chronic diseases represents the major challenge facing contemporary medical genetics. Examples of such polygenic diseases include the common diseases of adult life such as diabetes mellitus, hypertension, coronary artery disease, and schizophrenia, as well as a variety of common congenital defects such as cleft lip, cleft palate, and most congenital heart diseases. These diseases account for 25–50% of pediatric hospital admissions, approximately 25–35% of childhood mortality, and because of the chronicity of many of these conditions, perhaps an even greater component of disease burden in the adult population. Thus, the clinical impact of multifactorial diseases is important in both the neonatal period and in adult life (Fig. 1.1). Conceptually, this group of diseases poses the challenge of sorting out the ways in which the additive or interactive effects of several to many genes create the predisposition to disease, which in turn is manifest only in the presence of appropriate environmental triggers. It is hoped that a combination of molecular genetic approaches, gene mapping, and genetic epidemiology will allow a clearer definition of these genetic determinants and of the genetic heterogeneity underlying disease susceptibility. Models for how such interactions can cause disease, and methods for identifying the nature and contribution of genetic factors in such diseases will be discussed in chapter 4 and chapter 9.

SOMATIC CELL GENETIC DISORDERS

In contrast to the above three categories in which the genetic abnormality is found in the DNA of all cells in the body including germ cells (sperm and egg) and can be transmitted to subsequent generations, somatic cell genetic disorders arise only in specific somatic cells. The paradigm for somatic cell genetic diseases is cancer, in which development of malignancy is often the consequence of mutations in genes that control cellular growth. It is now clear that all human cancer results from mutations in DNA, making it the most common genetic disease. The various genetic mechanisms that can result in cancer are discussed in chapter 11.

Genetics and Medicine: The Dynamic Interface

The interaction between the basic science of genetics and the clinical science of medicine has been bidirectional and highly productive for the past several decades. In its early stages, genetics was more the province of the plant and animal breeders and the entomologists than the physician. Mendel, working in the 1860s, was able to formulate the concept of the gene from his experiments with pea plants, and his ability to perform planned matings and observe multiple generations provided crucial elements not so easily achieved when studying humans. Similarly, the work of Thomas Hunt Morgan and others on the fruit fly, *Drosophila melanogaster*, was much benefited by the short generation time and relatively simple genome (relative to mammals) of the fruit fly. However, as interest in human genetics began to blossom in the 20th century, important concepts began to be recognized and explored in greater depth for humans than they had been for other species. Prominent examples include population genetics, the study of polymorphism (see chapter 9), and biochemical genetics (see chapter 7). In more recent times, the trend has continued and the spin-offs from one discipline to another have multiplied. As will be described in chapter 11, for example, the newly emerging field of the genetics of human cancer has demonstrated that human cells carry a set of genes called "oncogenes," and another set called "tumor suppressor genes," which normally participate in growth control. Certain mutations of these genes can contribute to the uncontrolled growth pattern we recognize as cancer. The discovery of oncogenes and tumor suppressor genes has demonstrated an unexpected link between cancer, virology, and genetics and has brought together several diverse fields of biology and biochemistry. Many cancers are associated with consistent chromosomal rearrangements that have important diagnostic and prognostic significance. Cloning of these breakpoint regions has resulted in the discovery of new genes and a better understanding of the mechanisms of normal and abnormal growth control. Furthermore, several oncogenes or tumor suppressor genes have been identified in which inherited mutations may cause birth defects rather than cancer! Finally, the cloning and characterization of the genes involved in familial cancer syndromes have revealed unknown steps in regulation of cell growth. For example, cloning the gene for neurofibromatosis 1 (discussed in chapters 3 and 9) led to the surprising discovery that this gene is not only a tumor suppressor gene, but that its product, neurofibromin, plays a critical role in normal biochemical signal transduction pathways involving the oncogene *ras* and guanosine triphosphatases!

Thus, efforts in medicine have yielded continuing insights in genetics and basic biology. In the other direction, the contribution of research in genetics to medicine is even more apparent. It is easy to forget in today's technological medical care system that medicine for most of its history has been a descriptive discipline. Although the descriptive approach is a valuable one for determining the natural history of disease and describing the effects of various therapeutic maneuvers, fundamental advances in medicine generally have come instead from an elucidation of more basic scientific principles and their subsequent application to a clinical situation. Medical genetics deals with human disease at the most fundamental level—that of the gene itself. It is thus natural that developments in genetics have had profound implications for clinical medicine, and the magnitude of those implications will continue to grow.

A prime example is the concept of molecular disease, which was first clearly enunciated by Pauling with regard to sickle cell anemia. Known for centuries in West Africa as a lifelong disease causing anemia and pain in the bones, joints, and abdomen, the actual pathogenesis remained unknown until 1910 when James Herrick, a cardiologist in Chicago, first noted the abnormally shaped red blood cells in an affected individual. Four decades later Pauling demonstrated that hemoglobin from patients with sickle cell anemia was electrophoretically different from normal hemoglobin and that parents of affected children showed both normal and abnormal hemoglobins. In 1956, Ingram, using a peptide fingerprinting technique, showed that the difference was due to the substitution of valine for glutamic acid as the sixth amino acid of the β chain of hemoglobin. Subsequently the mutation has been identified at the nucleic acid level as a single base substitution of A to T, and prenatal diagnosis is now available based on DNA analysis (see chapter 6 for more details). The fact that such a severe and clinically complex disorder could be caused by alteration of only one nucleotide in 3 billion would not have been predicted by the descriptive approach that characterized medicine in previous centuries. This demonstration was powerful evidence that the genetic approach to medicine could be extremely revealing. It also illustrates an important paradigm: a single gene alteration can have complex clinical effects on multiple organ systems. Medical genetics is thus a broad specialty with wide areas of overlap with all other clinical disciplines.

The example of hemoglobin also demonstrates a second paradigm: the study of mutation can yield important insights about structure-function relationships. Subsequent to the description of sickle hemoglobin, which we now know creates its havoc by favoring the intracellular polymerization of hemoglobin, more than 300 other mutant hemoglobins have been described. Some of these, presumably located in noncritical parts of the hemoglobin polypeptide chain, have no functional consequences. Others, located near the site for heme binding, can lead to oxidation of the iron carried by the molecule (methemoglobinemia). Mutations that affect the equilibrium between the high and low oxygen affinity forms can lead to high-affinity hemoglobins, which release oxygen poorly. By determining the position of the mutations in these various conditions, the functional role of the various parts of the globin molecule begins to emerge. Detailed molecular analysis of other genetic diseases, such as glucose-6-phosphate dehydrogenase deficiency, cystic fibrosis, and hemophilia A and B, have indicated a similar multiplicity of mutations that can alter or disrupt the function of the relevant gene product.

The contribution of the study of hemoglobin to our understanding of human biology is difficult to overstate and is the reason for the dedication of an entire chapter of this text (chapter 6) to this topic. Another important principle is thus revealed: what one learns from an intensive study of a particular gene-protein system often provides critical insights for other systems.

The concept of molecular medicine has continued to broaden. For example, coronary artery disease is one of the leading causes of death in the Western world. The association of high serum cholesterol with an increased risk of coronary artery thrombosis has been noted for decades, but the inheritance pattern was not clear and the metabolic pathways leading to elevated cholesterol were obscure. Families with very high cholesterol levels, deposits of cholesterol in the skin and tendons, and an extremely high risk of heart attacks were discovered (see chapter 7). Focusing their studies on such families, which account for 5% of individuals with heart attacks, Goldstein and Brown were able to demonstrate the existence of a cell surface receptor for a cholesterol-rich lipoprotein called low-density lipoprotein (LDL) and found that the LDL receptor was defective in these patients. The elucidation of this important pathway by a genetic approach has contributed greatly to our understanding of cholesterol metabolism and of the cause of atherosclerosis in general. Even more than that, it has led to a rapid expansion in understanding of the whole phenomenon of cell surface receptor biology, including how such receptors are synthesized, how they are localized in the cell membrane, and how they carry their ligands into the cell interior (a process known as receptor-mediated endocytosis).

This example illustrates another important paradigm, one clearly recognized by William Harvey in the quotation that began this chapter: the study of rare genetic mutations provides a powerful way to understand normal function. Many examples of the success of this approach can be found in modern medicine.

Summary

Only a few years ago courses in medical genetics were given in only a small number of medical schools. Today most medical students are given some direct instruction in medical genetics, and the trend is to increase this emphasis. The direct relevance to clinical medicine, as well as the scientific undergirding of much of medical science that genetics provides, has made an understanding of this area essential to the modern physician. Fortunately, the grasp of a basic set of principles, which this text endeavors to present, allows the derivation of conclusions in complex situations. For the medical student burdened with a massive body of information to be memorized, genetics can be a welcome respite—a truly rational, logical, satisfying discipline. We live in an age of discovery in genetics comparable in excitement to that of Columbus and his contemporary explorers and cartographers 500 years ago. Our growing appreciation of the genetic diversity of our species underscores the uniqueness of each individual. Our expanding knowledge of the genetic basis of diseases positions us to play a central role in disease prevention, the focus of medicine of the future.

SUGGESTED READING

Harvey W, quoted by Garrod A. The lesson of rare maladies. Lancet 1928;1:1055–1066.

McKusick VA. Medical genetics. A 40-year perspective on the evolution of a medical specialty from a basic science. JAMA 1993;270:2351–2356.

Motulsky AG. Michael Brown and Joseph Goldstein. The 1985 Nobel Prize in Physiology or Medicine. Science 1986;231:126–129.

Neel JV. Physician to the gene pool. Genetic lessons and other stories. New York: J Wiley & Sons, 1994.

Stamatoyannopoulos G, Nienhuis AW, Majerus PW, Varmus H. The molecular basis of blood disease. 2nd ed. Philadelphia: WB Saunders, 1994.

Weatherall DJ. The new genetics and clinical practice. 3rd ed. New York: Oxford Univ Press, 1991.

Structure and Behavior of Genes and Chromosomes

"In the next day or so Crick and I shall send a note to Nature proposing our structure (of DNA) as a possible model, at the same time emphasizing its provisional nature and the lack of proof in its favor. Even if wrong, I believe it to be interesting since it provides a concrete example of a structure composed of complementary chains. If, by chance, it is right, then I suspect we may be making a slight dent into the manner in which DNA can reproduce itself."

—JAMES WATSON, FROM A LETTER TO MAX DELBRÜCK, MARCH 12, 1953

To begin a description of the basic principles of human genetics, we must start with DNA. DNA, or deoxyribonucleic acid, is the ultimate molecule of life. The instructions that direct human cells to grow, to differentiate into specialized structures, to divide, and to respond to environmental changes are all encoded within the elegant simplicity of the human DNA genome. Furthermore, the basis of all genetic disease ultimately is founded on changes in this DNA sequence. An understanding of the structure and behavior of DNA and of the chromosomes into which it is packaged is thus fundamental to medical genetics and to medicine in general, especially as these fields have moved from descriptive into molecular sciences.

Some readers of this text are already very familiar with the contents of this chapter and the next. We include this basic information, however, recognizing that those with an interest in medical genetics have diverse backgrounds.

DNA Is the Hereditary Material

That chromosomes contain DNA and are responsible for hereditary traits has been known since the 1860s. However, in the earlier part of the 20th century most biologists who were more familiar with the informational possibilities of proteins and their 20 amino acid building blocks tended to assume that a protein constituent of the chromosomes would be the true hereditary material. Resolution of this problem awaited the development of a biologic assay for genetic molecules, which was eventually provided by the pneumococcus, a bacterial agent that causes pneumonia. Pneumococci that cause human disease grow as smooth, glistening, mucoid colonies, whereas those that do not are rough in appearance (now known to be due to the presence or absence of the thick polysaccharide cell wall). Heat-killed smooth bacteria, when mixed with living rough cells, are able to transform a small percentage to a smooth appearance. By investigating the nature of this "transforming factor," Avery, MacLeod, and McCarty showed definitively in 1944 that it was not protein but DNA. This seminal observation provided a new fundamental paradigm and set the stage for the modern revolution in genetics.

Structure of DNA

With the demonstration that DNA itself carries genetic information, a number of laboratories at the end of World War II turned their attention to its physical structure. Using the careful x-ray crystallographic data of Wilkins and Franklin, Watson and Crick deduced the correct structure in 1953 (Fig. 2.1). That DNA was a long polymer was in itself not surprising. What no one had predicted was that DNA consists of *two* intertwined chains, running in opposite directions.

The molecular structure of DNA, depicted schematically in Figure 2.1 and in a space-filling model in Figure 2.2, consists of a double helix. The "backbone" of each strand of the helix consists of an invariant sugar-phosphate-sugar-phosphate polymer, with the sugar being deoxyribose and the phosphates being attached through ester bonds to its 3'- and 5'-hydroxyl groups. Attached to the 1' position of the sugar ring is one of four nitrogen-

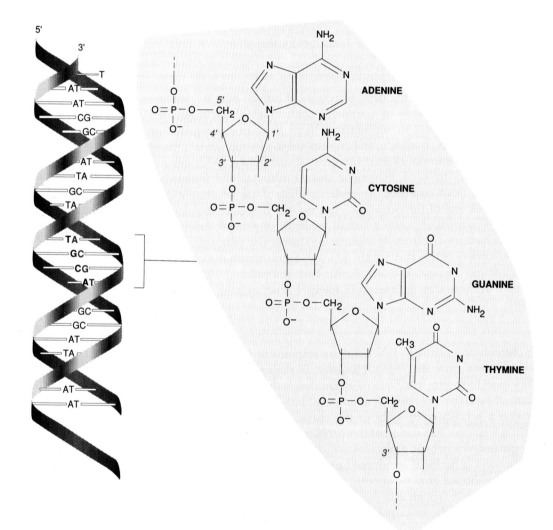

Figure 2.1.   The structure of DNA.   At the *left* is a schematic drawing of the DNA double helix, showing the sugar-phosphate backbone as a ribbon, with the bases arranged toward the middle. Note that A always pairs with T, and C always pairs with G. At the *right* is an expanded view of four nucleotides along one strand, showing the complete chemical structure of the sequence 5'-ACGT-3'. (A nucleotide consists of a sugar, a phosphate group, and an attached base.) Note that the 5' and 3' designations, used to indicate the polarity of a DNA strand, refer to the numbering of carbons on the deoxyribose ring.

STRUCTURE OF DNA

containing "bases." Two of these, adenine (A) and guanine (G), are purines, whereas the other two, cytosine (C) and thymine (T), are the less bulky pyrimidines. Watson and Crick correctly deduced that the bases lie almost flat within the interior of the double helix, like a stack of coins spaced 3.4 Å apart. The double helix is held together by hydrogen bonds, which can form between A and T bases and between G and C bases (Fig. 2.3), each of which is called a "base pair." Thus, the two strands of DNA are "complementary"; if one is 5′-ATGCCAG-3′, the other must be 5′-CTGGCAT-3′, with the full double-stranded structure of 7 base pairs (bp) being written as follows:

5′-ATGCCAG-3′

3′-TACGGTC-5′

This pairing of A with T and G with C explains the basis of Chargaff's rule, which was deduced before the structure of DNA was elucidated, and states that the percentage of A and T bases in a given species' DNA is the same, and the percentage of G and C is the same.

There are a number of features of this structure that should be carefully noted:

1. It provides a means of storing and coding vast amounts of information, based on the sequence of the bases present in the DNA strand; for a molecule N bases long, there are 4^N possible sequences. The complete DNA sequence of an organism, containing its complete genetic information, is called its genome. The smallest viruses have genomes of only a few thousand base pairs and contain only a small number of genes. The size and complexity of the genome increase in a nonlinear fashion, however, as one moves along the evolutionary tree, from 4×10^6 bp in a bacterium to 3×10^9 bp in humans. A representative sample of genome sizes is shown in Table 2.1.

2. As noted by Watson and Crick, the double helical complementary structure immediately suggests a mechanism of DNA replication. Each strand contains the full informational content of the DNA molecule and can serve as a template for synthesis of a new complementary strand as the helix unwinds and replicates (Fig. 2.4). This mode of replication is denoted "semi-conservative" because each daughter DNA strand contains one parental strand and one newly synthesized strand.

3. The complementary structure also provides a defense against information loss by DNA damage. A base on one strand that is damaged or lost can be replaced using the complementary strand to direct its repair. Similarly, a break in the sugar-phosphate backbone, which would be nearly impossible to correctly reconnect in a single-stranded molecule, can be repaired in a double-stranded molecule without any loss of contiguity.

4. The complementarity of DNA strands also allows them to find each other in a complex mixture of molecules. This "reannealing" or "hybridization" process is used in some situations by the nuclear machinery to regulate gene expression. Furthermore, this phenomenon has been heavily exploited in molecular biology, as we shall see in chapter 5, and is at the heart of its current success.

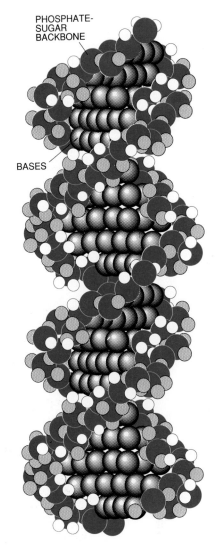

PHOSPHATE-SUGAR BACKBONE

BASES

Figure 2.2.   Space-filling model of DNA.

Even as early as the 19th century, another nucleic acid was known to exist within cells. This nucleic acid is present in the cytoplasm, particularly in association with polyribosomes, the protein synthesis factories of the cells. Chemical and structural analysis revealed this nucleic acid to be similar to

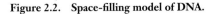

Transcription into RNA

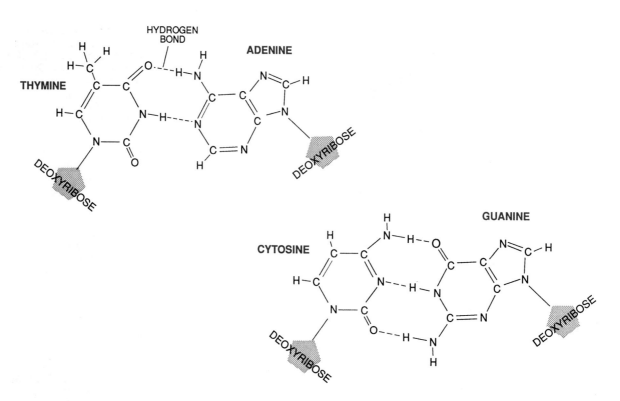

Figure 2.3. Hydrogen bonding between the adenine-thymine and guanine-cytosine base pairs.   Note that two hydrogen bonds can form in A-T pairs, and three in C-G pairs.

DNA, but with three crucial differences (Fig. 2.5): (*a*) it is single-stranded; (*b*) the sugar is ribose, not deoxyribose; and (*c*) the pyrimidine base uracil replaces thymine.

This ribonucleic acid (RNA) has many roles in the cell. Certain RNAs, called ribosomal RNAs, make up a part of the polyribosomes and are synthesized in the nucleolus. Small molecules called transfer RNAs (tRNAs) are crucial elements in the translation of genetic information into protein molecules (see below). Other RNAs are involved in transcript processing functions. But the major RNA species of concern to biologists and geneticists is messenger RNA (mRNA), which occupies the essential connecting link between information contained in a gene and its end result as the specific amino acid sequence of a protein.

We will save a complete presentation of the transcriptional process for chapter 5, where a description of the tools of the molecular biologist will allow

Table 2.1. Representative Genome Sizes in Base Pairs	
SV40, a mammalian DNA virus	4×10^3
λ, a bacterial virus	5×10^4
Escherichia coli, a bacterium	4×10^6
Saccharomyces cerevisiae, a yeast	1.2×10^7
Caennorhabitis elegans, a nematode	1×10^8
Drosophilia melanogaster, the fruit fly	1.2×10^8
Human chromosome 21	5×10^7
Human chromosome 1	3×10^8
Entire human genome[a]	3×10^9

[a] This is actually the *haploid* genome, or *half* the size of the number of base pairs of DNA in a human somatic cell. As will become clear in Chapter 3, the human is a *diploid* organism, with two copies of each chromosome, except for the sex chromosomes in males. Thus, there are actually 6×10^9 bp of DNA in each human somatic cell.

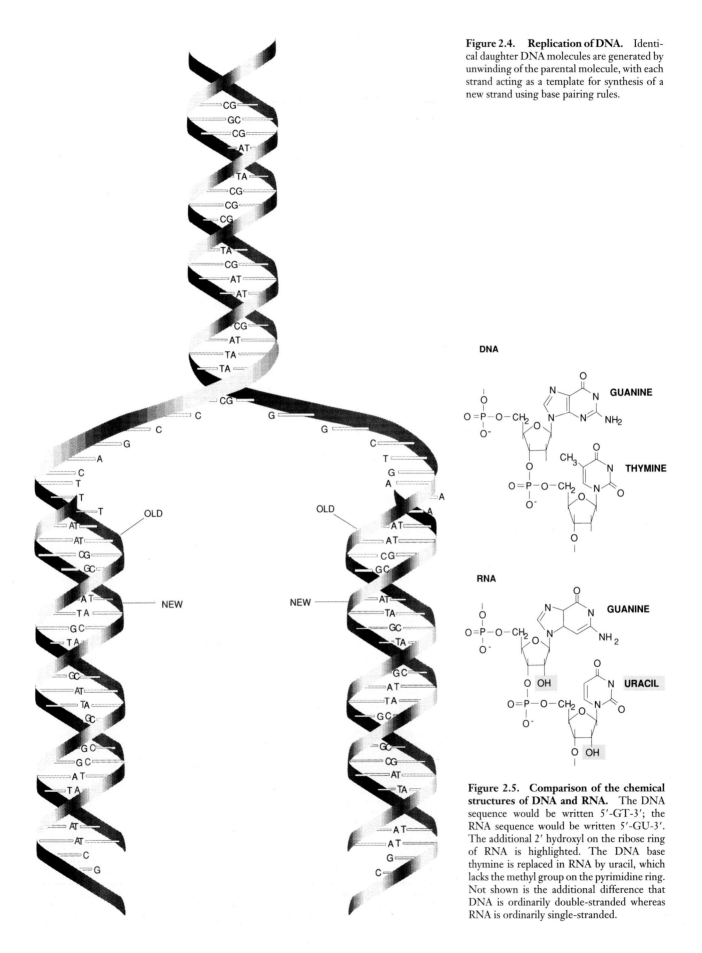

Figure 2.4. Replication of DNA. Identical daughter DNA molecules are generated by unwinding of the parental molecule, with each strand acting as a template for synthesis of a new strand using base pairing rules.

DNA

GUANINE

THYMINE

RNA

GUANINE

URACIL

Figure 2.5. Comparison of the chemical structures of DNA and RNA. The DNA sequence would be written 5'-GT-3'; the RNA sequence would be written 5'-GU-3'. The additional 2' hydroxyl on the ribose ring of RNA is highlighted. The DNA base thymine is replaced in RNA by uracil, which lacks the methyl group on the pyrimidine ring. Not shown is the additional difference that DNA is ordinarily double-stranded whereas RNA is ordinarily single-stranded.

more details to be included. For the time being, however, it is useful to consider transcription as the generation of a single-stranded RNA molecule from a double-stranded DNA template in the cell nucleus. This process, carried out by the enzyme RNA polymerase II, always occurs in the 5′ to 3′ direction; that is, new ribonucleotides are added to the 3′ end of the growing strand according to the DNA instructions (Fig. 2.6). In order for this process to be successful, some signal must be present in the DNA (the promoter) to indicate to the transcriptional machinery where to start. Similarly, transcription must not continue indefinitely, but must end after the necessary sequence has been transcribed.

Translation into Proteins

The messenger RNA produced by transcription must make its way out of the nucleus to ribosomes where it can be translated into a protein sequence. One of the great achievements of the past 30 years has been the deduction of the mechanism of translation and the "language" used in the process, commonly referred to as the genetic code. Because there are only 4 bases in DNA and RNA, but 20 amino acids in proteins, at least 3 bases ($4^2 = 16$, $4^3 = 64$) would be needed to unambiguously specify an amino acid. A series of careful experiments performed between 1961 and 1966 deduced that the 3-base word, or "codon," is correct and led to determina-

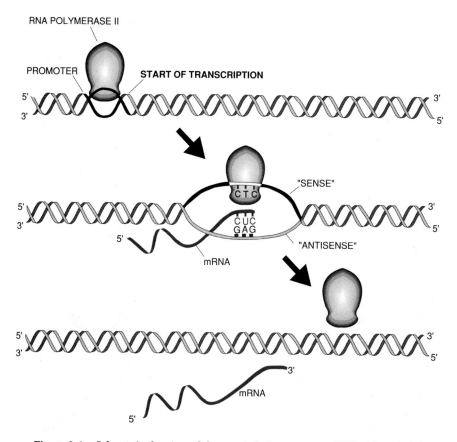

Figure 2.6.   Schematic drawing of the transcription process.   RNA polymerase II recognizes a specific sequence at the 5′ end of a gene (the promoter) and begins to transcribe it into messenger RNA (mRNA). The mRNA is synthesized in the 5′ to 3′ direction and has the same sequence as the 5′ to 3′ DNA strand, also known as the "sense" strand. The mechanism of RNA formation presumably depends on base pairing of the newly formed RNA with the "antisense" strand of the DNA, which acts as a template for copying.

Table 2.2. The Genetic Code [a]

First Position (5' end)	Second Position				Third Position (3' end)
	U	C	A	G	
U	Phe	Ser	Tyr	Cys	U
	Phe	Ser	Tyr	Cys	C
	Leu	Ser	STOP	STOP	A
	Leu	Ser	STOP	Trp	G
C	Leu	Pro	His	Arg	U
	Leu	Pro	His	Arg	C
	Leu	Pro	Gln	Arg	A
	Leu	Pro	Gln	Arg	G
A	Ile	Thr	Asn	Ser	U
	Ile	Thr	Asn	Ser	C
	Ile	Thr	Lys	Arg	A
	Met	Thr	Lys	Arg	G
G	Val	Ala	Asp	Gly	U
	Val	Ala	Asp	Gly	C
	Val	Ala	Glu	Gly	A
	Val	Ala	Glu	Gly	G

[a] Amino acid abbreviations are: Ala, alanine; Arg, arginine; Asn, asparagine; Asp, aspartic acid; Cys, cysteine; Gln, glutamine; Glu, glutamic acid; Gly, glycine; His, histidine; Ile, isoleucine; Leu, leucine; Lys, lysine; Met, methionine; Phe, phenylalanine; Pro, proline; Ser, serine; Thr, threonine; Trp, tryptophan; Tyr, tyrosine; Val, valine.

tion of the genetic code, as shown in Table 2.2. Note that there is "degeneracy" in this code, so that several codons may result in the same amino acid. Codons UUA, UUG, CUU, CUC, CUA, and CUG, for example, all code for leucine. Three codons, UAA, UAG, and UGA, do not encode amino acids but result in a termination of translation and are called stop codons.

The machinery that carries out the translation process on the ribosome is complex. An array of amino acid-specific adaptor molecules, called transfer RNAs, covalently bind a particular amino acid. The 3-base "anticodon" is complementary to the codon specifying that amino acid and allows it to be accurately added to the growing polypeptide chain, as depicted in Figure 2.7. This process continues until the stop codon is reached, which leads to release of the polypeptide chain from the ribosome. The order of addition of amino acids is such that the 5' end of the mRNA corresponds to the amino (NH_2) terminus of the protein, and the 3' end of the mRNA corresponds to the carboxy (COOH) terminus of the protein.

Higher Order Coiling of DNA

It is likely that each of the 46 chromosomes of humans is made up of a single molecule of double-stranded DNA. If stretched out, the DNA from a single cell would extend approximately 2 meters in length. Obviously an efficient method of packaging must be used by cells in order to deal with a molecule of such complexity. An elaborate system of coiling, which also seems to be involved in the control of gene expression in as yet poorly understood ways, is present in mammalian cells. Basic proteins called histones provide a core around which DNA is wound in a double loop composing approximately 146 bp of DNA (Fig. 2.8). This unit is referred to as a nucleosome; the tight evolutionary conservation of the histone structure implies an important functional role. The resulting "beads-on-a-string" DNA structure results in a compaction of length of about a factor of 7; further organization occurs by arrangement of the nucleosomes in a solenoid fashion and by higher order structural complexities (Fig. 2.8).

Figure 2.7. Translation of mRNA into protein by a ribosome. The mRNA sequence 5'-UACUUCUCCUUGGUC-3' is translated to the amino acid sequence Tyr-Phe-Ser-Leu-Val, using the tRNA molecules and their anticodons as adaptors.

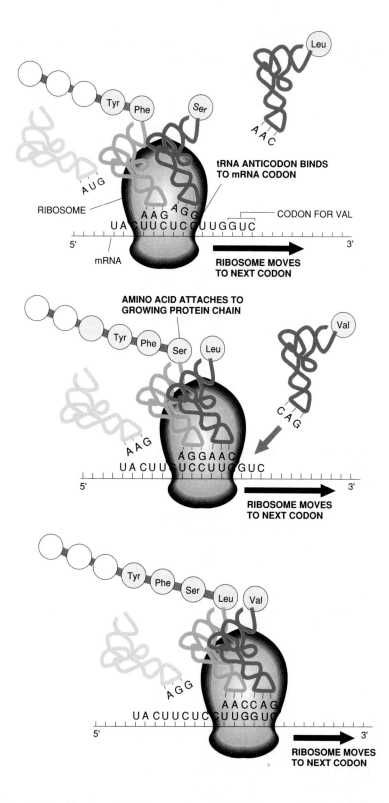

The mechanism by which factors responsible for regulation of gene expression interact with this monotonous histone-DNA complex represents an important area of current investigation. There is evidence that regions of the DNA molecule that are involved in regulation may be locally free of histones. For example, certain areas (especially the 5' ends) of actively expressed genes are unusually sensitive to cleavage by enzymes that cut DNA (nucleases), which do not efficiently cut histone-bound DNA.

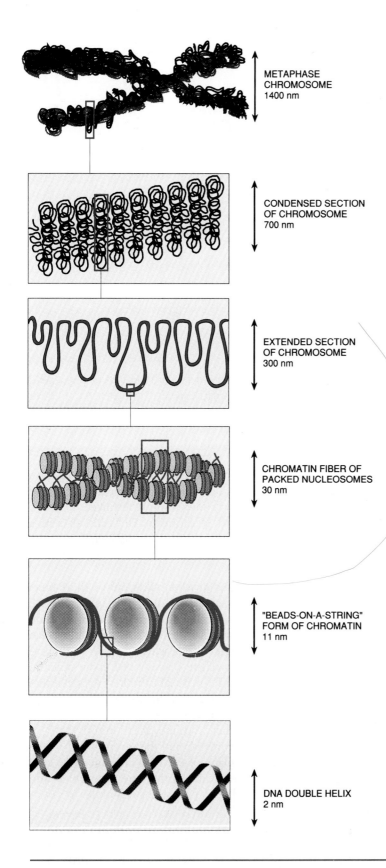

METAPHASE
CHROMOSOME
1400 nm

CONDENSED SECTION
OF CHROMOSOME
700 nm

EXTENDED SECTION
OF CHROMOSOME
300 nm

CHROMATIN FIBER OF
PACKED NUCLEOSOMES
30 nm

"BEADS-ON-A-STRING"
FORM OF CHROMATIN
11 nm

DNA DOUBLE HELIX
2 nm

Figure 2.8.   Coiling of DNA, arranged in increasing order of organization from *bottom* to *top*. In *each panel* a size marker in nanometers (nm) indicates the scale.

The highest order of DNA coiling is the chromosome. Each species has a characteristic number and size of chromosomes, known as the karyotype. The human karyotype, to be discussed in more detail in chapter 8, consists of 46 chromosomes (Fig. 2.9). As mentioned above, the human is a diploid

Human Chromosomes

Figure 2.9.   Karyotype of a normal human male, consisting of 22 pairs of autosomes, an X chromosome, and a Y chromosome.

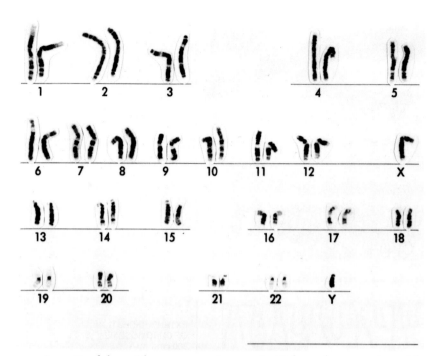

organism: 44 of these (the autosomes) occur in 22 homologous pairs, with each member of the pair containing the same genetic information. The remaining two chromosomes are the sex chromosomes; a female has two X chromosomes, and a male an X and a Y.

Mitosis

There are two kinds of cell divisions: mitosis and meiosis. Mitotic division is the process whereby one cell divides to give rise to two that are genetically identical to the parent. It is mitosis that allows a single fertilized oocyte to give rise to a complete human being with its estimated 10^{14} cells, all (with a few exceptions) genetically identical to the original single cell. In mitosis, each daughter cell must receive the complete chromosome complement of 46 chromosomes.

Mitosis itself, the process of nuclear division, takes only a short time. However, it is part of a carefully programed process, diagramed in Figure 2.10, called the cell cycle. Just after division, the cell that is destined to divide again enters a stage called G1 whereas one that will not enters a resting phase called G0. A cell in G1 next moves into S phase, during which time DNA replication occurs, by the semiconservative mechanism described above wherein each DNA strand serves as a template for its own replication. The result is that each of the 46 chromosomes is duplicated into "sister chromatids," held together by a central constriction called the centromere. At the end of S phase, another gap phase (G2) begins, which then leads into actual mitosis (M).

In mitosis (Fig. 2.11) the sister chromatids and the centromere become clearly visible and line up along the plane of eventual cleavage. The centromeres of all 46 chromosomes then divide, so that one sister chromatid from each ends up in the daughter cell, completing the cell cycle.

Meiosis and Gametogenesis

Meiosis, the variety of cell division that is used to generate the male and female gametes (sperm and oocytes, respectively) is different in crucial ways from mitosis. A little reflection suggests this must be so: if sperm and egg cells contained the full complement ("diploid") set of 46 chromosomes, the fertilized oocyte would have 92 chromosomes, including three Xs and a Y!

Meiosis, the special reduction process that is carried out in gameto-genesis to generate sperm and egg cells, each bearing 23 chromosomes (the "haploid" state), is diagramed in Figure 2.12. There are actually two divisions, meiosis I and meiosis II. In meiosis I, each chromosome replicates into sister chromatids, just as in mitosis. Unlike mitosis, however, the homologous chromosomes then align in pairs (a process called synapsis) and separate to *opposite* poles, with their sister chromatids still together. In meiosis II, the sister chromatids then separate, resulting in 23 chromosomes per gamete.

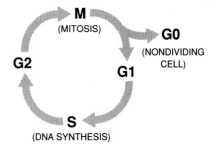

Figure 2.10.   The cell cycle.

MITOSIS

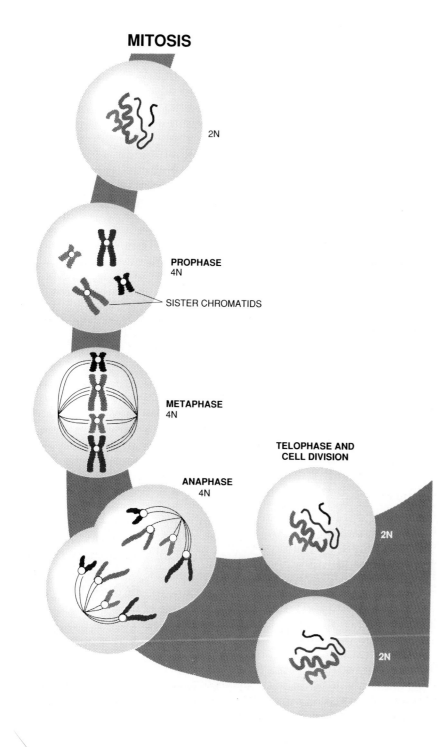

2N

PROPHASE
4N

SISTER CHROMATIDS

METAPHASE
4N

**TELOPHASE AND
CELL DIVISION**

ANAPHASE
4N

2N

2N

Figure 2.11.   Mitosis. For simplicity only four chromosomes, consisting of two pairs of autosomes, are shown. The "ploidy" of the cell is shown at each stage: 2N represents the diploid state. After formation of sister chromatids but before cell division, the cell contains an amount of DNA corresponding to 4N.

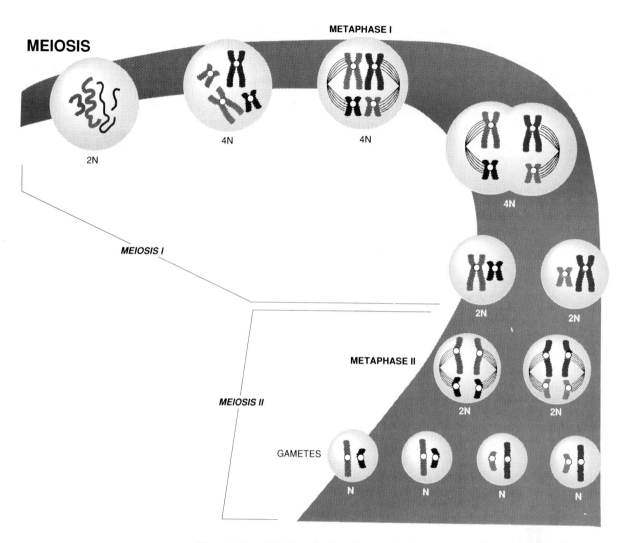

Figure 2.12. Meiosis. Again, only two pairs of autosomes are shown. Note that after meiosis I each cell retains only *one* of the homologous pair. Meiosis II then leads to sister chromatid separation. For simplicity, no crossing over is shown.

Crossing Over

An extremely important feature of meiosis I is that during synapsis, when homologous chromosomes are paired together, crossovers occur (Fig. 2.13). The practical result of this is that the chromosome retained in a gamete at the end of meiosis may be a patchwork of *both* homologous parental chromosomes. Genes that are close together on a chromosome, however (such as *A* and *B* in Fig. 2.13), are likely to be passed along together, whereas a crossover (or "recombination") is more likely to occur between genes that are far apart on a chromosome. On the average, about 30–40 crossovers (or 1–2 per chromosome) occur during a meiotic division.

Besides increasing enormously the potential genetic diversity of gametes, crossing over provides a quantitative estimate of the distance separating two genes on the same chromosome (called "syntenic" genes). As we shall see in chapter 9, this has provided a powerful means of mapping genes.

Mutation

Until now we have considered the DNA making up the human genome as unchanging and error-free. Were this the case, however, evolution would be impossible. On the other hand, mutations in DNA sequence, which must be

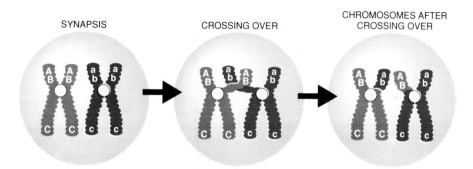

SYNAPSIS   CROSSING OVER   CHROMOSOMES AFTER CROSSING OVER

Figure 2.13. Crossing over in meiosis I.

possible to allow gradual selective change of organisms, must not be too frequent because the vast majority will be deleterious. As pointed out, many mutations are corrected using the undamaged DNA strand as a template to correct the damaged one. However, if damage occurs to both strands, or if it occurs just before or during DNA replication, the resulting alteration in DNA sequence becomes permanent for all the future progeny of that cell.

Considerable effort has been expended to attempt to determine the background mutation rate in humans. A new mutation in a given gene appears at a frequency of about one in a million as that gene is passed from parent to child. Because there are estimated to be about 80,000–100,000 genes in humans, this indicates that a surprising 8–10% of all newborns carry a new mutation. Fortunately, most of these are silent, because the balancing gene on the homologous chromosome is normal, so that their presence is not apparent. New mutations can take various forms at the molecular level. As we shall see throughout this text, the identification of an increasing number of mutations at the DNA level has borne out the principle that "whatever can go wrong, eventually will" (Murphy's law of the genome?). A few examples are shown in Figure 2.14. The simplest change is a substitution of one nucleotide for another, called a "point mutation." If this occurs in a coding region and changes

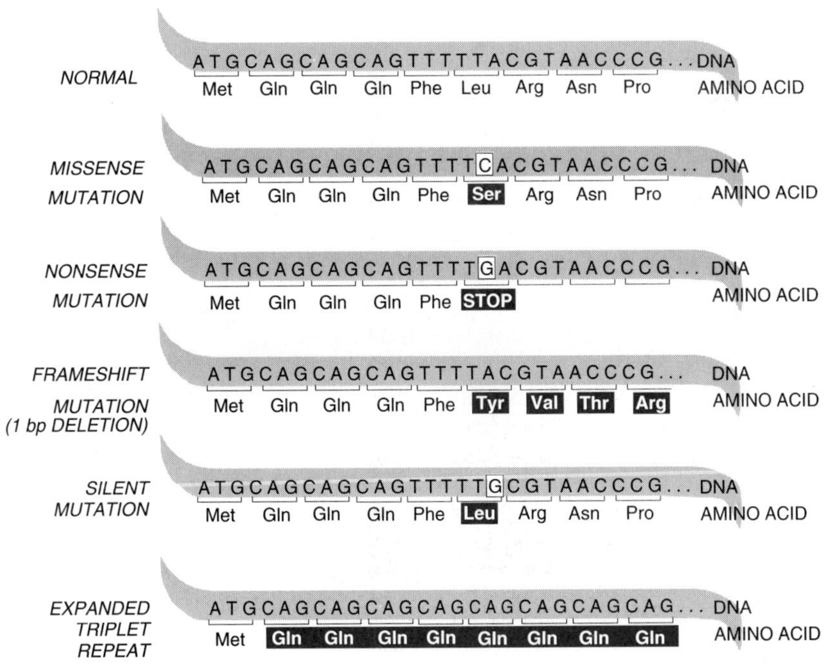

Figure 2.14. Examples of mutation. The "sense" strand DNA sequence of a coding region is shown, together with the encoded amino acid sequence. Four different mutations affecting a leucine codon, and an expansion of the normal (CAG)₃ sequence, are shown.

	DNA / AMINO ACID
NORMAL	A T G C A G C A G C A G T T T T T A C G T A A C C C G . . . DNA Met Gln Gln Gln Phe Leu Arg Asn Pro AMINO ACID
MISSENSE MUTATION	A T G C A G C A G C A G T T T T C A C G T A A C C C G . . . DNA Met Gln Gln Gln Phe **Ser** Arg Asn Pro AMINO ACID
NONSENSE MUTATION	A T G C A G C A G C A G T T T T G A C G T A A C C C G . . . DNA Met Gln Gln Gln Phe **STOP** AMINO ACID
FRAMESHIFT MUTATION (1 bp DELETION)	A T G C A G C A G C A G T T T A C G T A A C C C G . . . DNA Met Gln Gln Gln Phe **Tyr Val Thr Arg** AMINO ACID
SILENT MUTATION	A T G C A G C A G C A G T T T T T G C G T A A C C C G . . . DNA Met Gln Gln Gln Phe **Leu** Arg Asn Pro AMINO ACID
EXPANDED TRIPLET REPEAT	A T G C A G C A G C A G C A G C A G C A G C A G C A G . . . DNA Met **Gln Gln Gln Gln Gln Gln Gln Gln** AMINO ACID

the triplet codon to that for a different amino acid (a "missense mutation"), then the resultant protein will be structurally different. If the amino acid substitution occurs in a functionally important domain or alters the structure or stability of the protein, altered function will result. A particularly disruptive point mutation is one that converts the normal codon to UAA, UGA, or UAG, creating a premature stop codon. This is known as a "nonsense mutation."

If it does not represent a multiple of 3, insertion or deletion of a small number of nucleotides into a coding region will alter the reading frame of translation from that point onward, leading to a completely abnormal carboxy terminus of the protein. Such mutations are called "frameshifts."

Several other varieties of mutation alter transcription of a gene, but we will delay a discussion of these until chapter 5, when a more complete description of gene anatomy is given. First, we will delve into the effects of mutation in creating human disease and the inheritance patterns that can result.

SUGGESTED READINGS

History of Molecular Biology

Judson HF. The eighth day of creation: makers of the revolution in biology. New York: Simon & Schuster, 1979.
Watson JD. The double helix. New York: Athenum, 1968.

General Reference Texts

Alberts B, Bray D, Lewis J, Raff M, Roberts K, Watson JD. Molecular biology of the cell. 3rd ed. New York: Garland, 1994.
Darnell J, Lodish H, Baltimore D. Molecular cell biology. 2nd ed. New York: Scientific American Books, WH Freeman, 1990.
Watson JD, Tooze J, Kurtz DT. Recombinant DNA, a short course. New York: Scientific American Books, WH Freeman, 1983.
Watson JD, Hopkins NH, Roberts JW, Steitz JA, Weiner AM. Molecular biology of the gene. 4th ed. Menlo Park, CA: Benjamin/Cummings Publishing Co., 1987.

Classic Papers

Meselson M, Stahl FW. The replication of DNA in *E. coli*. Proc Natl Acad Sci USA 1958;44:671–682.
Nirenberg MW, Matthaei JH. The dependence of cell-free protein synthesis in *E. coli* upon naturally occurring or synthetic polyribonucleotides. Proc Natl Acad Sci USA 1961;47:1588–1602.
Watson JD, Crick FHC. A structure for deoxyribose nucleic acid. Nature 1953;171:737–738.

Mendelian Inheritance

"Those characteristics that are transmitted entire, or almost unchanged by hybridization, and therefore constitute the characters of the hybrid, are termed dominant, and those that become latent in the process, recessive."

—GREGOR MENDEL, 1865

In order to understand Mendelian inheritance, several essential terms must first be defined. A genetic **locus** is a specific position or location on a chromosome. Frequently, locus is used to refer to a specific gene. **Alleles** are alternative forms of a gene, or of a DNA sequence, at a given locus. If both alleles at a locus are identical, the individual is **homozygous** at that locus; if they are different, he or she is **heterozygous.** Such individuals are called **homozygotes** or **heterozygotes,** respectively. An individual with two different mutant alleles at a given locus is a **compound heterozygote,** whereas an individual with one mutant allele at each of two different loci is a **double heterozygote**.

The **genotype** is the genetic constitution or composition of an individual. Genotype also can refer to the alleles at a specific genetic locus. The **phenotype** is the observed result of the interaction of the genotype with environmental factors; more specifically, the observable expression of a particular gene or genes. The meaning of genotype and phenotype may be illustrated by a musical analogy. Figure 3.1 is a portion of the score of Mozart's Concerto in A Major for Piano and Orchestra, K. 488. The musical notation contains all of the necessary information or instructions for the notes to be played by each instrument and the temporal relationships of the various parts. This is the genotype. The phenotype is the sound we hear, which is strongly influenced by the environment, including the soloist, the conductor, the orchestra, and the hall in which it is performed, or the quality of the recording.

We define Mendelian diseases as diseases that are the result of a **single mutant gene** that has a large effect on phenotype and that are inherited in simple patterns similar to or identical with those described by Mendel for certain discrete characteristics in garden peas. Mendelian diseases are **autosomal** if they are encoded by genes on one of the 22 pairs of autosomes, or non-sex chromosomes, and **X-linked** if encoded by a mutant gene on the X chromosome. Following Mendel, we define as **dominant** those conditions that are expressed in heterozygotes, i.e., individuals who have one copy of a mutant allele and one copy of a normal, or wild-type, allele, and **recessive** those conditions that are clinically manifest only in individuals homozygous for the mutant allele (or compound heterozygotes for two different mutant alleles), i.e., carrying a double dose of an abnormal gene. It should be stressed that dominance and recessivity refer to traits, or phenotypes, and not to genes. Although we sometimes speak of dominant and recessive genes, this is a shorthand and should be understood to refer to traits. By now more than 5000 human phenotypes known to be inherited in a Mendelian

Figure 3.1.   The first page of the orchestral score of the Concerto in A Major for Piano and Orchestra, K. 488 by Wolfgang Amadeus Mozart.   (From Mozart WA. Piano Concertos Nos. 23–27 in Full Score. New York: Dover Publications, 1978:1.)

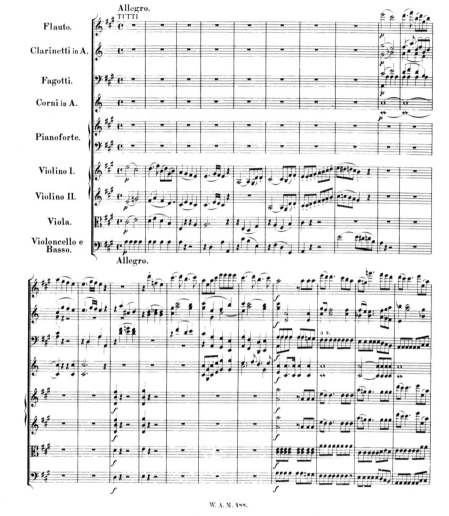

Piano Concerto No. 23 in A Major, K.488

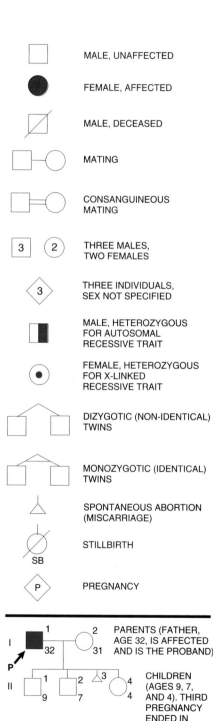

MALE, UNAFFECTED

FEMALE, AFFECTED

MALE, DECEASED

MATING

CONSANGUINEOUS MATING

3   2   THREE MALES, TWO FEMALES

3   THREE INDIVIDUALS, SEX NOT SPECIFIED

MALE, HETEROZYGOUS FOR AUTOSOMAL RECESSIVE TRAIT

FEMALE, HETEROZYGOUS FOR X-LINKED RECESSIVE TRAIT

DIZYGOTIC (NON-IDENTICAL) TWINS

MONOZYGOTIC (IDENTICAL) TWINS

SPONTANEOUS ABORTION (MISCARRIAGE)

STILLBIRTH

PREGNANCY

1   2   PARENTS (FATHER, AGE 32, IS AFFECTED AND IS THE PROBAND)

CHILDREN (AGES 9, 7, AND 4). THIRD PREGNANCY ENDED IN MISCARRIAGE.

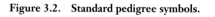

Figure 3.2.   Standard pedigree symbols.

fashion have been catalogued. More than half are autosomal dominant traits, 36% are autosomal recessive, and less than 10% are X-linked. Of these 5000 traits, approximately 4000 are associated with human diseases. In almost 600 of these, one or more disease-causing mutations have been identified.

The pattern of inheritance of most Mendelian traits has been deduced from observing the segregation or transmission of these traits within families. This information is expressed in the form of a pedigree, derived from the French expression "pied de grue" or crane's foot, from the branching pattern of the diagram. The standard symbols used for drawing a human pedigree are shown in Figure 3.2. More extensive recommendations for standardized human pedigree nomenclature, which take into account recent technical advances in medical genetics, have been published. The proband or index case, the first affected family member coming to medical attention, is indicated by an *arrow* and letter *P;* an arrow alone indicates the consultand, or individual(s) seeking genetic counseling or testing. The position of individuals within the pedigree is indicated by *Roman numerals* for the generation and *Arabic numerals* for an individual within a single generation. For pedigrees in physician records or hospital charts, it is useful to note the individuals' age next to or below, but not inside, the symbol.

Autosomal dominant diseases include many of the serious and more common genetic disorders of adult life including familial hypercholesterolemia, hereditary colon cancer, polycystic kidney disease, Huntington disease, and neurofibromatosis. The pedigree of a family with familial hypercholesterolemia is shown in Figure 3.3. This condition is characterized by an increased level of cholesterol in blood and by premature atherosclerotic cardiovascular disease with myocardial infarctions or heart attacks early in life. Although both men and women are affected, affected males tend to have coronary artery disease about a decade earlier than do women, just as is true for the general population without hypercholesterolemia. The basic defect in this condition has been defined as a deficiency in low-density lipoprotein receptors on the cell surface (see chapter 7). W.H. (II-4 in the pedigree in Fig. 3.3) is a 33-year-old white advertising executive. At the age of 25 years he began to experience recurrent chest pain on exertion and, at age 30, suffered a myocardial infarction. Coronary arteriography revealed extensive coronary artery disease and he underwent coronary artery bypass graft surgery. Physical examination revealed evidence of cholesterol deposits in extensor tendons, and laboratory evaluation indicated significant hypercholesterolemia. A family history revealed that his father had died at age 52 years of his second myocardial infarction and that a paternal uncle (I-1) had also died of a myocardial infarction at age 46 years. The patient's 50-year-old sister was asymptomatic but was found to have hypercholesterolemia. W.H.'s three children were entirely healthy and normal on physical examination, but all had significant hypercholesterolemia.

As seen in this pedigree, the characteristic pattern of inheritance is *vertical*; that is, the disorder is passed from one generation to the next in a vertical fashion. Both males and females are affected and can transmit the trait with equal probability, although the severity of manifestations can be affected by the sex of the individual. Each affected individual has one affected parent. Note that in pedigrees of dominantly inherited conditions, the unaffected spouse is often omitted.

The pattern of inheritance of autosomal dominant traits is best understood by observing the segregation of chromosomes bearing the mutant and normal alleles during meiosis (Fig. 3.4). Assuming for simplicity that there is only one normal allele and one mutant allele, there are three possible genotypes: homozygous normal, homozygous affected, and heterozygous. Because both males and females may have any of the three genotypes, there are six possible mating types; however, because both males and females may

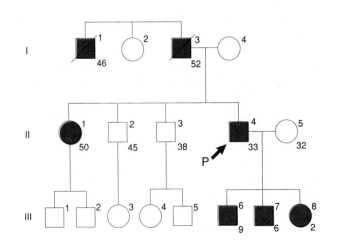

Figure 3.3. Pedigree of a family with autosomal dominant familial hypercholesterolemia. Affected individuals are indicated by the *solid red symbols*.

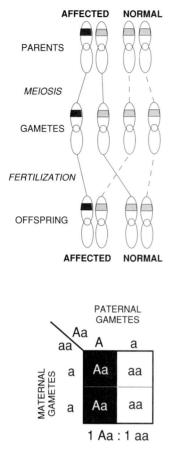

AFFECTED   NORMAL

PARENTS

MEIOSIS

GAMETES

FERTILIZATION

OFFSPRING

AFFECTED   NORMAL

PATERNAL
GAMETES

Aa
aa   A   a

MATERNAL
GAMETES

a | Aa | aa
a | Aa | aa

1 Aa : 1 aa

A = MUTANT, a = NORMAL

Figure 3.4. Autosomal dominant inheritance. The mating diagram *(top)* and Punnett square *(bottom)* show the outcome of a mating between a heterozygous affected individual and a homozygous normal individual. The mutant allele in the mating diagram is indicated in *red*, and affected offspring in the Punnett square are indicated in *red*.

transmit the abnormal gene with equal probability, sex differences will be ignored. Because homozygous affected individuals are very rare, the usual mating in dominantly inherited diseases is that between a homozygous normal individual and a heterozygous affected individual. Each gamete produced by these individuals will contain only one allele of the pair so that the possible gametes produced are shown in the mating diagram in the *top panel* of Figure 3.4. On the *bottom* is a Punnett square, an alternative method for showing the gametes produced and their possible combinations at fertilization. Each offspring of such a mating has a 50% probability of inheriting the chromosome bearing the mutant allele and a 50% probability of inheriting the chromosome bearing the normal allele, and thus, a 50% probability of being affected. On average, approximately half of the offspring of affected individuals will themselves be affected. An unaffected child, inheriting the chromosome bearing the normal allele, can have only normal offspring. In the pedigree shown in Figure 3.3, two offspring of four born to the affected parent I-3 are themselves affected, i.e., the expected 50% probability. Within any given sibship (set of siblings), however, the 50% prediction may not be met; all three children of W.H. (III-6, III-7, and III-8) are affected with familial hypercholesterolemia.

To understand this divergence from expectation, it is important to recall that each offspring represents an independent event with a 50% probability of being affected. According to the **independence principle,** the probability of the *joint* occurrence of two or more *independent* events is the *product* of their separate probabilities. Therefore, the probability of all three children being affected is the product of their independent probabilities or $(1/2) \times (1/2) \times (1/2) = 1/8$.

In summary, the typical pedigree pattern for an autosomal dominant trait or disease is quite striking, showing vertical inheritance and involvement of both sexes with equal probability with, on average, half of the offspring of an affected parent being affected, but none of the offspring of an unaffected parent. This pattern of inheritance of a rare disease or trait through three generations virtually defines that trait as being inherited in an autosomal dominant fashion.

VARIATIONS ON A THEME

There are a number of special characteristics of autosomal dominant inheritance that may be thought of as exceptions to the rule that all affected individuals have an affected parent. In these situations, patients with an autosomal dominant disease appear to be sporadic cases, that is, they have apparently unaffected parents. First, a sporadic case may arise as a result of a new **mutation** or change in the genetic material. The more severe a disorder is with respect to fertility, the more likely it is that patients with this disease are the result of a new mutation in one of the gametes that formed them. If an autosomal dominant disorder generally causes death before reproductive age or prevents the ability to reproduce, then cases of such a disease would arise only as the result of a new mutation. Osteogenesis imperfecta, type II (discussed in chapter 7), is a perinatal lethal autosomal dominant condition; all cases represent new mutations. Another example is achondroplasia, a common form of short-limbed dwarfism (Fig. 3.5), which significantly reduces reproductive fitness; more than 80% of cases represent new spontaneous mutations. There is evidence that increased paternal age may increase the risk of mutation. The gene that is mutated in achondroplasia encodes the type 3 fibroblast growth factor receptor, which mediates the effect of fibroblast growth factor on cartilage. Surprisingly, virtually

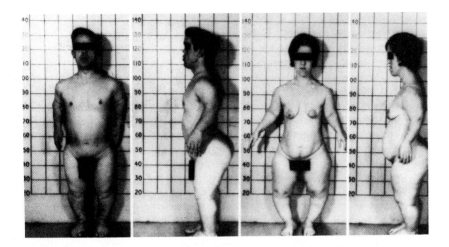

Figure 3.5. A man and a woman with achondroplasia. Note the short stature, relatively large head, short extremities especially in the proximal portion, and lordotic curvature of the spine. (From McKusick VA. Heritable disorders of connective tissue. 4th ed. St Louis: CV Mosby, 1972:758.)

all affected individuals have a mutation in exactly the same nucleotide in this gene, a highly unusual finding in human genetic disease. As discussed later in this and other chapters, it is far more usual to find multiple independent mutations causing a disease.

A second situation in which an affected child appears to have a normal parent can result from **decreased penetrance.** Penetrance is an all-or-none phenomenon that refers to the clinical expression, or lack of it, of the mutant gene. In a sense, penetrance is an artifact of our ability to recognize the expression or phenotype of a mutant gene. When the definition of expression is clinical disease, an individual carrying a mutant gene may not express the disease and thus the condition is nonpenetrant. We define penetrance quantitatively by determining the proportion of obligate gene carriers (heterozygotes) for a mutant allele who express the phenotype. Figure 3.6 shows the pedigree of a family with hereditary erythromelalgia, an unusual disease characterized by red, hot, painful feet and occasionally hands. It is clear from this pedigree that the disease is inherited as an autosomal dominant trait in this family. Individuals I-4, II-3, II-5, III-1, III-3, III-7, and IV-1 through IV-4 are heterozygotes for the mutant allele. All are affected except III-1. This woman is an *obligate* heterozygote because she has an affected mother and three affected children; but she herself gave no history of, nor showed any signs of, this disease. In this pedigree, 9 of 10 obligate heterozygotes

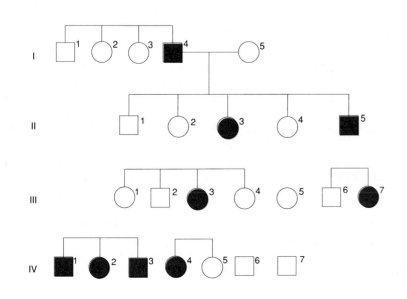

Figure 3.6. Pedigree of a family with autosomal dominant erythromelalgia illustrating nonpenetrance. Note that individual III-1 is clinically unaffected but is an obligate heterozygote for the mutant allele.

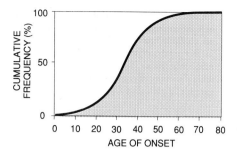

Figure 3.7.   Age of onset of Huntington's disease. Fifty percent of the patients in this study had onset of the disease by age 35 years. (From Conneally PM, Wallace MR, Gusella JF, Wexler NS. Huntington disease: estimation of heterozygote status using linked genetic markers. Genet Epidemiol 1984;1:81–88.)

manifested the disease, suggesting a penetrance of approximately 90%. If a disease is described as being 90% penetrant, it means that there is a probability of 90% that an individual carrying the mutant allele will express observable disease. The expression itself, however, is all-or-none.

Third, a number of important autosomal dominant diseases are not present at birth but have manifestations only later in life *(delayed onset)*. Polycystic kidney disease is characterized by bilateral enlargement of the kidneys with multiple cysts, blood in the urine, high blood pressure, abdominal pain, and progressive renal failure. Symptoms generally do not occur until the fourth decade of life or even later in many patients. The characteristic cysts in the kidney are not usually detectable by ultrasound or radiologic techniques until the second decade. Even more striking is Huntington disease, a degenerative neurologic disorder characterized by abnormal movements (chorea) and progressive loss of mental function (dementia). As shown in Figure 3.7, the average age of onset of this condition is about 35 years. Therefore, it is possible that an individual carrying the gene could have children and die from unrelated causes (for example, a motor vehicle accident) before reaching an age at which the disease is manifest. Thus, it would appear that the disease had skipped a generation or that an affected offspring had an unaffected parent, but this would simply reflect the delayed age of onset of this particular dominantly inherited disease. It should be noted that such late age of onset also allows the gene to spread within the population since individuals do not become ill until they have already borne children and passed the mutant gene on to the next generation. The examples described above also emphasize that "genetic" is not synonymous with "congenital" (present at birth); genetic diseases clearly need not be congenital. Conversely, congenital defects need not be genetic; the congenital malformations caused by the drug thalidomide are not known to have any genetic basis.

Fourth, occasionally two or more children affected with an autosomal dominant disease will be found in a family with *no prior history* of the disease. Because new mutations are rare events, it is unlikely that the affected individuals represent recurrent mutations. A more likely explanation is **germline mosaicism.** A mutation during embryonic life affecting precursors of gametes can result in some or all of that individual's gametes carrying a mutation, while an insufficient number of his or her somatic cells are affected to result in any clinical signs. Such a clinically unaffected individual could have multiple affected offspring. Germline mosaicism has been demonstrated by DNA analysis in the lethal perinatal form of osteogenesis imperfecta (see chapter 7) and in neurofibromatosis, as well as in the X-linked recessive diseases, Duchenne muscular dystrophy and hemophilia A.

Finally, a fifth source of apparent sporadic cases of an autosomal dominant disease is found in cases in which the putative father is not the actual biological father of the affected child. In one large study, the frequency of this event was approximately 5–10%.

GENETIC HETEROGENEITY

The majority of inherited human diseases exhibit **genetic heterogeneity.** Genetic heterogeneity means that different mutations can cause an identical or similar phenotype. We further distinguish **allelic heterogeneity,** which refers to different mutations at the same locus, from **locus heterogeneity,** which refers to mutations at different loci. Recent progress in understanding the molecular basis of several of the osteogenesis imperfecta (OI) syndromes, characterized by brittle bones that may spontaneously fracture before birth or fracture with minimal trauma later in life, has revealed a clear example of both allelic and locus heterogeneity. Mutations in either the gene encoding the α1 chain of type 1 collagen, on chromosome 7, or the α2 chain, on chromosome 17, can alter collagen structure and cause OI. This is *locus* heterogeneity. Furthermore, as discussed in chapter 7, different mutations in the *COL1A1* gene encoding the α1 chain can cause OI, often with varying degrees of severity; this is termed *allelic* heterogeneity. Other examples of locus heterogeneity include the hereditary colon cancer syndromes discussed in chapter 12. Allelic heterogeneity is virtually the rule among human Mendelian diseases (achondroplasia and sickle cell anemia are notable exceptions), and examples include the β-thalassemias (chapter 6), glucose-6-phosphate dehydrogenase deficiency (chapter 7), and familial hypercholesterolemia (chapter 7).

VARIABLE EXPRESSIVITY

Mutant genes with pleiotropic effects, i.e., affecting several organ systems and functions, frequently show **variable expressivity**. The expressivity of a trait, although often confused with penetrance, refers to the nature and severity of the phenotype. Variable expressivity is a frequent characteristic of autosomal dominant traits; the Marfan syndrome is a good example (Fig. 3.8). This disorder is the result of a mutation in the gene for fibrillin, the main component of extracellular microfibrils. It affects the connective tissues of the body, primarily in the skeletal system (long, thin extremities and fingers, lax joints, bony deformities of the spine and sternum), the eye (severe nearsightedness and dislocation of the lens), and the heart (valvular incompetence, widening of the root of the aorta, and sometimes dissection of the aorta and sudden death). An individual affected with the Marfan syndrome may have involvement of only two or all three major systems, and the severity of the manifestations may vary widely. Furthermore, as shown in the pedigree in Figure 3.9, this variability occurs among affected individuals within the same family who presumably carry the same mutant allele. This pedigree is particularly informative because DNA analysis has been carried out in four affected and five unaffected members of the family. These studies confirm that the same mutation was found in all four affected individuals tested; despite this, the age of onset of clinical signs, and distribution and severity of organ system involvement in affected family members was quite varied. These observations indicate that the Marfan phenotype is not determined *solely* by the mutant genotype at the fibrillin locus. The variable expressivity must be caused either by environmental influences and/or by the effects of other genes that modify the expression of the mutant gene for the Marfan syndrome. The virtually identical phenotype of the affected monozygotic twins in generation V indicates that alleles at other loci influence the expression of the mutant fibrillin allele.

An even more striking example of variable expressivity is seen in neurofibromatosis 1 (NF1) or von Recklinghausen disease (Fig. 3.10). This autosomal dominant condition is characterized by brownish spots on the skin called café au lait spots, benign hamartomatous nodules on the iris of the eye (Lisch nodules), and cutaneous and subcutaneous neurofibromas, fleshy benign tumors often arising along the course of nerves. The characteristic neurofibromas usually appear about the time of puberty and may increase during a lifetime to number in the thousands. In addition, this disease has protean manifestations affecting almost every system in the body. Highly vascular plexiform neurofibromas, which infiltrate surrounding tissues, can cause serious growth abnormalities and deformities. Manifestations of this disease can range from the mere presence of café au lait spots and Lisch

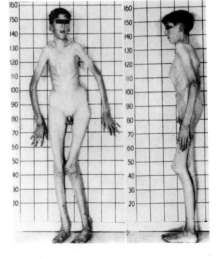

Figure 3.8. A 17-year-old boy with the Marfan syndrome.   Note the long thin extremities, thin spiderlike fingers (arachnodactyly), flat feet, and deformities of the breastbone and spine. (From McKusick VA. Heritable disorders of connective tissue. 4th ed. St. Louis: CV Mosby, 1972:67.)

Figure 3.9. Pedigree of autosomal dominant Marfan syndrome illustrating variable expressivity. DNA was analyzed from individuals IV-1, 2, and 3, V-1, 2, 3, 4, and 5, and VI-1. All affected individuals demonstrated the same fibrillin gene mutation, and all tested family members who carry the mutation show manifestations of the Marfan syndrome in at least one organ system. However, there is marked variability in age of onset of clinical signs and in distribution and severity of organ system involvement. Individuals I-2, II-2, and III-3 all died at a young age of severe cardiovascular involvement, but had mild eye and/or skeletal involvement. In contrast, individuals IV-4 and V-3 had severe skeletal involvement with mild, or no, eye or cardiac involvement. (Redrawn from Dietz HC, Pyeritz RE, Puffenberger EG, et al. Marfan phenotype variability in a family segregating a missense mutation in the epidermal growth factor-like motif of the fibrillin gene. J Clin Invest 1992;89:1674–1680.)

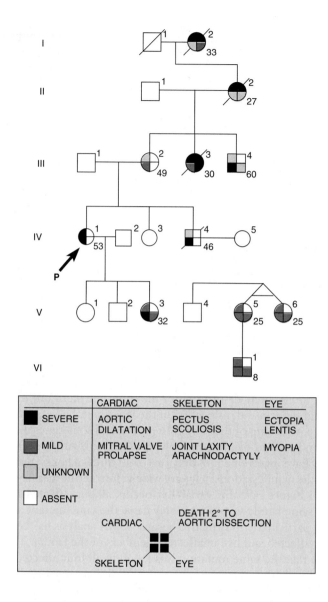

nodules to cosmetically disfiguring cutaneous neurofibromas, to severe deformities and functional impairment in a few less fortunate patients. All affected individuals have mutations at the same neurofibromin locus; therefore, interfamilial variability is not because of locus heterogeneity. There is no way to predict how severe the manifestations will be in any affected individual nor is there any evidence that the severity "breeds true" in any given family.

GENETIC INSTABILITY AND ANTICIPATION

It has been observed for several decades that some dominantly inherited diseases manifest an earlier age of onset and increasing severity in successive generations. The most striking example of this phenomenon, called **anticipation,** is myotonic dystrophy, the most common muscular dystrophy affecting adults. Myotonic dystrophy is characterized by muscle wasting, beginning in the face (and causing the characteristic masklike facies with ptosis or drooping eyelids [Fig. 3.11]), neck, and hands, but gradually becoming generalized, and by myotonia, or the inability of a muscle to relax after contraction. Myotonic dystrophy also affects cardiac and smooth mus-

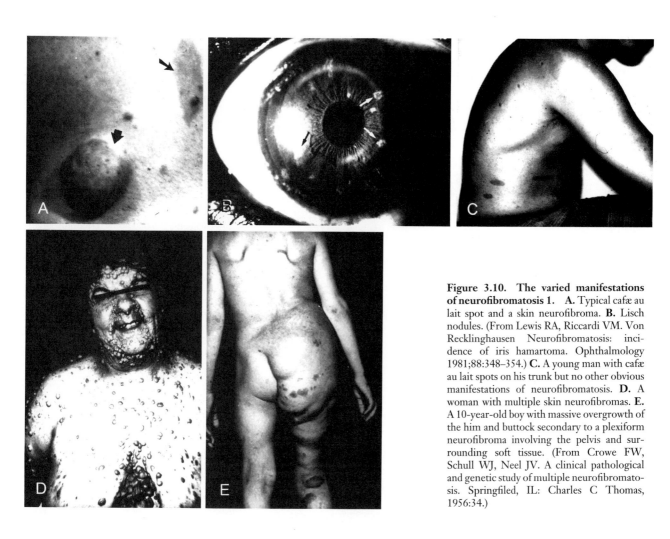

Figure 3.10. The varied manifestations of neurofibromatosis 1. A. Typical cafæ au lait spot and a skin neurofibroma. **B.** Lisch nodules. (From Lewis RA, Riccardi VM. Von Recklinghausen Neurofibromatosis: incidence of iris hamartoma. Ophthalmology 1981;88:348–354.) **C.** A young man with cafæ au lait spots on his trunk but no other obvious manifestations of neurofibromatosis. **D.** A woman with multiple skin neurofibromas. **E.** A 10-year-old boy with massive overgrowth of the him and buttock secondary to a plexiform neurofibroma involving the pelvis and surrounding soft tissue. (From Crowe FW, Schull WJ, Neel JV. A clinical pathological and genetic study of multiple neurofibromatosis. Springfiled, IL: Charles C Thomas, 1956:34.)

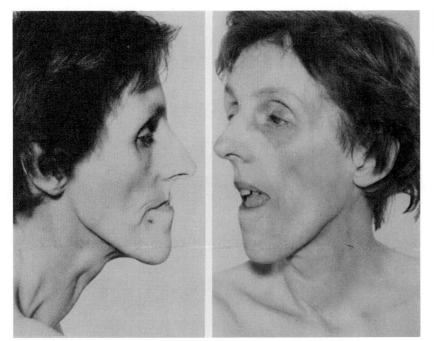

Figure 3.11. Adult patient with myotonic dystrophy. Note the ptosis, facial weakness, and wasting of the jaw and sternocleidomastoid muscles.

A.

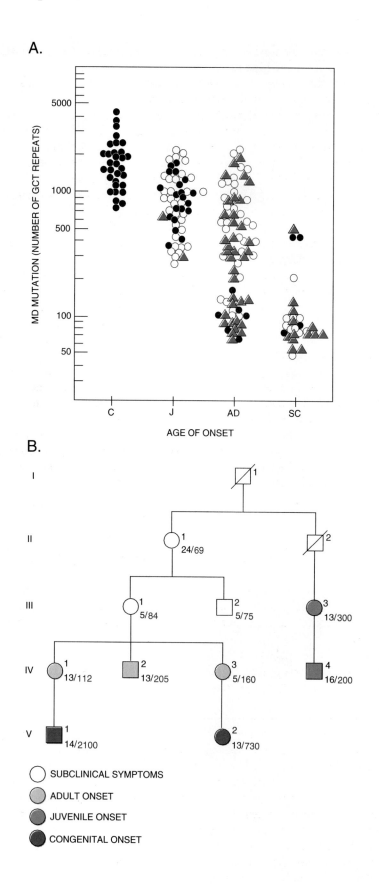

B.

○ SUBCLINICAL SYMPTOMS

◑ ADULT ONSET

◑ JUVENILE ONSET

● CONGENITAL ONSET

Figure 3.12.   Relationship between trinucleotide repeat length and severity and/or age of onset of myotonic dystrophy. A. Size of the myotonic dystrophy GCT repeat and the age of onset of disease in 197 patients. The size of the GCT repeat expansion, expressed in number of repeats, is plotted with age of onset of disease and, where known, the sex of the transmitting parent. The categories for age of onset are congenital (C) for symptoms up to 1 year of life, juvenile (J) for onset from 1 to less than 20 years, adult (AD) for onset at 20 years or older, and subclinical (SC) indicating no signs other than cataracts or an abnormal, but nondiagnostic electromyogram. The sex of the transmitting parent is noted as a black circle (mother), an open circle (father), or a red triangle (unknown). (Reproduced with permission from Redman JB, Fenwick RG, Fu Y-H, Pizzuti A, and Caskey CT. Relationship between parental trinucleotide GCT repeat length and severity of myotonic dystrophy in offspring. JAMA 1993;269:1960–1965). **B.** Pedigree of a family with myotonic dystrophy illustrating anticipation. The size of the normal allele (number of trinucleotide repeats) is indicated to the left of the diagonal line; the size of the expanded allele to the right. (Redrawn from Redman JB, Fenwick RG, Fu Y-H, Pizzuti A, and Caskey CT. Relationship between parental trinucleotide GCT repeat length and severity of myotonic dystrophy in offspring. JAMA 1993;269:1960–1965.)

cle, and is associated with early cataracts, immunoglobulin abnormalities, and often mild mental retardation.

Before the cloning of the myotonin gene, there was no biological explanation for anticipation, and it was thought to reflect an artifact of ascertainment of clinically affected patients. Analysis of the myotonin gene, however, revealed the presence of multiple repeats of a GCT (or CTG) triplet in the 3'-untranslated region of the gene. Normal individuals were found to have 5 to 35 copies of the triplet; affected individuals have > 50 and sometimes hundreds to > 1000 copies. Significantly, this region of the gene is unstable, making it susceptible to undergo dynamic mutation manifested by an increase in number of repeats in successive generations (Fig. 3.12). Furthermore, the severity and age of onset of myotonic dystrophy is highly correlated with the number of triplet repeats (Fig. 3.12). The highest number of repeats is found in infants with the rarer congenital form of myotonic dystrophy, characterized by severe hypotonia (floppiness) and mental retardation. The congenital form occurs only in infants, of either sex, born to affected mothers, and the greatest increase in number of repeats appears to occur in female meioses. Thus the long-established clinical observation of anticipation in myotonic dystrophy now has a molecular basis in genetic instability and expansion of a triplet repeat. The mechanism of this genetic instability and the basis for the sex-specific expansion resulting in congenital myotonic dystrophy remains to be determined. Expansion of triplet repeats has also been described in the fragile X syndrome (discussed in chapter 8), and in several dominantly inherited, adult-onset neurodegenerative diseases, including Huntington's disease. In the latter group of diseases, a stretch of 10–30 CAG triplets, encoding a polyglutamine tract, is expanded approximately two- to fourfold in affected individuals. Anticipation, with age of onset related to the number of repeats, is also observed, though less strikingly than in myotonic dystrophy.

HOMOZYGOUS AFFECTED INDIVIDUALS

For most relatively rare autosomal dominant diseases, affected individuals are heterozygotes. However, when the gene is sufficiently common, matings between heterozygous affected parents resulting in homozygous affected offspring are seen. In most cases, affected homozygotes are much more severely affected than are heterozygotes. This is well illustrated by familial hypercholesterolemia, in which homozygotes have much higher elevations of cholesterol and develop atherosclerotic cardiovascular disease in childhood. Similarly, homozygous achondroplasia and Marfan syndrome are lethal in infancy. In contrast, homozygotes for Huntington disease appear to be no more severely affected than heterozygous individuals.

Autosomal Recessive Inheritance

Autosomal recessive diseases are characterized by clinical manifestations only in individuals homozygous for the mutant gene (or compound heterozygotes for two different mutant alleles at the same locus). The characteristic pedigree pattern (Fig. 3.13) is *horizontal* rather than vertical in that affected individuals tend to be limited to a single sibship and the disease is not found in multiple generations. Males and females are affected with equal probability. The usual mating (Fig. 3.14) is that between two individuals who are clinically normal but heterozygous for the mutant allele. There is a 1 in 4 chance that each offspring will be homozygous for the mutant allele and affected; a 1 in 4 chance that he or she will be homozygous for the normal or wild-type allele and clinically normal; and 2 chances in 4 that he or she will be heterozygous for the mutant allele and a clinically normal carrier like each parent.

The probability that two individuals heterozygous for the same mutant allele will mate depends upon the frequency of heterozygotes in the population and this in turn is a function of the mutant allele frequency. A more detailed discussion of gene frequencies will be presented in chapter 4. It is intuitively apparent, however, that if the mutant allele is rare in the population, then the probability will be very low that any two individuals carrying this same mutant allele will marry. This probability would be increased if they were related and had inherited the same mutant allele from a common ancestor. Thus, **consanguinity,** or the mating between close relatives, is

Figure 3.13.   Pedigree of an autosomal recessive trait.   Affected individuals, indicated by *solid red symbols*, are found in only one generation. Note that both parents of an affected child are obligate heterozygotes (designated by *half-shaded red symbols*), as are all of the offspring of a mating between an affected individual and a homozygous normal individual.

Figure 3.14.   Autosomal recessive inheritance.   The mating diagram and Punnett square illustrate the outcome of a mating of two individuals who are clinically normal but are heterozygous for the mutant allele. As in Figure 3.4, the mutant allele is indicated in *red* and affected individuals are indicated by the *solid red box*. Heterozygous carriers are indicated by the *light red boxes*.

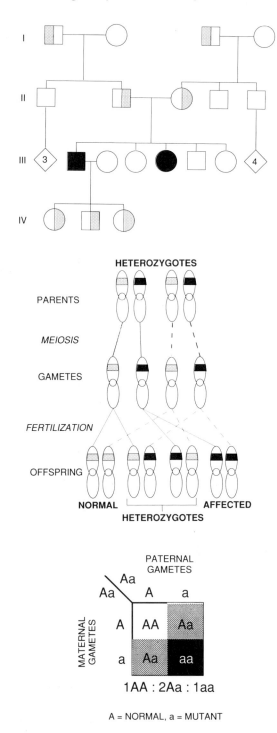

found more frequently among parents of children with rare autosomal recessive diseases. On the other hand, if the mutant gene is common in a population, such as cystic fibrosis in the white population, Tay-Sachs disease among Ashkenazi (European) Jews, or sickle cell anemia among African-Americans, the mating of heterozygotes would be more common and parental consanguinity would not be expected to be found as frequently.

Because the risk is only 1 in 4 that a child will be affected if both parents are carriers and because most American families are small (two to three children), most affected individuals with autosomal recessive diseases will appear to be sporadic cases. That is, there will be only one affected member in the family. If two or more children are affected, the disease is more likely to be recognized as a genetic disorder. Nevertheless, it should be kept in mind that most autosomal recessive diseases will appear as sporadic cases, and it is important that their genetic etiology not be overlooked because of the lack of a positive family history.

This point is illustrated in Figure 3.15. If one were able to ascertain all 3-child families in which both parents were carriers of the same mutant allele, nearly half (42%) of these families would have no affected children. Because, in practice, we recognize matings between heterozygous carriers only by the presence of an affected child, such families would not be ascertained in the absence of a screening program for detecting heterozygous carriers. Another 42% of 3-child families of this sort would have a single affected child; whereas 14% would have two affected children and only 2% of such families would have all three

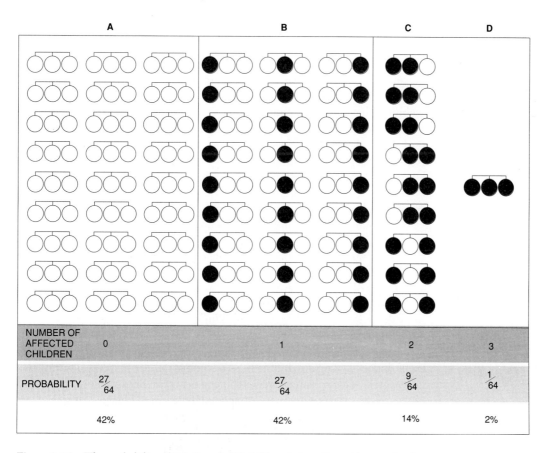

Figure 3.15.   The probability of 0, 1, 2, or 3 of 3 children being affected in a mating between heterozygotes for an autosomal recessive trait.   In this diagram, *circles* represent offspring of either sex; *red symbols* indicate affected individuals. The probabilities can be calculated using the binomial formula. Note that for families with three offspring, nearly half of the matings (42%) will result in no affected offspring and nearly half will result in a single affected offspring. (From Li CC. Human genetics. New York: McGraw-Hill, 1961.)

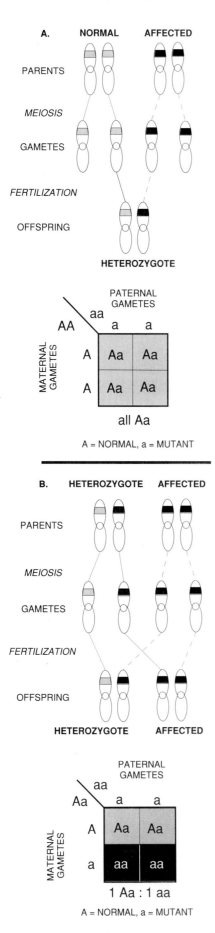

A.

NORMAL AFFECTED

PARENTS

MEIOSIS

GAMETES

FERTILIZATION

OFFSPRING

HETEROZYGOTE

PATERNAL
GAMETES

	aa	
AA	a	a
A	Aa	Aa
A	Aa	Aa

MATERNAL GAMETES

all Aa

A = NORMAL, a = MUTANT

B.

HETEROZYGOTE AFFECTED

PARENTS

MEIOSIS

GAMETES

FERTILIZATION

OFFSPRING

HETEROZYGOTE **AFFECTED**

PATERNAL
GAMETES

	aa	
Aa	a	a
A	Aa	Aa
a	aa	aa

MATERNAL GAMETES

1 Aa : 1 aa

A = NORMAL, a = MUTANT

offspring affected. Even among the families ascertained because they have at least one affected offspring, nearly 3 of 4 (27/37 or 73%) would have a single affected child and thus the disease would appear to be sporadic in these families.

How then do we recognize autosomal recessive traits? Obviously the appearance of multiple affected siblings within large sibships and the presence of parental consanguinity suggest the presence of a rare recessive disease. Stronger evidence, however, is the demonstration of a partial defect in obligate heterozygotes. Tay-Sachs disease (or GM$_2$ gangliosidosis) is a degenerative neurological disorder in which there is virtual absence of the activity of a lysosomal enzyme, hexosaminidase A, in affected children. The clinically normal parents of a child with Tay-Sachs disease usually have approximately half the normal amount of this enzyme, confirming the autosomal recessive nature of the disease that was suggested by pedigree analysis. Such heterozygote detection techniques also allow for efficient screening programs in populations in which carriers are frequent, as is the case for Tay-Sachs disease among Ashkenazi Jews (approximately 3%) and sickle cell anemia among African-Americans (8%). The molecular definition of many recessive disorders now allows a more precise identification of carriers.

Sickle cell anemia also demonstrates that it is traits, not genes, that are dominant or recessive. Sickle cell anemia (discussed in detail in chapter 6) is an autosomal recessive disease in that it occurs only in individuals homozygous for the mutant β^S globin gene. Expression of the mutant β^S gene, however, is readily detected in heterozygous carriers, i.e., individuals with sickle cell trait, who are clinically normal. Thus, sickle cell trait is an autosomal dominant trait.

All of the offspring of an individual homozygous for a mutant allele causing an autosomal recessive disease are obligate heterozygous carriers, assuming that the mating is between a homozygous affected and a homozygous normal individual (Fig. 3.13, generation IV, and Fig. 3.16A). However, when a homozygous affected individual marries a heterozygous carrier, there is a 50% probability that any offspring will also be homozygous for the mutant allele, resulting in a pattern of inheritance that resembles autosomal dominant but is known as quasi-dominance (Fig. 3.16B). Such a mating is unlikely by chance, but is made more likely if the homozygous affected individual marries a close relative such as a first cousin, or if the mutant allele is common.

The mating of two individuals homozygous for the same mutant allele results in all of the offspring being homozygous affected. The pedigree shown in Figure 3.17 shows an example of this latter type of mating involving individuals with autosomal recessive congenital deafness. All the offspring of individuals I-3 and I-4 and of II-10 and II-11 are congenitally deaf like their parents. However, none of the offspring (IV-1 through IV-6) of individuals III-7 and III-9 are deaf. The simple explanation for this apparent paradox is that each of these parents (III-7 and III-9) is homozygous for a *different nonallelic* mutant gene causing congenital deafness. Therefore, all six of their offspring are double heterozygotes, i.e., are heterozygous for two different, nonallelic mutant genes causing deafness. Because they are not homozygous for either one, they are normal in hearing. This pedigree is an example of locus heterogeneity, i.e., mutations at different loci causing the same phenotype, congenital deafness.

Figure 3.16.   Mating diagram and Punnett square illustrating the outcome of a mating between a homozygous affected individual and a homozygous normal indivdiual (A) and between a homozygous affected individual and a clinically normal heterozygous individual (B). Note that all of the offspring in **A** are obligate heterozygotes, and that there is a 50% probability that each offspring in **B** will be homozygous affected.

X-linked diseases are caused by mutant genes on the X chromosome. X-linked mutant genes are fully expressed in males, who have only a single X chromosome, i.e., are **hemizygous** for X-linked genes. All somatic cells in human females contain two X chromosomes; however, only one X chromosome is genetically active. One of the two X chromosomes is randomly and permanently inactivated early in embryonic development, a process called lyonization (see chapter 8 for discussion). Because of this random X-inactivation, X-linked traits are variably expressed in women who are heterozygous for an X-linked mutant gene. A disease encoded by a mutant X-linked gene may or may not be expressed clinically in a heterozygous female. Diseases that are rarely expressed clinically in heterozygous females are called **X-linked recessive.**

Typical X-linked recessive disorders are hemophilia A and Duchenne muscular dystrophy. The former is the result of a deficiency of an essential clotting factor, factor VIII, and is characterized by soft tissue bleeding, often into joints (see chapter 7). Duchenne muscular dystrophy is a form of muscular dystrophy that has its onset in boys younger than 5 years of age and causes progressive muscle weakness, usually terminating in death in the 20s from respiratory complications. A characteristic pedigree for Duchenne muscular dystrophy is shown in Figure 3.18. Only males are affected, but the disease is transmitted by healthy females who are heterozygous carriers. Thus, one can trace the disease among male relatives on the mother's side of the family.

The pattern of inheritance of X-linked recessive traits is so characteristic that it has been recognized since antiquity. The Talmud makes reference to hemophilia and provides dispensation from circumcision in families with this bleeding disorder. Another example is the legend of the water drinker's curse from 18th century Nova Scotia. On a hot summer day, a gypsy stopped at a farmhouse seeking water for his thirsty young son. The farmer's wife refused them water and sent them away, whereupon the gypsy placed a curse upon her: "May your sons be afflicted with a terrible craving for water and may the curse be revisited upon the sons of your daughters, for generation upon generation." And so it came to pass. The disease traced to early settlers in this area is nephrogenic diabetes insipidus, which is caused by an insensitivity of the kidney to antidiuretic hormone, resulting in the passage of large volumes of dilute urine, dehydration, and thirst.

X-linked inheritance can be best understood by paying attention to the X chromosome and remembering that these conditions are X-linked and not "sex-linked." The usual mating is that between a heterozygous carrier woman and a normal man (Fig. 3.19A). Each son has a 50% chance of receiving the X chromosome bearing the mutant gene and of being affected. Daughters have the same 50% chance of inheriting the mutant gene, but will inherit a normal X chromosome from the father and will generally be clinically unaffected, although they will have a 50% chance of being a carrier. A second typical mating (Fig. 3.19B) is that between an affected man and a homozygous normal woman, as for example in hemophilia. In such a mating, all the sons are normal because they receive from the affected father his Y chromosome rather than the X chromosome, and they receive a normal X chromosome from the mother. However, all the daughters are *obligate* carriers because they receive an X chromosome carrying the mutant gene from their father. Thus, there is no transmission of an X-linked recessive trait from a father to his sons; this lack of male-to-male transmission is a hallmark of X-linked inheritance.

The pedigree, shown in Figure 3.20, of a family with an inherited chronic renal disease, focal glomerular sclerosis, was thought by the physicians caring for these patients to represent "sex-linked inheritance." A consideration of the points made above, however, indicates that this cannot represent X-linked inheritance because there is male-to-male transmission. This pedigree illus-

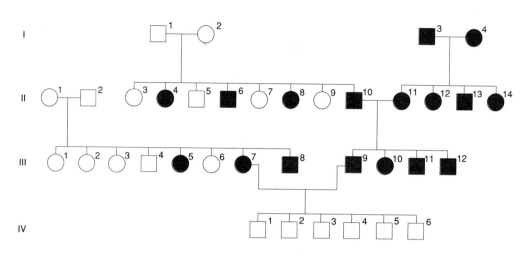

Figure 3.17.   Pedigree of a family with autosomal recessive congenital deafness. All of the individuals in generation IV have normal hearing and are presumably double heterozygotes for two nonallelic mutant genes. (From Li CC. Human genetics. New York: McGraw-Hill, 1961.)

trates that the designation sex-linked inheritance can be misleading and should not be used. In this family, the trait is likely to be autosomal dominant, possibly sex-limited or sex-influenced, i.e., being expressed in males more than, or rather than, in females even though the mutant gene is on an autosome rather than the X chromosome. A common sex-influenced autosomal dominant trait is male pattern baldness, which affects males predominantly and is transmitted from generation to generation, often in a male-to-male fashion.

Apparent male-to-male transmission of an X-linked trait can occur when the gene is sufficiently common, as for example the gene for deficiency of the enzyme glucose-6-phosphate dehydrogenase (G6PD) in African-American and Mediterranean populations (see chapter 7). In African-Americans, approximately 18% of women are heterozygous carriers of G6PD A⁻ deficiency and approximately 10% of men are hemizygous deficient. Thus, the apparent transmission of G6PD deficiency from father (II-4) to son (III-1), shown in Figure 3.21, is in fact due to the transmission of the gene on an X chromosome from the heterozygous carrier mother (II-3) and is independent of the fact that the father is also affected. It should be noted that when an X-linked gene occurs at such a high frequency, homozygous affected females may also be seen with reasonable frequency.

Figure 3.18.   Pedigree of a family with X-linked recessive Duchenne muscular dystrophy. Obligate heterozygotes are indicated by the *red dot inside the circle.*

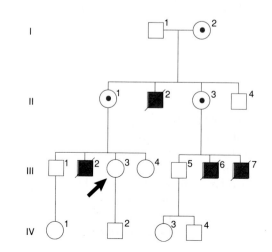

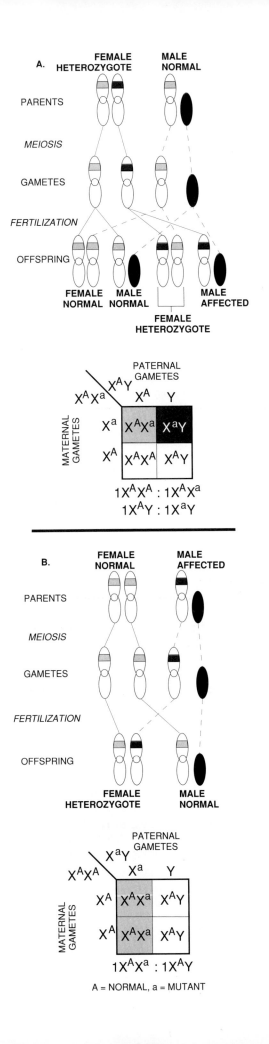

Figure 3.19. X-linked recessive inheritance. The mating diagram and Punnett square illustrate the outcome of a mating between a clinically normal female heterozygous for the mutant allele (shown in *red*) and a normal male (**A**) and between a homozygous normal female and a hemizygous affected male (**B**). The Y chromosome is indicated in *black*. Note that there can be no male-to-male transmission of the mutant allele on the X chromosome, but that all of the daughters of an affected male are obligate heterozygotes.

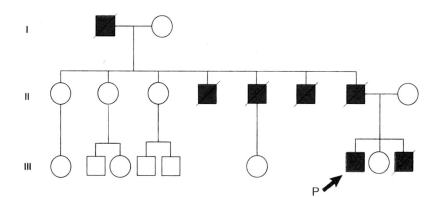

Figure 3.20.   Pedigree of a family with focal glomerular sclerosis. Note the male-to-male transmission that rules out X-linked inheritance. This pedigree is most consistent with autosomal dominant inheritance despite the fact that only males are affected in this family.

Rarely, women or girls are observed to express diseases thought to be inherited as X-linked recessive traits. There are several reasons for this. First, as noted above, the mutant allele may be sufficiently common so that homozygous females are observed with reasonable frequency. For example, deficiency of G6PD (G6PD A⁻) occurs in approximately 1% of African-American women. Such women are homozygous for the mutant allele, inheriting one copy from an affected father and the other from a carrier mother. Second, a female will occasionally express even a rare X-linked gene such as hemophilia because she is hemizygous for the X chromosome. This can occur in Turner syndrome in which there are 45 rather than 46 chromosomes and only one X chromosome (to be described in chapter 8). Third, rare chromosomal rearrangements involving exchange of material (translocations) between the X chromosome and an autosome and resulting in deletion of X-chromosomal material can result in expression of X-linked diseases such as Duchenne muscular dystrophy in females. This occurs because the normal, nontranslocated X-chromosome is preferentially inactivated (chapter 8), and the translocation chromosome with the deleted gene is active in all cells. These accidents of nature were critical in localizing the gene for this disease, as discussed in chapter 9. Fourth, because of differences in the degree of lyonization (discussed in chapter 8), it is possible that a heterozygous female will express clinical manifestations of an X-linked "recessive" disease. Finally, a girl may appear to have an X-linked recessive disease such as Duchenne muscular dystrophy, but in fact have a similar clinical phenotype caused by homozygosity for a mutant autosomal gene. This is another example of locus heterogeneity in which a different mutant gene can cause a similar phenotype.

Figure 3.22 shows a typical pedigree for an **X-linked dominant** trait, hypophosphatemic (or vitamin D-resistant) rickets, characterized by low blood and high urinary phosphate, short stature, and bony deformities. A characteristic of this pattern of inheritance is, once again, the absence of male-to-male transmission because the mutant gene is on the X chromosome. In this case, however, females are also affected and the ratio of affected females to males is approximately 2 to 1, reflecting the ratio of X chromosomes in females to males. Characteristically, the clinical expression of X-linked dominant diseases is more constant and more severe in hemizygous affected males than in heterozygous affected females, in whom the expression of the disease is often quite variable. All of the daughters of an affected man will be affected because all receive the X chromosome bearing a mutant gene from their father. All of the sons of an affected father, however, must be normal because they receive only the father's Y chromosome. Both daughters and sons of an affected woman have a 50% chance of receiving the X chromosome bearing the mutant allele and hence of being affected.

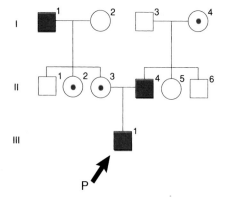

Figure 3.21.   Pedigree of a family with X-linked recessive glucose-6-phosphate dehydrogenase deficiency. Despite the apparent male-to-male transmission, III-1 must have received the mutant allele from his mother (II-3) who is an obligate heterozygote.

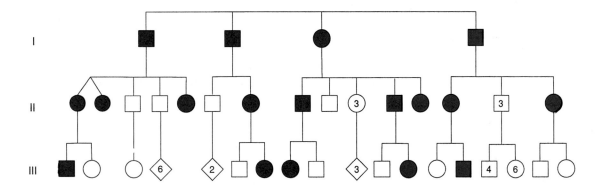

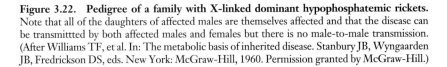

Figure 3.22. Pedigree of a family with X-linked dominant hypophosphatemic rickets.
Note that all of the daughters of affected males are themselves affected and that the disease can be transmittted by both affected males and females but there is no male-to-male transmission. (After Williams TF, et al. In: The metabolic basis of inherited disease. Stanbury JB, Wyngaarden JB, Fredrickson DS, eds. New York: McGraw-Hill, 1960. Permission granted by McGraw-Hill.)

Mitochondrial Inheritance

Mendelian inheritance describes the transmission of genes encoded by chromosomes in the nucleus of cells; however, DNA is also found in mitochondria residing in the cytoplasm of cells. Each cell contains 2–100 mitochondria, each of which contains 5–10 circular chromosomes. The 16.5-kb mitochondrial chromosome encodes two ribosomal RNA genes, 22 tRNAs, and 13 polypeptides that are parts of multi-subunit enzymes involved in oxidative phosphorylation. The mutation rate of mitochondrial DNA (mtDNA) is approximately 20 times higher than that of nuclear DNA, probably secondary to the generation of mutagenic oxygen radicals in mitochondria and their limited DNA repair capacity. Because of its cytoplasmic location, the inheritance of mtDNA is exclusively maternal (mature sperm contain very little cytoplasm with few mitochondria). Thus only females can transmit mitochondrial diseases, and they pass the mutation to all of their offspring of either sex (Fig. 3.23). Because mitochondrial DNA replicates autonomously from nuclear DNA, and mitochondria segregate in daughter cells independently of nuclear chromosomes (a process called replicative segregation), the proportion of mitochondria carrying an mtDNA mutation can differ among somatic cells and tissues. This heterogeneity is termed **heteroplasmy** and plays an important role in the variable and tissue-specific phenotype of mitochondrial disease. Furthermore, tissues differ in their dependence on oxidative phosphorylation, with heart, skeletal muscle, and central nervous system being the most dependent. Therefore mitochondrial diseases are often characterized by myopathies and encephalopathies (disorders of muscle and brain, respectively). Finally, oxidative phosphorylation declines with age, perhaps related to accumulation of mtDNA mutations. Thus, clinical phenotype in mitochondrial diseases is not simply or directly related to mtDNA genotype, but reflects several factors, including the inherent capacity for oxidative phosphorylation determined by both nuclear and mitochondrial genes, the accumulation of somatic mtDNA mutations and degree of heteroplasmy, tissue-specific requirements for oxidative phosphorylation, and age.

One of the best-characterized mitochondrial diseases is Leber's hereditary optic neuropathy (LHON), in which there is loss of central vision secondary to optic nerve degeneration. Precipitous vision loss usually occurs in the 20s and, for unknown reasons, men are affected far more commonly than women. The

Figure 3.23. Pedigree of a family with mitochondrial encephalomyopathy with ragged-red muscle fibers (MERRF). Note the maternal transmission to all male and female offspring and the absence of male transmission that is characteristic of mitochondrial inheritance. The severity of clinical manifestations among affected members correlates with the deficiency in mitochondrial energy generating capacity, and the variability among affected members reflects heteroplasmy for the mitochondrial mutation. (Redrawn from Wallace DW, Zheng X, Lott MT, et al. Familial mitochondrial encephalomyopathy (MERRF): genetic, pathophysiological, and biochemical characterization of a mitochondrial DNA disease. Cell 1988;56: 601–610.)

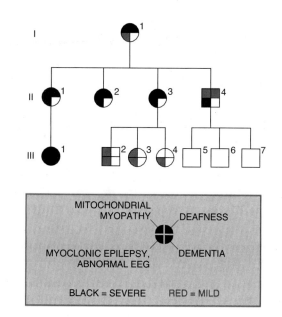

disease is maternally inherited. Eleven different missense mutations in three different mitochondrial genes encoding respiratory chain enzyme subunits have been described. Although the phenotype, blindness, is the same in each, the propensity to become blind and the age of onset varies considerably. Other mitochondrial diseases tend to involve various combinations of muscle and nervous system involvement and manifest highly variable clinical phenotypes.

One noncoding region of the mitochondrial chromosome (the D-loop) manifests a high degree of sequence variation (polymorphism, discussed in chapter 4) and has been used in anthropologic and evolutionary studies to trace human origins and connections. Because mtDNA polymorphisms allow accurate identification of individuals and their maternal relatives, they have been applied to a unique human rights problem; mtDNA polymorphisms were used to match maternal grandmothers with orphaned children whose parents were among "the disappeared" during Argentina's military dictatorship.

SUGGESTED READINGS

Bennett RL, Steinhaus KA, Uhrich SB, et al. Recommendations for standardized human pedigree nomenclature. Am J Hum Genet 1995;56:745–752.

Dietz HC, Pyeritz RE. Review. Mutations in the human gene for fibrillin-1 (*FBN1*) in the Marfan syndrome and related disorders. Hum Mol Genet 1995;4:1799–1809.

Francomano CA. Clinical implications of basic research. The genetic basis of dwarfism. N Engl J Med 1995;332:58–59.

Gusella JF, MacDonald ME. Huntington's disease and repeating trinucleotides. N Engl J Med 1994;330:1450–1451.

Harper PS, Harley HG, Reardon W, Shaw DJ. Review. Anticipation in myotonic dystrophy: new light on an old problem. Am J Hum Genet 1992;51:10–16.

Johns DR. Review. Mitochondrial DNA and disease. N Engl J Med 1995;333:638–644.

King MC. An application of DNA sequencing to a human rights problem. In: Friedmann T, ed. Molecular genetic medicine, vol. 1. Orlando: Academic Press, 1991:117–131.

McKusick VA. Mendelian inheritance in man. 11th ed. Baltimore, Johns Hopkins University Press, 1994. *This valuable reference source is also available on the World Wide Web (or internet) at http://www.ncbi.nlm.nih.gov/Omim/.*

Nawrotzki R, Blake DJ, Davies KE. Review. The genetic basis of neuromuscular disorders. Trends Genet 1996;12:294–298.

Sutherland GR, Richards RI. Review. Simple tandem DNA repeats and human genetic disease. Proc Natl Acad Sci USA. 1995;92:3636–3641.

Warren ST. The expanding world of trinucleotide repeats. Science 1996;271:1374–1375.

Population Genetics and Multifactorial Inheritance

"Almost all disorders in man are familial in that they are more likely to afflict someone with an affected relative than someone with an equivalent set of unaffected relatives."

—J.H. EDWARDS (FROM FAMILIAL PREDISPOSITION IN MAN. BR MED BULL 1969;25:58–64).

In this chapter we will consider two topics that require a more quantitative approach to genetics: population genetics and multifactorial inheritance. Population genetics is the study of the distribution of genes in populations and of the factors that maintain or change the frequency of genes and genotypes from generation to generation. It is a central part of the discipline of human genetics and the study of evolution, as well as human gene mapping. Understanding population genetics is essential for the application of DNA testing in forensics. In medical genetics, population genetic data are used primarily in genetic counseling and in planning genetic screening programs. Multifactorial inheritance deals with traits and diseases that are not inherited in a simple Mendelian fashion nor associated with chromosomal abnormalities, but in which there is considerable evidence that genetic factors play an important role in their causation. Examples include common diseases, such as hypertension and diabetes mellitus, and common birth defects, such as cleft lip and cleft palate. Multifactorial models provide a framework for understanding genetic predisposition to disease and for providing genetic counseling to patients and families with these conditions.

Population Genetics

For the medical geneticist, the most important concept in population genetics is the Hardy-Weinberg equilibrium. Independently described in 1908 by the English mathematician G. H. Hardy and the German physician W. Weinberg, it was derived to explain why dominant traits do not automatically replace recessive traits in the population. Its utility for medical genetics, however, is in explaining why, in a large population with random mating, allele frequencies do not change from generation to generation and how, for any genetic locus, the genotype frequencies are determined by the relative frequencies of the alleles at that locus.

HARDY-WEINBERG EQUILIBRIUM

Consider a single autosomal locus with two alleles (A and a), whose population frequencies in both sperm and eggs are p = frequency of allele A, and q = frequency of allele a. Because there are only two alleles, $p + q = 1$. Random mating (mating without regard to genotype) is mathematically equivalent to random mixing and union of sperm and eggs as shown in Table 4.1. The frequency of each genotype is shown in parentheses. The genotype frequencies in the progeny are thus:

genotype:	AA	Aa	aa
frequency:	p^2	$2pq$	q^2

Table 4.1.   Genotype Frequencies in Progeny

		Paternal Gametes	
		A (p)	a(q)
Maternal Gametes	A (p)	AA (p^2)	Aa (pq)
	a (q)	Aa (pq)	aa (q^2)

In the next generation, each of the three paternal genotypes can mate with each of the three maternal genotypes as indicated in Table 4.2. The frequency of each mating type is in parentheses. The genotypes of the offspring for each mating type are shown in Table 4.3. Thus, the frequency of each genotype (AA, Aa, and aa) is stable over successive generations and the population is said to be in Hardy-Weinberg equilibrium.

Applications of the Hardy-Weinberg Equilibrium

The most important medical application of the Hardy-Weinberg equilibrium is the determination of allele frequency and heterozygote carrier frequency in a population for which the frequency of a trait is known. For example, cystic fibrosis occurs in approximately 1 in 2000 whites of Northern and Central European origin. Thus q^2, or the frequency of homozygous affected individuals, is 1/2000, and q, the frequency of the mutant allele, is $\sqrt{2000}$ = 1/45 or 0.022. The frequency of the normal allele is p = 44/45 or 0.978. The heterozygote carrier frequency is 2pq = 2 × 44/45 × 1/45 ≈ 1/23 or 0.043. Thus, more than 4% of whites are heterozygous for the cystic fibrosis allele, a fact of considerable importance in genetic counseling of families with cystic fibrosis.

For rare recessive traits (q^2 ≤ 0.0001), p approximates 1, so that the heterozygote carrier frequency (2pq) is approximately 2q, or twice the frequency of the mutant allele. It is clear that for any rare autosomal recessive disease the number of heterozygous carriers in the population (2pq) is much larger than the number of homozygous affected individuals (q^2), and, as shown in Table 4.4, this ratio (Aa/aa or 2pq/q^2) increases as the disease frequency (q^2) decreases.

This relationship, in turn, has important implications for genetic screening programs. For example, the frequency of Tay-Sachs disease in the Ashkenazi Jewish population, before the establishment of screening programs, was approximately 1 in 3600 or 0.0003; therefore, the frequency of

Table 4.2.   Frequency of Mating Types

		Paternal Genotypes		
		AA (p^2)	Aa (2pq)	aa (q^2)
Maternal Genotypes	AA (p^2)	AA × AA (p^4)	AA × Aa (2p^{3}q)	AA × aa (p^{2}q^2)
	Aa (2pq)	Aa × AA (2p^{3}q)	Aa × Aa (4p^{2}q^2)	Aa × aa (2pq^3)
	aa (q^2)	aa × AA (p^{2}q^2)	aa × Aa (2pq^3)	aa × aa (q^4)

Table 4.3. Frequency of Different Genotypes in Offspring from Each Mating Type

Mating Type	Frequency	Offspring		
		AA	Aa	aa
AA × AA	p^4	p^4		
AA × Aa	$4p^3q$	$2p^3q$	$2p^3q$	
AA × aa	$2p^2q^2$		$2p^2q^2$	
Aa × Aa	$4p^2q^2$	p^2q^2	$2p^2q^2$	p^2q^2
Aa × aa	$4pq^3$		$2pq^3$	$2pq^3$
aa × aa	q^4			q^4

AA offspring = $p^4 + 2p^3q + p^2q^2 = p^2(p^2 + 2p + q + q^2) = p^2(p + q)^2 = p^2(1)^2 =$ **p^2**.

Aa offspring = $2p^3q + 4p^2q^2 + 2pq^3 = 2pq(p^2 + 2pq + q^2) = 2pq(p + q)^2 = 2pq(1)^2 =$ **$2pq$**.

aa offspring = $p^2q^2 + 2pq^3 + q^4 = q^2(p^2 + 2pq + q^2) = q^2(p + q)^2 = q^2(1)^2 =$ **q^2**.

the mutant allele (q) is approximately 0.017 and the frequency of heterozygous carriers (2pq) is 0.033. The frequency of matings between Ashkenazi heterozygotes, and thus of couples at risk of having a child with Tay-Sachs disease, is 2pq × 2pq or approximately 1 in 1000. Assuming each couple has two children, one would have to screen approximately 2000 couples in this population (and offer prenatal diagnosis and selective pregnancy termination to those couples who choose it) to avoid the birth of a child with Tay-Sachs disease. In contrast, the frequency of Tay-Sachs disease in the non-Ashkenazi population is approximately 1 in 360,000; thus, q = 0.0017 and 2pq = 0.003. The number of matings between non-Ashkenazi carriers of Tay-Sachs disease is approximately 1 in 100,000, so that one would have to screen 200,000 couples to avoid the birth of a single child with Tay-Sachs disease. Clearly, screening the Ashkenazi Jewish population is a far more cost-effective program than screening the entire population for this otherwise rare disease. In fact, screening programs have decreased the incidence of Tay-Sachs disease in the North American Ashkenazi population by > 90% (chapter 13).

For X-linked genes, estimation of allele frequencies is different from that for autosomal genes because males are hemizygous for X-linked genes, and thus the frequency of affected males is *equal* to the frequency of the mutant allele, q. For a relatively rare X-linked recessive disease such as hemophilia A (where q, the disease frequency, is approximately 1 in 5000 and p ≈ 1), the frequency of heterozygous carriers is only twice the frequency of affected males (2q = 1/2500). However, the ratio of affected males to homozygous

Table 4.4. Effect of Genotype Frequency on the Ratio of Heterozygotes to Homozygotes

Disease	Disease Frequency	Allele Frequency		Genotype Frequency			Ratio of Heterozygotes to Homozygotes
		A(p)	a(q)	AA(p^2)	Aa(2pq)	aa(q^2)	Aa/aa (2pq/q^2)
Alkaptonuria	1/1,000,000	0.999	0.001	0.998	0.002	0.000001	2000
TSD (nA)	1/360,000	0.998	0.0017	0.997	0.003	0.000003	1071
OCA I	1/40,000	0.995	0.005	0.990	0.010	0.000025	400
PKU	1/10,000	0.990	0.010	0.980	0.020	0.0001	200
TSD (A)	1/3600	0.983	0.017	0.966	0.033	0.0003	110
CF	1/2,000	0.978	0.022	0.956	0.044	0.0005	88
SCA	1/400	0.950	0.050	0.902	0.095	0.0025	38

TSD (nA); Tay Sachs disease (non-Ashkenazi); TSD (A); Tay Sachs disease (Ashkenazi) OCA I; oculocutaneous albinism, type I (tyrosinase-negative); PKU: phenylketonuria; CF; cystic fibrosis; SCA; sickle cell anemia

affected females is very high because $q \geqslant q^2$ (1/5000 versus 1 in 25 million for hemophilia). In contrast, for rare X-linked dominant diseases, the frequency of affected males is about half that of affected females, q:2q.

FACTORS THAT ALTER GENE FREQUENCIES

The Hardy-Weinberg principle is at best an approximation, because it is absolutely true only under certain very specific conditions, rarely met in human populations. Fortunately for medical geneticists, however, it "works" and allows estimation of clinically useful allele frequencies as described above. The Hardy-Weinberg equilibrium holds exactly only for large populations in which there is random mating and in which there is no selection, mutation, or migration. Deviation from any of these conditions can alter allele frequency in a population and lead to an increase or decrease in allele frequencies from one generation to another.

Nonrandom Mating

In human populations, mating is seldom random. It is usually assortative in that members of a particular subpopulation are more likely to mate with other members of that same subpopulation, whether it is defined by racial, ethnic, religious, or other criteria. For example, congenitally deaf individuals marry congenitally deaf partners more often than would be expected by chance. A special form of nonrandom mating in the human population is **consanguinity,** or mating among close relatives. Although consanguinity (or inbreeding) does not change allele frequencies per se, it does increase the proportion of homozygotes in the next generation at the expense of heterozygotes, thereby exposing disadvantageous recessive phenotypes to selection. Such selection may in turn alter allele frequencies in subsequent generations. Consanguineous marriages not only have a greater risk of producing offspring homozygous for a deleterious recessive gene, but also offspring with increased susceptibility for polygenic or multifactorial diseases or birth defects. As discussed later in this chapter, the risk is proportional to the degree of relationship of the parents. The degree of consanguinity can be described by the **coefficient of relationship (r),** which is the probability that two persons have inherited a particular allele from a common ancestor. It also represents the proportion of all genes that are identical by descent from a common ancestor (Table 4.5.)

As discussed in chapter 3, consanguinity increases the probability of a mating between two individuals heterozygous for the same mutant allele. Therefore, one might expect an increased frequency of consanguinity among the parents of children with rare autosomal recessive disease. In fact, this is found, and the frequency of such consanguinity is inversely related to the frequency of the mutant allele; the more rare the disease, the more likely is parental consanguinity. The relationship between the frequency of con-

Table 4.5. Coefficient of Relationship with Different Degrees of Relationship		
Relationship	Degree	Coefficient of relationship (r)
Parent-child	First	1/2
Siblings	First	1/2
Uncle-niece	Second	1/4
First cousins	Third	1/8
Second cousins	Fifth	1/32

sanguinity and the frequency of a recessive disease is illustrated by comparing Tay-Sachs disease in the Ashkenazi and the non-Ashkenazi populations. In the latter, q = 0.0017 and the frequency of consanguinity among parents is approximately 4%, whereas in the Ashkenazi population, in which q = 0.017, it is less than 0.4%. In the general United States population the frequency of first cousin marriages is less than 0.1%; however, in certain isolates such as the Hutterites or the old-order Amish, the frequency of consanguineous matings is considerably higher.

Small Populations

For political, religious, or geographic reasons, a small subgroup of the population may become physically and/or socially isolated from the rest of the population, forming a genetic isolate. The founder members of such an isolate may, by chance, be carriers of mutant alleles for certain recessive traits, so that the frequency of these alleles will be higher within the isolate than within the population at large. Furthermore, the actual frequency in such a small population will vary widely from one generation to the next, a phenomenon called **genetic drift.** By chance, one allele may fail to be passed on to the next generation and thus disappear from that line of descent, leaving only the alternative allele. Such a mechanism, called **founder effect,** may account for the high frequency of certain rare diseases among genetic isolates. An example is the autosomal recessive Ellis-van Creveld syndrome, characterized by short-limbed dwarfism, polydactyly (extra fingers and toes), and congenital heart disease (Fig. 4.1), which has an allele frequency of q = 0.07 in the old-order Amish in Pennsylvania, but is extremely rare in the general population. Another example of such a possible founder effect is the high frequency of variegate porphyria, an autosomal dominant disease characterized by attacks of acute abdominal pain, weakness, and sun-induced skin problems, among the Afrikaner population in South Africa. This mutant allele is thought to have been introduced by Dutch settlers into a very small population in the Cape colony in the late 17th century and the disease now has a frequency of 1 in 400. The high frequency of certain genetic disorders in the Ashkenazi Jewish population is also thought to reflect a founder effect.

Selection

Selection represents the action of environmental factors on a particular phenotype, and hence its genotype, and may be positive or negative. It is the consequence of differences in the **biological fitness** (f) of individual phenotypes. Biological fitness is a measure of fertility and therefore of the contribution to the gene pool of the succeeding generation. Thus, selection may operate at any time from conception to the end of the reproductive period. A mutant allele may be a "genetic lethal" if it interferes with fertility, even though it causes no illness.

Most deleterious dominant mutations have a fitness value between 0 (a genetic lethal) and 1 (the fitness of the normal allele). Mutant alleles encoding autosomal dominant traits are expressed in heterozygotes and thus exposed to direct selection; therefore, a change in selective forces can rapidly alter the allele frequency for a dominant mutation.

In contrast, selection against mutant alleles encoding autosomal recessive diseases operates very slowly. As described above (Table 4.4), the frequency of heterozygous carriers of rare recessive disorders is much higher than the frequency of affected homozygotes; thus, the great majority of mutant alleles are carried by heterozygotes rather than homozygotes. For a lethal autosomal

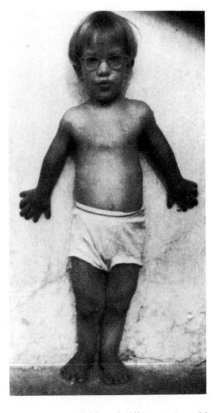

Figure 4.1. Child with Ellis-van Creveld syndrome. (From McKusick VA, et al. Trans Assoc Am Physicians 1964;77:154.)

recessive disease with a frequency of approximately 1 in 15,000, restoring the biological fitness of the affected homozygote from 0 to 1 would lead to a doubling in the gene frequency only after 50 generations. Conversely, a small increase in the fitness of the clinically normal heterozygous carrier could have a large effect on the frequency of the mutant allele. In the case of X-linked recessive diseases such as Duchenne muscular dystrophy and hemophilia A, one-third of the mutant alleles in the population are in hemizygous males and exposed to direct selection. Increasing the biological fitness of affected males, for example, by improved therapy of hemophilia A, would be expected to significantly increase the frequency of the mutant allele.

Mutation

A mutation is a change in the genetic material. The **mutation rate (μ)** is the frequency of such change and is expressed as the number of mutations per locus per gamete per generation. Most information on human mutation rates comes from studies of rare autosomal dominant traits for which it is much easier to estimate mutation rates than for recessive traits. For rare autosomal dominant traits, the mutation rate is $\mu = n/2N$, where n is the number of affected patients with unaffected parents and N is the total number of births. The denominator is 2N rather than N, because mutation of either allele at an autosomal locus could result in the mutant phenotype. Locus heterogeneity (mutations at different genetic loci resulting in a similar phenotype) and decreased penetrance in an affected parent may both lead to erroneously high estimates of mutation rate.

Estimates of mutation rates for a variety of autosomal dominant diseases have yielded rates that vary from 10^{-6} to as high as 10^{-4}. For most human genes, the best estimates for mutation rates lie between 10^{-6} and 10^{-5} mutations per locus per gamete per generation. There is evidence that the frequency of mutations for certain autosomal dominant traits increases with increasing paternal age.

Two important genetic disorders are noteworthy for having extremely high calculated rates of mutation. One is type 1 neurofibromatosis (NF1) with an estimated rate of 10^{-4}. Although it had been suggested that this is because several different genetic loci may contribute to NF1, this explanation has now been excluded (see chapter 9). Duchenne muscular dystrophy is also thought to have a very high mutation rate of approximately 0.2 to 1.0 $\times 10^{-4}$. In this case the high rate may be a reflection of the very large size of the gene (> 2400 kilobases [kb]), making it the largest human gene known and perhaps presenting a large "target" for putative mutagenic agents.

At equilibrium, the birth frequency for a rare autosomal dominant trait with reduced fitness, such as achondroplasia, represents a balance between the introduction of new mutant alleles by mutation and their removal by negative selection. The more severe the reduction in biological fitness, the greater the proportion of patients whose disease is the result of new mutations. In the case of lethal osteogenesis imperfecta type II, all cases of the disease represent new mutations. In contrast, in Huntington disease, in which the age of onset of clinical disease is late and biological fitness is only marginally impaired, new mutations account for very few of the total cases of this disease. In genetically lethal X-linked recessive disorders such as Duchenne muscular dystrophy (DMD), all the alleles in affected hemizygous males, representing one-third of the mutant alleles in the population, are lost in each generation. According to the Haldane hypothesis, if the population is at equilibrium with respect to the incidence of the disease, the number of new mutations must equal the number of alleles lost. Thus, one-third of affected males with DMD represent new mutations.

Among the probable environmental causes of mutations in humans are ionizing radiation and chemical mutagens. Although there is good experimental evidence on the relationship between radiation dose and mutation rate in other mammals and in lower organisms, there are fewer data in human populations. Long-term studies on the genetic effects of radiation exposure due to nuclear bombings or radiation accidents have provided a major source of information on this topic. The assessment of possible mutagenic risk to humans from the tremendous number of both natural and synthetic chemicals known to be mutagenic in other biological systems is a major area of public health concern.

Migration and Gene Flow

Migration of populations into new regions and intermarriage with indigenous populations can result in a change in allele frequencies in both populations, a phenomenon known as **gene flow.** This may account for the high frequency of the allele for blood group B in Asia, with a gradual decline as one moves westward across Europe.

POLYMORPHISM

The discussion up to this point has dealt primarily with rare mutant alleles at genetic loci where the vast majority of the population carries a single normal (or wild-type) allele. However, at many loci in humans, two or more alleles occur with appreciable frequency in the same population. A polymorphism is defined as the occurrence of two or more genetically determined alternative phenotypes in a population at such a frequency that the rarest could not be maintained by recurrent mutation alone. In practice, a genetic locus is considered polymorphic if one or more of the rare alleles has (have) a frequency of at least 0.01, with the result that heterozygotes carrying this allele occur at a frequency greater than 2%. More than one-third of human genetic loci coding for proteins that have been studied have been found to be polymorphic. Examples include the loci coding for common blood groups such as the ABO, MN, and Rh systems, for a variety of red blood cell enzymes and serum proteins, and for the cellular antigens encoded by the major histocompatibility complex. Polymorphisms, as markers of genetic diversity, are also valuable tools for mapping the human genome, as is discussed in detail in chapter 9. DNA polymorphisms affecting restriction enzyme recognition sites or involving tandem repeats of short DNA sequences (discussed in chapter 5) are particularly valuable in this regard.

The extensive polymorphism in the human genome allows for multiple combinations of alleles at different loci and hence tremendous genetic diversity in the population and genetic uniqueness of individuals. This genetic diversity is thought to account for differences in genetic susceptibility to a variety of diseases, as discussed later in this chapter for diabetes. One of the best studied examples of this phenomenon is the major histocompatibility complex, or MHC, a cluster of highly polymorphic genes important in the regulation of the immune response. Two of the three classes of genes found in this region, Class I (HLA-A, HLA-B, and HLA-C) and Class II (DP, DQ, and DR), are known as human leukocyte antigen (HLA) genes, and encode integral membrane proteins essential in the presentation of antigens to immune cells known as T-lymphocytes. Because the MHC loci are tightly linked, occupying just under 4000 kb of chromosome 6, HLA alleles on a given chromosome are generally transmitted together as a haplotype and show strong linkage disequilibrium (discussed in chapter 9). Certain HLA antigens show striking association with specific diseases, usually autoimmune diseases in which the body appears to mount an immune reaction against its own tissues. The best known of these associations is that of HLA-B27 with ankylosing spondylitis, a chronic, inflammatory arthritis involving the spine and sacroiliac joints. Whereas only 7% of whites are HLA-B27-positive, the frequency is 95% in patients with ankylosing spondylitis, and although not all individuals who are B27-positive will develop the disease, their risk is 90 times higher than that of B27-negative individuals.

It is generally believed that most stable polymorphisms involving expressed genes are the result of selection for advantageous mutant alleles, although the selective pressures responsible for such so-called balanced polymorphisms have in most cases remained elusive. The best understood example of selection resulting in a balanced polymorphism is that of the sickle cell allele. Individuals homozygous for this mutant allele are affected with sickle cell anemia, a severe hemolytic anemia, and often die before reproductive age. Nevertheless, the frequency of sickle cell anemia at birth in United States blacks is approximately 1/400, and in parts of equatorial Africa, up to 1/25 of the population are affected with this disease. Because the affected homozygote obviously has decreased fitness, the high frequency of the mutant allele must be the result of the increased fitness of individuals heterozygous for this allele. Sickle cell anemia is most frequent in regions of the world in which falciparum malaria (caused by infection with *Plasmodium falciparum*) was common in the past (Fig. 4.2). In such regions, many people are ill with malaria and have reduced fertility. Heterozygous carriers of the sickle cell allele (individuals with sickle cell trait) are more

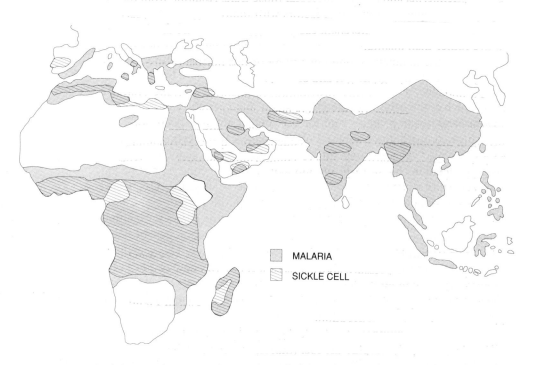

MALARIA

SICKLE CELL

Figure 4.2. Geographic distribution of falciparum malaria prior to 1930 and of sickle cell anemia. (Redrawn from Friedman MJ, Trager W. The biochemistry of resistance to malaria. Sci Am 1981;244:154–164.)

resistant to malarial infection, apparently because their red cells, when parasitized by *P. falciparum*, are more effectively removed from the circulation than are parasitized red cells in normal individuals without sickle cell trait. Because the number of heterozygotes for an autosomal recessive trait is much greater than the number of affected homozygotes (Table 4.4), a relatively small selective advantage in the heterozygote can outweigh a large selective disadvantage in the homozygote. In the case of sickle cell anemia, it has been calculated that a 20% increase in fitness of sickle cell trait individuals could balance an 85% decrease in the fitness of individuals with sickle cell anemia. One might expect that, with the control of malaria in many parts of the world, the frequency of this allele should decline. The thalassemias, a group of autosomal recessive anemias discussed in chapter 6, and G6PD deficiency, discussed in chapter 7, are also found in the same geographic distribution as is sickle cell anemia, and resistance to malaria may also be the positive selective force accounting for the high frequency of these diseases.

Multifactorial Inheritance and Quantitative Traits

Although many human diseases are inherited as simple Mendelian traits or are associated with chromosomal abnormalities, most of the common diseases of adult life (e.g., diabetes mellitus, hypertension, schizophrenia) and most common congenital malformations (e.g., cleft lip, cleft palate, neural tube defects) are not. Yet, as is discussed below, there is considerable evidence that genetic factors are important in their etiology. This genetic predisposition to disease is thought to reflect the cumulative effect of genetic variation at several and possibly multiple loci, each with a relatively small effect on phenotype. We define as **polygenic** those traits or diseases caused by the impact of many different genes, each having only a limited individual impact on phenotype, and as **multifactorial** those traits resulting from the interplay of multiple environmental factors with multiple genes. In practice, the terms are often used interchangeably. Polygenic traits are usually quantitative rather than qualitative in nature and are frequently distributed continuously in the population, often in a more or less normal (Gaussian) frequency distribution, e.g., height and blood pressure.

To understand the normal distribution of quantitative traits, consider the hypothetical example of two independent genetic loci, A and B, which affect systolic blood pressure. Each has two alleles, A and a, and B and b, occurring in the population with equal frequency (p = q = 0.5). Assuming that the population is in Hardy-Weinberg equilibrium, the three genotypes at each locus (AA, Aa, aa and BB, Bb, bb) will occur in the ratio of $p^2:2pq:q^2$ = (1/4):(1/2):(1/4). The frequencies for the two-locus genotypes are obtained by multiplication of the separate probabilities for the single locus genotypes (independence principle) as shown in Table 4.6. Assume that the allele designated by the capital letter (A or B) contributes one unit (an increment of 10 mm Hg pressure) to the hypothetical quantitative trait of interest (systolic blood pressure above a basal level of 100 mm Hg) and that the allele designated by the lower case letter (a or b) contributes zero units (Table 4.6). The population distribution of the trait, shown in Figure 4.3, approximates a normal distribution.

The larger the number of individual genetic loci contributing to a trait and/or the more polymorphic the loci (that is, the more different alleles at any given locus) the more likely that the distribution of the trait will be a smooth normal curve. The effects of environmental factors may further modify the shape of the frequency distribution.

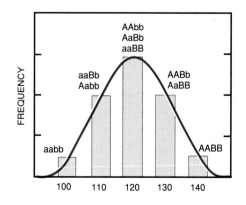

Figure 4.3. Frequency distribution of systolic blood pressure determined by a two-locus two-allele model. See text for explanation.

Table 4.6.   Frequency Distribution of Systolic Blood Pressure Determined by a Two-Locus Two-Allele Model[a]

	AA 1/4	Aa 1/2	aa 1/4
BB 1/4	1/16 (40)	2/16 (30)	1/16 (20)
Bb 1/2	2/16 (30)	4/16 (20)	1/16 (10)
bb 1/4	1/16 (20)	2/16 (10)	1/16 (0)

[a] The numbers in parentheses indicate the increment (in mm Hg pressure) to the systolic blood pressure above a basal level of 100 mm Hg contributed by each genotype.

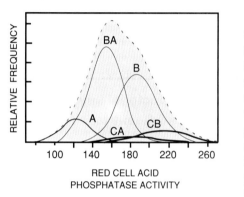

Figure 4.4.   Distribution of red cell acid phosphatase activities in the general population (*broken red line*) and in individuals with the separate phenotypes. The *solid* curves are constructed from the data on the different phenotypes as found in the British population. (From Harris H. The principles of human biochemical genetics. 3rd ed. Amsterdam: Elsevier/North-Holland, 1980:186.)

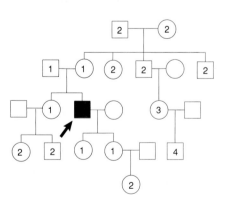

Figure 4.5.   Pedigree showing degree of relationship. In this figure, the *numbers inside the symbols* indicate the degree of relationship to the proband (*red symbol*).

As suggested by the hypothetical example above, an apparently continuous unimodal distribution of a quantitative trait may, in fact, represent the summation of several discrete phenotypes. This is illustrated by studies on red cell acid phosphatase activity shown in Figure 4.4. Six different phenotypes, distinguishable by differences in the electrophoretic mobility of the enzyme and determined by three alleles at a single autosomal locus, occur in the British population. The six phenotypes represent the three homozygous genotypes, AA, BB, and CC, and the three heterozygous genotypes, BA, CA, and CB. Each type is associated with a characteristic range of enzyme activity. Although there is considerable variation in the amount of acid phosphatase activity between individuals with the same acid phosphatase genotype, significant differences in the mean level of activity between types is apparent. Figure 4.4 shows the individual distributions of enzyme activity (*black curves*) of the five common acid phosphatase phenotypes (CC is relatively rare), as well as the general population distribution of acid phosphatase activity (*red curve*) in the British population. The apparently unimodal distribution in the whole population is a composite of the five separate but overlapping distributions.

Polygenes and Relationship

Although each individual, except monozygotic (or identical) twins, is genetically unique, each is more like his/her relatives than he/she is like unrelated individuals. As discussed below, polygenic disorders run in families; therefore, it is important to define the genetic relationship between relatives. This relationship is shown in the pedigree in Figure 4.5. The *number* inside the symbol indicates the degree of relationship with the proband, indicated by the *arrow* and *solid symbol*. First-degree relatives share 1/2 of their genes with the proband; second-degree relatives share 1/4 of their genes; and third-degree relatives share 1/8 of their genes. Note that the fraction of genes shared is the same as the coefficient of relationship (r) (Table 4.5). Spouses and other relatives by marriage are presumably unrelated and do not share any greater genetic relationship with the proband than any individual picked at random from the population.

In humans, the best example of a "pure" polygenic trait is the fingertip ridge count. This is the total number of ridges on the 10 fingertips, counted according to specific rules. The fingertip ridge pattern is determined early in development and there is apparently minimal influence from environmental factors. Its polygenic character is suggested by its normal distribution in the population and by the fact that the degree of correlation of fingertip ridge count among relatives corresponds very closely to the number of genes they share in common (Table 4.7).

EVIDENCE FOR GENETIC FACTORS IN COMMON DISEASES AND MALFORMATIONS

The evidence that genetic factors are important in common diseases and malformations comes mainly from epidemiologic studies comparing the frequency of disease among genetically related individuals with that in the general population. First, there is a higher frequency of specific diseases or malformations among relatives of affected individuals (a "familial tendency") that is proportional to the degree of relatedness. This is illustrated in large-scale family studies on the frequency of cleft lip with or without cleft palate (Fig. 4.6) from both Europe and North America, where the frequency of this anomaly is approximately 1/1000 (Table 4.8). It is clear that the frequency of cleft lip among relatives is much higher than in the general population; yet, the proportion of affected relatives is not consistent with either autosomal dominant or recessive inheritance. The sharp decline in frequency of affected second-degree relatives compared with first-degree relatives, and to a lesser extent, third-degree relatives compared with second-degree relatives, is greater than would be predicted by autosomal dominant inheritance, in which the frequency is expected to decrease by 1/2 with each step. The similar proportion of affected siblings and children of affected probands is inconsistent with autosomal recessive inheritance. The increased risk to relatives of affected individuals is often described by the parameter λ_R, defined as the risk for a relative of an affected proband divided by the risk in the general population. The subscript R defines the type of relative; e.g., λ_S refers to the risk to siblings.

It should be noted, however, that not everything that is familial is necessarily genetic; families also share common environments. The percentage

Table 4.7. Correlation of Fingertip Ridge Counts among Relatives Compared with Expectations Based on the Proportion of Shared Genes[a]

Relationship	Observed Correlation	Expected Correlation
Monozygotic twins	0.95 ± 0.07	1.00
Dizygotic twins	0.49 ± 0.08	0.50
Siblings	0.50 ± 0.04	0.50
Parent-child	0.48 ± 0.04	0.50
Spouses	0.05 ± 0.07	0.00

[a] From Carter CO: Genetics of common disorders. Br Med Bull 25:52–57, 1969.

Table 4.8. Family Studies of the Incidence of Cleft Lip (± Cleft Palate)[a]

Relatives	Pecentage of Relatives Affected	Incidence Relative to General Population
First degree		
Sibs	4.1	× 40
Children	3.5	× 35
Second degree		
Aunts and uncles	0.7	× 7
Nephews and nieces	0.8	× 8
Third degree		
First cousins	0.3	× 3

[a] From Carter CO: Genetics of common disorders. Br Med Bull 25:52–57, 1969.

Figure 4.8. Multifactorial threshold model: distribution of genetically determined liability among relatives. The distribution of genetic liability in relatives of an affected proband is indicated by the *lightly shaded red area below* the *red curve. X* is the difference in mean genetic liability between affected probands and the general population. See text for details. (From Carter CO. Multifactorial genetic disease. Hosp Pract 1970;5:45–59.)

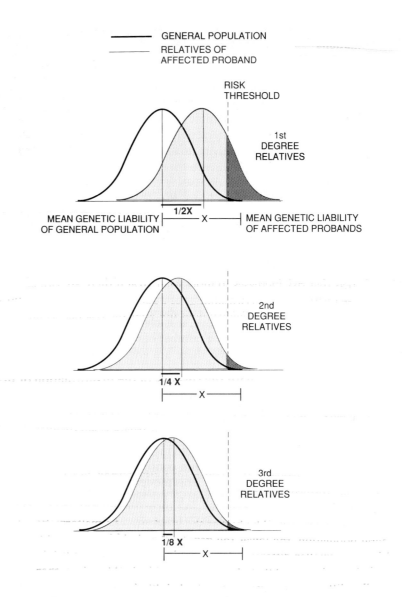

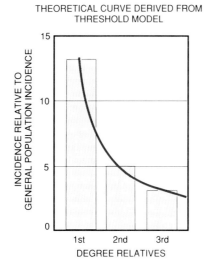

Figure 4.9. Multifactorial threshold model: predicted recurrence risks for relatives. (From Carter CO. Multifactorial genetic disease. Hosp Pract 1970;5:45–59.)

1. Recurrence risks represent average risks and will vary among different families. The multifactorial threshold model assumes that affected individuals fall above a certain threshold in the population distribution of genetically determined liability, but that their exact position cannot be directly defined. The average recurrence risks predicted are derived from empirical data such as those shown in Table 4.8, as opposed to being determined by specific models or patterns of inheritance, as is the case for Mendelian traits. The model also predicts that recurrence risks for relatives will decline sharply as the degree of relatedness decreases, as shown in Figures 4.8 and 4.9. That this is indeed the case is shown in Table 4.8 for the recurrence risk to first-, second-, and third-degree relatives of individuals affected with cleft lip ± cleft palate, and in Table 4.10 for several common congenital malformations.

2. The risk increases with the number of affected relatives. For an autosomal recessive disease such as cystic fibrosis, the recurrence risk for a sibling of an affected child is 25%, whether that family has previously had one, two, or several affected children. In contrast, the recurrence risk for a sibling of a child with cleft lip, with or without cleft palate, is approximately

Table 4.10. Family Patterns in Some Common Congenital Malformations[a]

Malformation	Incidence in General Population	Incidence Relative to General Population			
		Monozygotic Twins	First Degree Relatives	Second Degree Relatives	Third Degree Relatives
Cleft lip (± cleft palate)	0.001	×400	×40	×7	×3
Club foot	0.001	×300	×25	×5	×2
Neural tube defects	0.002		×8		×2
Congenital dislocation of hip (females only)	0.002	×200	×25	×3	×2
Congenital pyloric stenosis (males only)	0.005	×80	×10	×5	×1.5

[a] From Carter CO: Genetics of common disorders. Br Med Bull 25:52–57, 1969 and Smith DW, Aase JM: Polygenic inheritance of certain common malformations. J Pediatr 76:653–659, 1970.

Table 4.11. Proportion of Children Affected with Pyloric Stenosis[a]

Proband	Children	
	Sons	Daughters
	%	
Father	5.5	2.4
Mother	19.4	7.3
Population incidence	0.5	0.1

[a] From Carter CO: Genetics of common disorders. Br Med Bull 25:52–57, 1969.

4%; whereas that risk increases to more than 10% if there are two affected first-degree relatives such as two siblings or a parent and a sibling. The presence of a second affected individual does not alter the risk per se; however, it suggests that the family is further to the right in the distribution of genetic liability. Therefore, this family can be identified as having a higher than average recurrence risk.

3. **The risk increases with the severity of the malformation or disease.** The recurrence risk for a sibling of a child with unilateral cleft lip without cleft palate is approximately 2.5%, whereas the recurrence risk for a sibling of a child with bilateral cleft lip and cleft palate is approximately 6%. This reflects the assumption that the more severe the defect, the greater the underlying genetic liability, and, therefore, the placement of the severely affected individual further to the right on the distribution curve.

4. **The differential risk to relatives of an affected proband increases as the frequency of the disease or malformation in the general population decreases.** The higher the incidence of a malformation in the general population, the lower the genetic threshold is presumed to be, resulting in a smaller difference between the average genetic liability of the population at large and that of affected individuals. Therefore, there will be a smaller difference in average genetic liability between relatives of an affected proband and the general population; and the increase in risk with close relationship to a proband will be relatively less.

5. **When the sex ratio of affected probands deviates significantly from unity, offspring of affected probands of the less frequently affected sex are at higher relative risk.** Congenital pyloric stenosis, an obstruction to the stomach outlet caused by muscular hypertrophy, is five times more common in boys than in girls. This suggests that the threshold for genetic liability for girls is higher than for boys (Fig. 4.10). Therefore, an affected girl might be expected to have a higher degree of genetic liability, and her relatives should have higher recurrence risks than those of an affected boy. In fact, children of affected females are three times more likely to have this same malformation than children of affected males. However, male offspring are still at higher absolute risk than are female offspring (Table 4.11).

Although the above considerations do not prove the validity of the threshold model, and indeed other, nonthreshold models of multifactorial disease have been developed, the multifactorial threshold model provides a useful framework for providing genetic counseling for families with common congenital malformations and common diseases. In the absence of

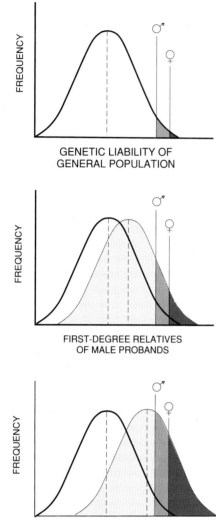

FREQUENCY

GENETIC LIABILITY OF
GENERAL POPULATION

FREQUENCY

FIRST-DEGREE RELATIVES
OF MALE PROBANDS

FREQUENCY

FIRST-DEGREE RELATIVES
OF FEMALE PROBANDS

Figure 4.10. Multifactorial threshold model: explanation for sex differences in incidence of pyloric stenosis in probands and their relatives. The risk thresholds for males and females are indicated by the *solid vertical lines.* The distribution of genetic liability in relatives of male and female probands is indicated by the *red shaded areas below* the *red curve.* Affected individuals are indicated by the *darker red areas.* See text for details. (Redrawn from Thompson M. Genetics in medicine. 4th ed. Philadelphia: WB Saunders, 1986:217.)

known Mendelian inheritance, such patients are all too often counseled erroneously, either being told that they have a high risk of recurrence (when they do not) or that they have no risk at all (when they do). For most multifactorial conditions, such as insulin-dependent diabetes mellitus, cleft lip, or congenital heart disease, the recurrence risk for children or siblings of an affected proband is approximately 5% or less.

THE IDENTIFICATION OF GENETIC FACTORS IN COMMON COMPLEX DISEASES

With the characterization of highly polymorphic markers scattered throughout the human genome, it has become possible to search for the genes responsible for susceptibility to common multifactorial diseases (see chapters 5 and 9 for more detailed discussion). The two major approaches are **association** and **linkage** analysis. The first approach seeks the correlated occurrence of specific alleles at a genetic locus and the disease in a **population.** Usually this involves the use of **candidate genes,** genes that encode proteins known or thought to be involved in the disease process. Finding that a specific allele is present in significantly higher frequency in individuals with the disease than in unaffected individuals suggests that the product of that allele plays a role in the pathogenesis of the disease. For example, the epsilon 4 (ϵ4) allele of the apolipoprotein E gene may be an important risk factor for late-onset Alzheimer disease. Linkage studies, in contrast, search for the cotransmission, in **families,** of a marker locus, regardless of the specific allele at that locus, with the disease. Linkage analysis provides direct evidence for the role of a genetic locus, or one very close to it, in the disease process. Finally, animal models of human multifactorial diseases have also been used to identify genetic factors, whose human homologues can then be studied.

Insulin-Dependent Diabetes Mellitus

Type 1 diabetes (insulin-dependent diabetes, IDDM) has become a paradigm for the genetic analysis of multifactorial diseases. IDDM, formerly called juvenile-onset diabetes, affects 0.4% of the population with a peak age of onset at 12 years. It is characterized by an autoimmune destruction of the β-cells of the pancreatic islets, resulting in an absolute deficiency of insulin and a requirement for exogenous insulin to survive. IDDM is a major risk factor for heart disease, kidney failure, and blindness. IDDM clearly runs in families: 10% of patients have an affected sibling; the risk to siblings of a diabetic or to the offspring of an IDDM father is more than 10 times the population risk; and the concordance of IDDM in monozygotic twins is 25–30%, approximately 5 times higher than the concordance of dizygotic twins.

The major approach to identifying the genetic factors in insulin-dependent diabetes mellitus has involved analysis of affected sib pairs in families to see how often a particular allele at a chromosomal locus is shared identical-by-descent (IBD), that is, inherited from a common ancestor, i.e., a parent. The frequency of IBD sharing at a genetic locus can then be compared with random expectation. Two siblings would be expected to show IBD sharing for zero, one, or two copies of any locus, with a probability of 25%, 50%, and 25% under random segregation (Fig. 4.11).

Both association and linkage studies have identified a locus, called *IDDM-1,* in the HLA region as having a major role in determining susceptibility to IDDM. Especially important are genes encoding class II molecules,

HLA-DQ and HLA-DR, which are involved in presenting peptide antigens to T lymphocytes and thus play a key role in the immune response. Individuals heterozygous for HLA DR3 and DR4 are at particularly high risk. A second important locus, called *IDDM-2*, is the insulin gene itself (*INS*); susceptibility alleles appear to be associated with increased expression of the insulin gene. Using genome scanning methods (discussed in chapter 9), at least 11 additional genetic loci affecting susceptibility to IDDM have now been identified. Analysis of the non-obese diabetic (NOD) mouse has identified at least 10 loci involved in susceptibility to IDDM in the mouse, but thus far none of these have resulted in the identification of novel human susceptibility genes.

By analyzing polymorphisms at the HLA and INS loci, it might be possible to identify individuals in the general population (without a family history of IDDM) at increased risk of developing diabetes. In diabetic families, these same analyses can identify children with a 25% risk of developing IDDM. Finally, by combining these genetic marker studies with assays for pancreatic islet autoantibodies and of β-cell function, children in families of diabetics can be identified with a very high risk of developing IDDM.

IMPLICATIONS OF MULTIFACTORIAL INHERITANCE

The multifactorial threshold model suggests that environmental triggers of disease are most likely to have a major impact on genetically predisposed individuals. Therefore, searching for environmental triggers of multifactorial diseases should be most fruitful when it is focused on those at highest genetic risk. Identification of these individuals should aid in identifying the environmental components in multifactorial illnesses. Correspondingly, medical intervention in the form of altering the environment of such individuals can then be focused on those at highest risk and thus most likely to benefit from such intervention. Perhaps more important in the long run, it will be possible to identify genetic markers of liability to common diseases, and thus gain insight into the pathogenetic mechanisms of these diseases. This, in turn, may lead to novel therapies.

Although the discussion of the genetics of multifactorial diseases often assumes multiple genes, each with a small effect, it is likely that some non-Mendelian diseases, such as IDDM, are primarily the result of the effects of relatively few genes, some of which have rather large effects on phenotype. Thus, these diseases may be oligogenic rather than polygenic. As discussed above, this has important implications for genetic counseling and for population screening to identify susceptible individuals.

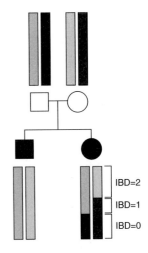

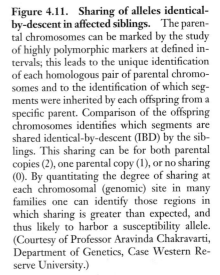

Figure 4.11. Sharing of alleles identical-by-descent in affected siblings. The parental chromosomes can be marked by the study of highly polymorphic markers at defined intervals; this leads to the unique identification of each homologous pair of parental chromosomes and to the identification of which segments were inherited by each offspring from a specific parent. Comparison of the offspring chromosomes identifies which segments are shared identical-by-descent (IBD) by the siblings. This sharing can be for both parental copies (2), one parental copy (1), or no sharing (0). By quantitating the degree of sharing at each chromosomal (genomic) site in many families one can identify those regions in which sharing is greater than expected, and thus likely to harbor a susceptibility allele. (Courtesy of Professor Aravinda Chakravarti, Department of Genetics, Case Western Reserve University.)

SUGGESTED READINGS

Bell JI. Polygenic disease. Curr Opin Genet Devel 1993;3:466–469.
Carter CO. Genetics of common disorders. Br Med Bull 1969;25:52–57.
Carter CO. Multifactorial genetic disease. Hosp Pract 1970;5:45–59.
Cavalli-Sforza LL, Bodmer WF. The genetics of human populations. San Francisco: WH Freeman, 1971.
Emery AEH. Methodology in medical genetics. An introduction to statistical methods. 2nd ed. Edinburgh: Churchill Livingstone, 1986.
Harris H. The principles of human biochemical genetics. 3rd ed. Amsterdam: Elsevier/North-Holland, 1980.
Keats B. Population genetics. In: Rimoin DL, Connor JM, Pyeritz RE, eds. Emery and Rimoin's principles and practice of medical genetics. 3rd ed. New York: Churchill Livingstone, 1996:347–357.
King RA, Rotter JI, Motulsky AG, eds. The genetic basis of common disease. New York: Oxford University Press, 1992.
Lander ES, Schork NJ. Genetic dissection of complex traits. Science 1994;265:2037–2048.

Lathrop GM, Terwilliger JD, Weeks DE. Multifactorial inheritance and genetic analysis of multifactorial disease. In: Rimoin DL, Connor JM, Pyeritz RE, eds. Emery and Rimoin's principles and practice of medical genetics. 3rd ed. New York: Churchill Livingstone, 1996:333–346.

Risch NJ. Genetic epidemiology. In Rimoin DL, Connor JM, Pyeritz RE, eds. Emery and Rimoin's principles and practice of medical genetics. 3rd ed. New York: Churchill Livingstone, 1996:371–382.

Todd JA. Genetic analysis of type 1 diabetes using whole genome approaches. Proc Natl Acad Sci USA 1995;92:8560–8565.

Vogel F, Motulsky AG. Human genetics. 3rd ed. Berlin: Springer-Verlag, 1996.

Molecular Genetics: Gene Organization, Regulation, and Manipulation

"Just as our present knowledge and practice of medicine relies on a sophisticated knowledge of human anatomy, physiology and biochemistry, so will dealing with disease in the future demand a detailed understanding of the molecular anatomy, physiology and biochemistry of the human genome. We shall have to have physicians who are as conversant with the molecular anatomy of chromosomes and genes as the cardiac surgeon is with the structure and workings of the heart and circulatory tree."

—PAUL BERG, M.D. NOBEL LECTURE, 1981

The flow of information from DNA to RNA to protein is described in general terms in chapter 2. An understanding of the true nature of human genetic disease requires a more detailed grasp of the structure and function of human genes. This also requires us to delve more deeply into the techniques of genetic analysis, which are together and sometimes rather loosely referred to as "recombinant DNA technology."

There are an estimated 50,000 to 100,000 genes dispersed throughout the 23 pairs of human nuclear chromosomes. The smallest of these genes may occupy no more than a few hundred base pairs of DNA, whereas the largest known human gene (dystrophin) is more than 2 million base pairs in length. Figure 5.1 shows the structure of an idealized gene, modeled after the genes for adult human hemoglobin, about which we will have much more to say in chapter 6. Hemoglobin is a tetramer composed of two α-protein chains and two β-protein chains. The genes for these proteins are on different chromosomes, with α being on chromosome 16 and β on chromosome 11 (Fig. 5.2). The α gene is approximately 800 bp in length whereas the β gene is nearly twice this long. The protein products, however, are similar: α is 141 amino acids long, and β is 146.

A striking feature of most eukaryotic genes is the presence of **introns,** which are stretches of DNA located within the gene, transcribed into RNA, but then spliced out before the RNA is translated into protein. These are shown as open areas in Figure 5.1. The solid red areas of the gene diagram indicate regions that contain coding information. There are also untranslated regions at either end of the gene, which are marked as dark stippled boxes in Figure 5.1. The 5'-untranslated region represents a sequence that is transcribed into messenger RNA by RNA polymerase but is not translated. In general, translation does not begin until the first AUG that appears in the RNA, referred to as the initiation codon, and sequences that are located 5' to this therefore do not appear in the protein. The 3'-untranslated region represents a sequence that appears in the mRNA but occurs after the stop codon (UAG, UGA, or UAA, see Table 2.2) and therefore also does not get translated into protein. Together, the coding segments and the 5'- and 3'- untranslated regions constitute the **exons,** which are spliced together to

General Structure of Genes and Gene Families

make the mature messenger RNA (mRNA). In the case of the hemoglobin α gene, exon 1 encodes the 5′-untranslated region and amino acids 1–31, exon 2, amino acids 32–99, and exon 3, amino acids 100–141 and the 3′-untranslated region. The number of introns interrupting a gene is highly variable, with occasional genes confined to a single exon and others interrupted by as many as 100 introns.

Genes sometimes occur in clusters, with genes of similar function located near each other. In Figure 5.2 are shown the α- and β-globin gene clusters of humans. Located near the β-globin gene are four other functional genes, namely ε, Gγ, Aγ, and δ, which also code for hemoglobin proteins but are expressed at different times during development. Similarly, the α-

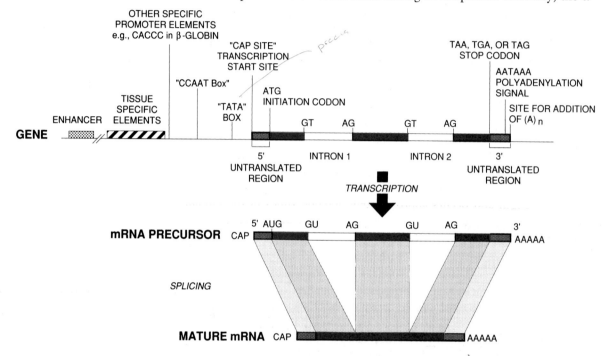

Figure 5.1.   Structure and expression of an idealized gene, including various promoter elements, an enhancer, and the transcribed region of the gene.   The example shown is modeled after the hemoglobin genes. The two introns each begin with GT and end with AG; these are spliced out to generate the mature mRNA. As described in the text, not only promoter elements but also enhancers can be tissue specific.

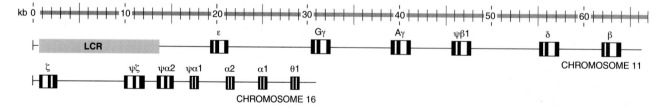

Figure 5.2.   Map of the β-globin gene cluster on the short arm of chromosome 11 and the α-globin gene cluster on the short arm of chromosome 16.   In each case the genes are arranged from 5′ to 3′ in order of their developmental activation. The ζ and ε genes are embryonic genes. ψζ, ψα2, ψα1, and ψβ1 are pseudogenes, which have acquired a number of inactivating mutations that prevent their giving rise to a functional globin chain. θ1 is a globin-like gene without inactivating mutations, whose function remains unknown. Hemoglobin F, the predominant hemoglobin in fetal life, consists of α and γ chains; the two α genes (α1 and α2) code for identical proteins and the two γ genes (Gγ and Aγ) differ by a single amino acid at codon 136. In adulthood the major hemoglobin is α2β2, with a minor contribution from α2γ2. *Open blocks* within the genes indicate introns. Note that there is a large amount of "spacer" DNA between the genes, some of which contains repetitive sequences. The LCR, locus control region, is discussed in chapter 6.

globin genes (there are actually two, α1 and α2, with identical coding regions) are also part of a gene cluster. The ζ gene is an embryonic gene, and the gene marked θ1 remains to have its function determined. In the β-globin cluster, an additional gene marked ψβ1 is shown, and in the α-globin cluster, a ψζ, a ψα1, and and a ψα2 gene are indicated. These so-called **pseudogenes**, designated by ψ, are DNA sequences that have some of the structures of expressed genes and were presumably once functional but have acquired one or more mutations during evolution that render them incapable of producing a protein product.

As evident for the globin gene cluster shown in Figure 5.2 there are often relatively long stretches of DNA in between transcribed genes. In the 80 kb (1 kb = 1000 bp) of DNA analyzed around the β-globin genes, only about 12% is actually transcribed and only 2.5% codes for protein. The nontranscribed DNA is termed "**intergenic**" DNA. Some of the sequences in intergenic DNA close to expressed genes are crucial for control of gene expression (as we shall see shortly), but a large amount of intergenic DNA seems to be rather dispensable and of no known function. Similarly, many genes contain very large introns much of which also appear to be dispensable. For example, introns account for more than 99% of the 2400-kb dystrophin gene. Located within intergenic DNA, and sometimes also within introns, are repetitive sequences that occur dispersed throughout the genome in many thousands of copies and of no apparent known function. The most ubiquitous of these, the so-called *Alu* repetitive sequence, is about 300 bp in length and occurs approximately 500,000 times in the human genome. Since their dispersal into the genome millions of years ago, the *Alu* sequences have diverged, so that one *Alu* repeat is about 80% identical to another one. It is unusual to find a stretch of DNA longer than about 30 kb that does not contain at least one of these sequences.

Control of Gene Expression

With a few notable exceptions, all of the cells of the human body contain the complete genome. Yet, in any given tissue only a subset of these genes are being expressed. Therefore, the control of gene expression is fundamental to understanding virtually all aspects of human biology.

In general, it is the mature protein product of a gene that carries out its function. The level of this mature protein can be altered by (*a*) the rate of transcription of the gene into RNA; (*b*) the processing of this RNA; (*c*) the transport of the mRNA from nucleus to cytoplasm; (*d*) the rate of translation of the mRNA into protein on cellular ribosomes; (*e*) the rate of degradation of the mRNA; (*f*) posttranslational modifications of the protein; and (*g*) the rate of degradation of the protein. All of these control mechanisms have been implicated in specific instances. Perhaps the most economical method of control, however, and one that is widespread in eukaryotes, is to control the protein production at its earliest level, namely that of transcription of the gene. Figure 5.1 shows a schematic diagram of the control elements of an idealized human gene. The important sequence elements have been identified by a variety of methods, including mutational analysis, evolutionary comparison, and functional assays using gene transfer into cultured cells or transgenic mice.

THE PROMOTER

The promoter is somewhat loosely defined as the sequence elements located immediately 5′ to the gene that interact with RNA polymerase and other components of the transcription machinery. These elements fix the site of transcription initiation and control mRNA quantity and sometimes tissue specificity. While in some situations the promoter may extend for several kilobases, the important promoter elements are generally located in the region 100–200 bp 5′ to the gene.

Many human genes contain a conserved "**TATA box**" sequence, which is located 25–30 bp 5′ to the start of transcription, and seems to be involved in the precise localization of the start. Further upstream, there is often a "**CCAAT** box" sequence located 75–80 bp 5′ to the start site, although this is less commonly present than the TATA box. In those genes with a CCAAT box, its presence seems to be required for quantitatively efficient transcription, at least in gene transfer experiments. Notably, some "housekeeping" genes, which encode enzymes that are present in virtually all cells, are usually lacking both of these boxes and contain promoters that are highly enriched in C and G nucleotides. The start site of transcription in genes lacking a TATA box often shows heterogeneity within a 10–20-bp region. A particular modified nucleotide, 7-methylguanosine, called a "cap," is added to the 5′ end of the growing mRNA chain. Thus, the site of initiation of transcription is also often called the "**cap site**."

SPLICING

As noted previously, most eukaryotic genes have their coding regions interrupted by introns, which must be removed in a process called splicing to generate a mature mRNA that can be translated into a functional protein. While the function of introns remains unclear, the mechanism of splicing is beginning to be understood. At the beginning and end of an intron, certain nucleotide sequences are found (Fig. 5.1). The intron almost always begins with a GT (the splice donor) and ends with an AG (the splice acceptor), and other adjacent bases tend to follow a certain sequence (referred to as a consensus [Fig. 5.3]). However, these consensus sequences, while necessary, are not entirely sufficient for recognition by the splicing apparatus; one can find consensus splice donor or acceptor sequences in transcribed genes that are not used. Interestingly, inactivation of the normal splice signal by mutation occasionally activates one of these "cryptic" splice signals.

The mechanism by which a particular splice donor "finds" the correct acceptor remains unclear. A 5′ to 3′ scanning model would be one possibility, but is not consistent with the pattern of splicing seen in the presence of certain splice acceptor mutations. A random search mechanism, however, is not tenable, given the fact that some genes such as collagen (chapter 7) contain up to 50 separate introns and yet always connect the correct donor to the correct acceptor.

POLYADENYLATION

Most messenger RNAs that code for protein are characterized by the addition of a string of about 200 adenosine residues at their 3′ end (polyadenylation). A hexanucleotide signal AAUAAA in the 3′-untranslated region is a

Figure 5.3. Consensus sequences found at 5′ and 3′ splice sites. The GT at the beginning of the intron and the AG at the end are nearly invariant, whereas some deviation from the rest of the consensus sequence is often seen. The position marked N can be any nucleotide (A, C, G, or T).

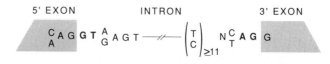

consistent feature of such mRNAs, although other sequences in the vicinity also may play a role in correct polyadenylation. The A residues are added at a point 18–20 bp downstream from this AAUAAA signal. The "poly-A tail" appears to play a role in transport out of the nucleus and the regulation of mRNA stability.

ENHANCERS

Enhancers are DNA sequences defined by the following properties: (a) they increase transcription from a nearby gene; (b) they can operate over considerable distances and are relatively unaffected by altering this distance; and (c) they are effective even if inverted. The first enhancers characterized were those of certain DNA viruses such as SV40, which bears a 72-bp twice-repeated sequence meeting these criteria, capable of increasing transcription from a large number of genes in almost any tissue tested. More recently, tissue-specific enhancers have been discovered. An example of the latter is the enhancer located in the immunoglobulin gene, which has been shown to be functional in B cells (which synthesize immunoglobulin) but not in other tissue types.

TRANSCRIPTION FACTORS

Considerable progress has been made over the past few years in understanding the intricate regulation of gene expression at the level of transcription. The transcription initiation complex, which contains RNA polymerase and a number of associated molecules, binds at the promoter and synthesizes the RNA copy. The process of transcription is also controlled by a number of other transcription factors. Transcription factors are proteins that act by binding to specific DNA sequences within the promoter or enhancer of the target gene to increase, decrease, or otherwise modulate the level of gene expression. Powerful techniques have been developed for studying the binding of transcription factors to DNA and for characterizing their function. These proteins often contain specific domains that bind directly to DNA as well as segments involved in interaction with other proteins.

The interactions of numerous large families of transcription factors with their specific DNA target sequences in promoters and enhancers, as well as with each other, is what determines the complex developmental and tissue-specific patterns of gene expression required in all higher organisms. Recently, genetic abnormalities in several transcription factors have been shown to play important roles in some human diseases.

A general understanding of recombinant DNA technology is essential to the study of modern medical genetics. It may be difficult to appreciate the full power of these techniques as they are initially presented; however, throughout the remainder of this textbook, it will be apparent that all of these techniques have played major roles in defining the nature of human genetic disease. It is also important to point out that the revolution in our understanding of human genetics resulting from the development of recombinant DNA technology is all quite recent. The polymerase chain reaction (PCR), which is central to nearly any experiment in modern medical genetics, was only discovered about 10 years ago. The methods used to identify disease genes by positional cloning, and to disrupt specific genes in experimental animals, are even more recent (Fig. 5.4).

The Tools of the Trade: Recombinant DNA Technology

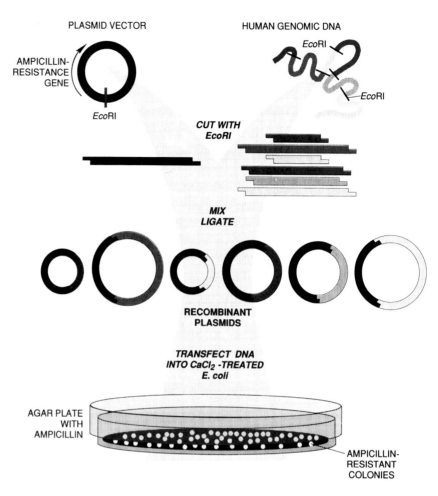

Figure 5.6.   Diagram of the process of generating a specific recombinant DNA molecule.   In this example, the vector, a bacterial plasmid carrying an ampicillin-resistance gene, is cut with the restriction enzyme *Eco*RI, as is the genomic DNA, which contains within it the desired fragment. The sticky ends can be ligated together to generate a series of recombinant molecules, in which different genomic fragments have been inserted into the vector. This mixture is then transfected into ampicillin-sensitive *E. coli*, which have been treated with calcium chloride to promote their uptake of DNA. Only those bacteria that have taken up a plasmid will form colonies when plated on ampicillin. Each of the ampicillin-resistant colonies is a plasmid clone derived from a single recombinant plasmid molecule. A number of different approaches can be used to identify and isolate the specific recombinant clone of interest from the large collection, or library, of clones on the plate, including hybridization with a specific DNA probe as illustrated in Figure 5.9.

COMPLEMENTARY DNA (cDNA)

Sometimes it is desirable to start with the RNA transcribed from the gene rather than the genomic DNA sequence itself. To take advantage of the recombinant DNA strategy, single-stranded RNA first must be converted to double-stranded DNA. This is accomplished by means of an enzyme called **reverse transcriptase**. This conversion of single-stranded mRNA to double-stranded DNA (so-called complementary DNA or cDNA) is diagrammed in Figure 5.7.

MOLECULAR HYBRIDIZATION

The detection of a specific desired DNA or RNA sequence among a large collection of different sequences is often based on molecular hybridization.

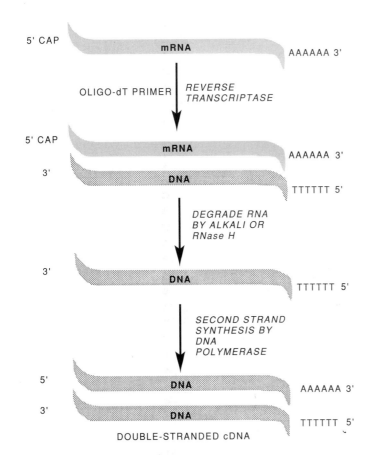

Figure 5.7. Steps involved in making a double-stranded cDNA from single-stranded messenger RNA. RNase H is an enzyme that will cut and degrade the RNA strand of an RNA-DNA heteroduplex.

Simply stated, hybridization is the ability of a single-stranded DNA or RNA to anneal by base-pairing to its complementary single strand, while failing to anneal to an unrelated sequence. This process is illustrated in Figure 5.8. The probe DNA is usually labeled with a tag such as a radioisotope, so that its fate can be followed. If a large number of independent clones are fixed to a nitrocellulose filter, for example, hybridization with labeled probe, followed by placing the filter against x-ray film, will detect the specific clone bearing a complementary DNA sequence. As we will see, identification of specific nucleic acid sequences by hybridization is also the principle underlying Northern and Southern blotting.

CLONING A GENE

Cloning a cDNA by hybridization, as depicted in Figure 5.9, requires the availability of a reagent (the "**probe**") that is capable of recognizing the desired clone in a complex mixture of many different DNA sequences. If one is trying to clone a mutant β-globin gene, for example, this is not really a problem because the normal β-globin sequence can be used. However, if this is a gene that has never previously been cloned, designing the probe is a challenging task. If the gene is expressed at very high levels in a particular tissue, making cDNA clones from this tissue is likely to yield some that have the right insert. Red blood cells, for example, contain α and β globin as their major protein component; thus reticulocytes, which are young red blood cells still containing mRNA, were used successfully to obtain the first hemoglobin cDNAs. If no such abundantly expressing tissue is available, then one must know something about the gene. Often, limited amino acid sequencing of the protein

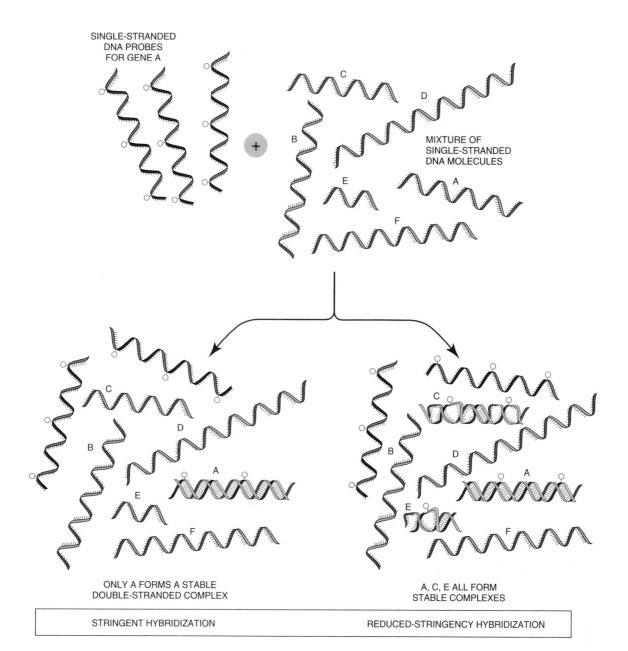

SINGLE-STRANDED
DNA PROBES
FOR GENE A

MIXTURE OF
SINGLE-STRANDED
DNA MOLECULES

ONLY A FORMS A STABLE
DOUBLE-STRANDED COMPLEX

A, C, E ALL FORM
STABLE COMPLEXES

STRINGENT HYBRIDIZATION

REDUCED-STRINGENCY HYBRIDIZATION

Figure 5.8. Nucleic acid hybridization. This process of matching between two independent strands is based on the intrinsic structure of nucleic acid, which favors precise base pairing between complementary DNA or RNA strands. This property is the basis for the fundamental processes of DNA replication and transcription, as reviewed in chapter 2. In this example, the single-stranded DNA probe for gene A, shown in red, is labeled to allow detection of its matching sequences. When mixed with a complex collection of target DNA molecules, the probe will only form a stable duplex with its exactly complementary strand or a closely related sequence. The conditions of hybridization can be adjusted to break apart complementary strands that are partially matched and only permit perfectly matched sequences to stay together in a stable, double-stranded form. The latter is referred to as stringent hybridization. Under more relaxed conditions, referred to as reduced stringency, closely related but not identical complementary strands can remain associated. Reduced stringency of hybridization is useful for identifying homologous genes across species, or members of closely related gene families, in which sequences are similar but not identical. (Adapted from Alberts B, Bray D, Lewis J, Raff M, Roberts K, Watson JD. Molecular Biology of the Cell. New York: Garland Publishing, 1994:306.)

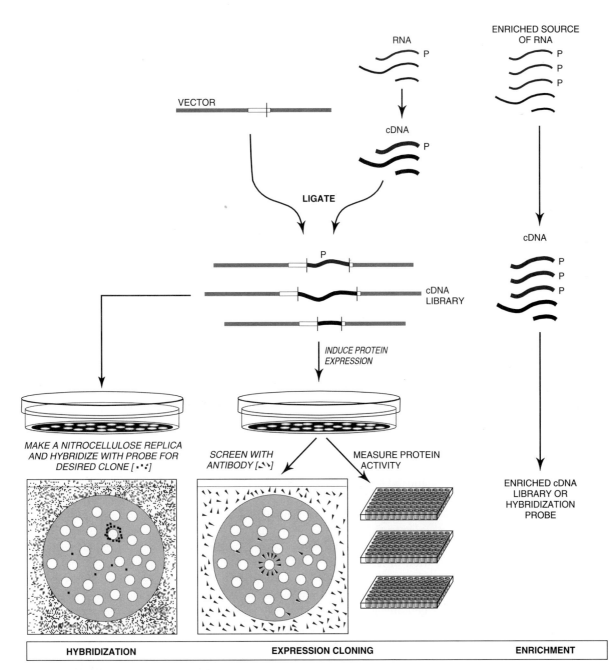

Figure 5.9.   Methods for cloning the cDNA for a specific gene.   cDNA is prepared from a tissue where the gene (P) is expressed and inserted into a cloning vector (gray hatched bar) that is subsequently transformed into bacteria, as in Figure 5.6. The resulting collection of bacteria, each carrying a copy of the vector with a different inserted cDNA, is called a "cDNA library." The cDNA library can be transferred to a nitrocellulose filter and screened by hybridization with an oligonucleotide or other DNA probe, as shown at the left. Alternatively, an "expression cloning" vector can be used that carries the sequences (white box) to direct the expression of the protein encoded by the cloned cDNA. This approach is depicted in the middle of the figure. The protein product, sometimes fused to a carrier bacterial or other protein, can be detected by a specific antibody, if available, or an assay that measures the known function of the target protein. Large numbers of cDNA clones from the library can be screened on nitrocellulose filters, or as individual colonies or pools of colonies grown in liquid culture. For simplicity, only a few clones are shown; in practice, several hundred thousand to 1 million are often screened. A number of additional approaches, represented on the right, rely on enrichment of the mRNA or cDNA for the specific sequence of interest. Enrichment has been accomplished in a number of ways including selection by hybridization, size fractionation, and antibody selection of mRNA-ribosome complexes. In a particular type of enrichment called subtraction, common sequences between two cell types can be removed by hybridization, leaving behind sequences unique to one of the cells. Enriched mRNA or cDNA can be used to construct a specific cDNA library or to prepare a hybridization probe.

product is performed. Using the genetic code (Table 2.2), a short single-stranded DNA molecule (14–30 nucleotides long, called an **oligonucleotide**), which is predicted to match the sequence coding for this protein, can be chemically synthesized. Because of the degeneracy of the genetic code, it usually is not possible to predict the exact sequence, so a mixture of oligonucleotides that covers all of the possibilities is often made. An example of this strategy is shown in Figure 5.10. If no specific DNA or protein sequence is available to generate a probe that can detect the desired cDNA by hybridization, an alternative strategy must be employed. A host of clever strategies for cloning cDNAs have been developed over the years, most fitting into one of the general categories outlined in Figure 5.9. To begin, a large collection of cDNAs is generated as depicted in Figure 5.7, using mRNA prepared from the desired cell type and ligated or cloned into a specific vector. This collection of cDNA clones is referred to as a cDNA **library.** For one group of approaches collectively referred to as "expression cloning," the vector is designed to express the actual protein product encoded by the cDNA by joining it to other sequences required for RNA transcription and protein translation. The desired cDNA can then be identified by the presence of the corresponding protein sequence, detected either with an antibody or by a functional property of the protein. In another set of approaches, a variety of tricks are used to enrich the hybridization probe, or the cDNA library itself, for sequences corresponding to the particular clone of interest.

Once a particular cDNA has been successfully cloned by one of the approaches outlined in Figure 5.9, the cDNA itself can be analyzed in a number of ways, as we will now see, including determination of its entire DNA sequence and prediction of the corresponding amino acid sequence from knowledge of the genetic code. The cDNA can also be used as a hybridization probe to identify related DNA or RNA sequences, such as in Southern and Northern blotting. In addition, the cDNA can be used as a probe to clone the complete structural gene, including all the exons and introns and the adjacent promoter sequences. For this latter purpose, a genomic library is constructed from total cellular DNA, as depicted schematically in Figure 5.6. In practice, specialized vectors are generally used to facilitate the isolation of large pieces of DNA and the rapid screening of large numbers of clones. Recombinant clones containing the desired genomic sequences can be identified by hybridization using the cDNA as probe. Comparison of the genomic and cDNA sequences identifies the position of the introns within the gene. (Compare the mature mRNA to the intact gene in Figure 5.1.) The distinction between genomic and cDNA clones can be confusing. Remember that genomic DNA contains all of the components of the gene including exons and introns whereas the cDNA, being derived from mRNA, contains only the transcribed and processed exons.

In the past, it has generally been more straightforward to begin with the cloning of a cDNA, based on knowledge of a protein's structure or function. However, recent advances in molecular genetics have now made it possible to clone a gene based only on genetic information, with no knowledge of the corresponding protein. When a genomic clone is identified in this way, it can then be used as a hybridization probe to screen a cDNA library. The cDNA in turn can be used to study the protein's function and its possible role in the corresponding human disease. The identification of a gene based only on knowl-

Figure 5.10. Constructing a DNA probe from amino acid sequence information. If limited amino acid sequence is available on a protein, it is possible to construct a synthetic oligonucleotide that will hybridize with the gene encoding that protein, allowing cloning of the gene. Using the genetic code dictionary (see Table 2.2), the codons for each amino acid can be predicted; because of the degeneracy of the code, many amino acids have more than one codon, so in practice one synthesizes a mixture of oligonucleotides to cover all the possibilities. In the example above, a mixture of eight (2^3) 17-mers should include the correct sequence and allow cloning of the gene.

AMINO ACID SEQUENCE: — Phe — Trp — Met — Asp — Cys — Ala —

OLIGONUCLEOTIDE: — TT$_C^T$ — TGG — ATG — GA$_C^T$ — TG$_C^T$ — GC —

edge of its position within the genome is generally referred to as **positional cloning,** an approach that is discussed in more detail in chapter 9.

SOUTHERN BLOTTING

Once a DNA segment has been cloned, that segment can be used as a hybridization probe to identify variability among individuals. One such technique is the **Southern blot,** which derives its name from its originator, Edwin M. Southern, and not from any geographic considerations. In this procedure, diagrammed in Figure 5.11, genomic DNA from an individual is digested with a restriction enzyme. The resulting myriad of fragments is separated by size on an electrophoretic gel and the DNA is then transferred to a nitrocellulose filter and hybridized with a labeled probe. Only those DNA fragments containing sequences complementary to the probe will be detected. When the result is compared with a normal pattern, two sorts of mutational differences can be discovered: (*a*) any rearrangement, such as a deletion or insertion, that is larger than 50–100 bp usually can be detected by a change in size of a fragment (Fig. 5.12); and (*b*) a single base difference that creates or destroys a restriction site for the enzyme used to digest the DNA will result in an altered band size (Fig. 5.13). Detection of these types of mutational differences by Southern blotting are illustrated in Figures 5.12 and 5.13, using the FVIII gene as an example. The structure of the FVIII gene is shown in Figure 5.14.

NORTHERN BLOTTING

A similar hybridization approach can be used to identify the specific mRNAs complementary to a labeled probe. In this procedure, called a **Northern blot,** messenger RNA is prepared from the tissue of interest, separated on a gel by size, transferred to a filter, and hybridized with the DNA probe (Fig. 5.11). As it happens, DNA-RNA hybrids are even more stable than DNA-DNA hybrids. The resulting band identified by the probe indicates the size of the mRNA, and demonstrates that the corresponding gene is being transcribed ("expressed") in the tissue from which the RNA was prepared. The intensity of the band is also a rough indication of its abundance. In searching for mutation, this approach can uncover mRNAs of abnormal size as well as alterations in the level of expression (Fig. 5.15).

THE POLYMERASE CHAIN REACTION (PCR)

An important development in DNA technology, with far-reaching consequences for basic research and genetic diagnostics, is the ability to amplify a short sequence of DNA from a complex mixture. This allows the study of a particular DNA fragment without first having to clone it, which greatly increases the speed of analysis. The principle of the method is diagrammed in Figure 5.16. It is necessary to chemically synthesize two short oligonucleotide primers (usually 15–30 nucleotides long), based upon the known sequence of the region (A and B in Fig. 5.16). The primers are added to double-stranded DNA, which is then heated to denature ("melt") it into single-stranded DNA. Because the primers are present in great excess, each primer will "find" its complementary sequence in the total DNA mix and hybridize to it. An enzyme capable of withstanding temperatures as high as 95°C, called *Taq* polymerase, is also added, which synthesizes a DNA strand from the end of the annealed primer, using the original DNA as a template. The mixture is then denatured again, additional primers are annealed, and the polymerase reaction is carried out again. This entire process can easily

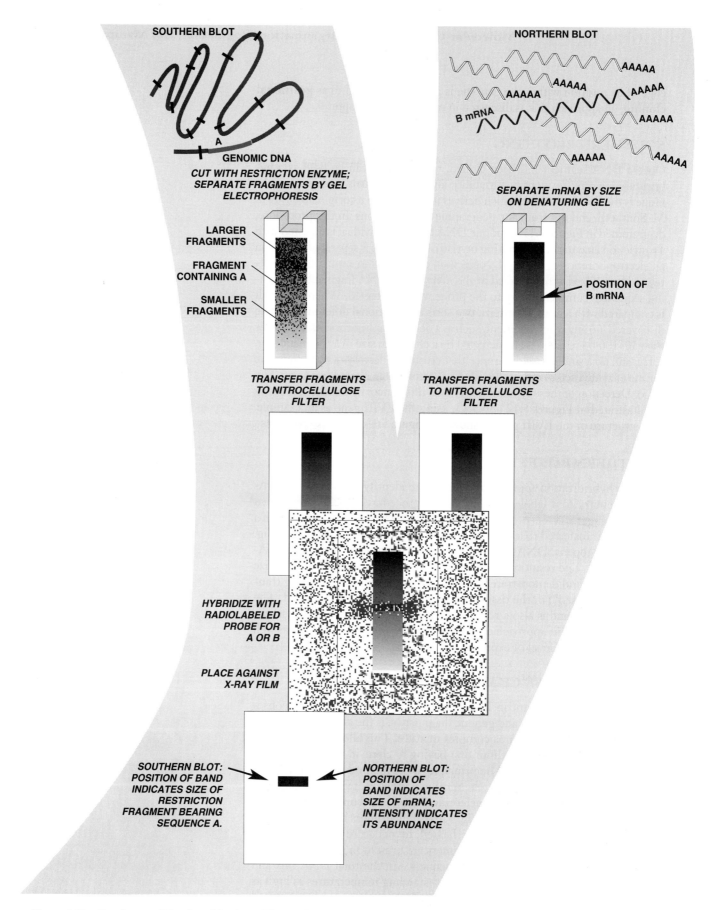

Figure 5.11. Southern and Northern blotting. These techniques allow detection of specific genomic DNA fragments or specific mRNA in complex mixtures. A Southern blot can visualize a specific, single genomic fragment (here denoted as gene *A*) in a mixture of about a million such fragments. The precise size of the fragment of interest can also be determined from how far it has migrated in the gel. In a Northern blot, a specific mRNA molecule (here denoted as *B*) can be detected in a complex mixture of 10,000 or more mRNAs derived from a tissue sample. The size of the mRNA can be determined by how far it has migrated in the gel, and its abundance by the intensity of the band.

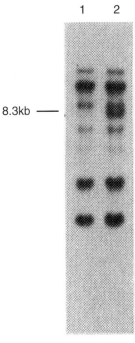

Figure 5.12. Hemophilia A caused by deletion in the factor VIII gene, detected by Southern blot analysis.   This Southern blot was performed on DNA digested with the restriction enzyme *Sst*I and probed with the complete factor VIII cDNA. Multiple bands are seen from many different regions of the factor VIII gene detected by the cDNA. The DNA in lane 1 carries a 39-kb deletion within the factor VIII gene removing all of exons 23–25, leading to hemophilia A in the patient. Comparison of the pattern in lane 1 to the pattern in a DNA sample that does not have a deletion in lane 2 reveals the absence of an 8.3-kb band. This band contains the deleted exons detected by the cDNA probe, which are only present in the nondeleted DNA sample. (Adapted from Gitschier J, Wood WI, Tuddenham EGD, Shuman MA, Goralka TM, Chen EY, Lawn RM. Detection and sequence of mutations in the factor VIII gene of haemophiliacs. Nature 1985;315:427–430.)

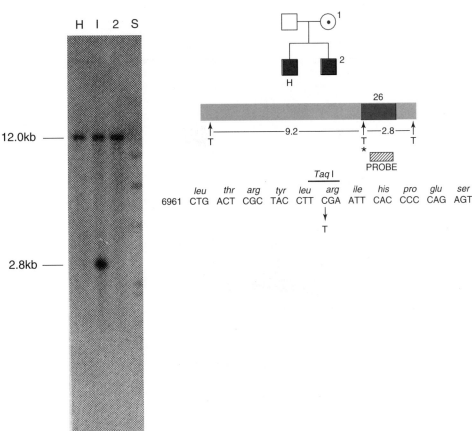

Figure 5.13. Hemophilia A caused by a single base-pair mutation in the factor VIII gene, detected by Southern blot analysis.   The DNA sequence in the region of the mutation is shown at the bottom, with the mutation indicated as a single base change from C to T. Since the recognition sequence for the restriction enzyme *Taq*I is TCGA (see Fig. 5.5), the mutation, which changes the TCGA to TTGA, results in loss of this restriction site. This particular *Taq*I restriction site is indicated by the asterisk in the gene diagram with the next *Taq*I site on either side also indicated by a T. The location of the probe for the Southern blot is also indicated. This probe detects a 2.8-kb *Taq*I fragment on a normal X chromosome. Note that this probe does not detect the normal 9.2-kb fragment. However, since the mutation destroys the asterisked *Taq*I site, the mutant chromosome gives rise to a 12-kb band. The mother, individual 1, can be seen to carry both one copy of the normal gene, accounting for the 2.8 kb-band, and one copy of the mutant X chromosome giving rise to the 12-kb band. Her two hemophilic sons, whose DNAs are shown in lanes H and 2, both inherited the abnormal copy of the gene and thus have only the 12-kb band. (Adapted from Gitschier J, Wood WI, Tuddenham EGD, Shuman MA, Goralka TM, Chen EY, Lawn RM. Detection and sequence of mutations in the factor VIII gene of haemophiliacs. Nature 1985;315:427–430.)

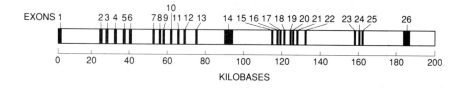

Figure 5.14.   A map of the factor VIII gene on the X chromosome.   Each exon is numbered, and the large size of the gene is apparent. Defects in the factor VIII gene, which produces a protein involved in blood clotting, result in hemophilia A. (Reprinted with permission from Lawn RM, Vehar GA: The molecular basis of hemophilia, Sci Am 1986;254:48–54.)

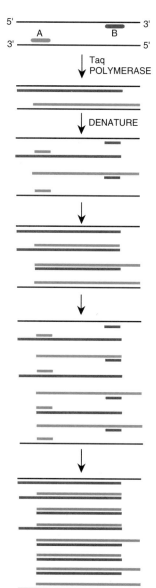

Figure 5.16.   Diagram of the polymerase chain reaction.   Repeated cycles of DNA synthesis using the A and B primers build up an exponential amount of DNA located between these primers. Analysis of a large number of cycles (not shown) reveals that the major product after 20–30 cycles is DNA that begins precisely at the beginning of the A primer and ends precisely at the end of the B primer, as shown in the third and sixth duplexes of the last panel.

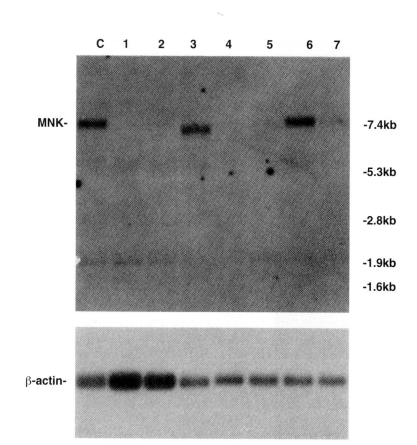

Figure 5.15.   Mutations in the MNK gene leading to Menkes' syndrome, as detected by Northern blot analysis.   The RNA for this Northern blot was prepared from fibroblasts obtained from a normal control (Lane C) and 7 unrelated affected boys with Menkes' syndrome, an X-linked recessive disorder (lanes 1–7). The probe is an MNK cDNA for the upper panel and a β-actin cDNA for the bottom panel. As expected, the β-actin mRNA is seen to be expressed in all of the RNA samples. The size and abundance of the MNK mRNA in normal fibroblast is evident in lane C. No detectable MNK mRNA is seen in lanes 1 and 4 whereas only lane 6 also shows an MNK mRNA of normal size and abundance. Though the abundance of the MNK mRNA in lane 3 appears normal, it is a smaller size than expected, whereas the mRNA in lane 7 is of normal size but markedly decreased quantity. The samples in lanes 2 and 5 have markedly decreased amounts of two hybridizing mRNAs, one of normal size and another of larger size. (Adapted from Vulpe CB, Levinson S, Whitney S, Packamn S, Gitschier. Isolation of a candidate gene for Menkes disease and evidence that it encodes a copper-transporting ATPase. Nat Genet 1993;3:7–13.)

be cycled, with each cycle requiring only a few minutes, and as many as 30 or 40 cycles can be carried out without the need to add fresh enzyme or primers. As shown in the figure, the result is an exponential increase in the amount of DNA in the region between the two primers. The amount of this material doubles with each cycle; therefore, at the end of 30 cycles, the original target sequence has been amplified 2^{30} times, or about 1 billion-fold. These repeated cycles of melting, annealing, and polymerase copying are performed automatically in a device called a thermocycler that has been programmed to cycle through the desired temperatures for specific times. The practical consequence of this is that one can start with nanogram amounts of DNA, carry out the PCR, and then run the sample on a gel to visualize a specific band corresponding precisely to the distance between the A and B primers (including the length of the primers themselves).

PCR can also be used to amplify specific RNA sequences. First the RNA must be copied into cDNA by reverse transcriptase, identical to the first step in the synthesis of double-stranded cDNA illustrated in Figure 5.7. In the first cycle of the PCR reaction, the single-stranded cDNA is copied by one of the primers into double-stranded cDNA, which can now be amplified by PCR in a manner identical to double-stranded DNA as illustrated in Figure 5.16. PCR products amplified from genomic DNA, messenger RNA, or any other DNA source, can then be analyzed in a variety of ways. Amplified DNA can be used as a specific probe for Northern and Southern blot analysis as discussed above, or analyzed for its specific DNA sequence content by a variety of methods, as described below. PCR has revolutionized recombinant DNA technology. Procedures to identify human genetic disease defects, which used to take many weeks to perform, can often now be accomplished in a matter of minutes to hours.

DNA SEQUENCING

The exact nucleotide sequence of a PCR product or a cloned fragment of DNA can readily be determined. In the most commonly employed technique, the Sanger method (Fig. 5.17), an enzymatic approach is used. The end result is a ladder of bands from which the DNA sequence can be directly read. A region of approximately 500 bp can routinely be sequenced in a single set of reactions. Automated DNA sequenators can now perform this procedure very rapidly on large numbers of samples. The DNA template is subjected to a standard set of enzyme reactions and loaded on to the sequenator, which then automatically separates and analyzes the DNA fragments, depositing the final DNA sequence result in a computer disk file. Continued advances in this technology have made determination of the entire human genomic sequence a practical goal, leading to the establishment of the human genome project (see chapter 10).

POLYMORPHISMS

Another area in molecular genetics technology that has far-reaching consequences for the identification of human disease genes (as we shall see in chapter 9) is the analysis of common DNA sequence variations or polymorphisms. This phenomenon may at first seem like only a curiosity, but as we consider examples of the applications of molecular genetics to human disease, it will become clear that these tools provide the opportunity to follow human disease genes in families in ways that would otherwise be impossible.

As previously pointed out, the majority of human DNA is not involved in coding sequences and is therefore not subject to tight selection. Perhaps for this reason, differences in DNA sequence between individuals are not a

large background of other *Eco*RI fragments generated from other places in the genome. Figure 5.18 shows the pattern that one would see, depending on whether probe 1, probe 2, or probe 3 was used. Note that the pattern differs as a function of which fragments are overlapped by the labeled probe. (A genomic fragment will be detected if even part of its DNA sequence is shared with the probe because these can then hybridize; it is not necessary for the entire probe sequence to overlap the genomic fragment.) In the figure are shown the results that one would obtain for an individual who has two A chromosomes, one A and one B chromosome, or two B chromosomes. DNA sequence polymorphisms of this type, resulting in variations in the length of specific restriction fragments, are generally referred to as **restriction fragment length polymorphisms** or RFLPs. If the DNA sequence surrounding the polymorphic site is known, it is generally easier and faster to analyze an RFLP by PCR, as also shown in Figure 5.18. For this analysis, PCR is performed with primers flanking the polymorphic restriction site, the PCR product is digested with the corresponding restriction enzyme, and the sizes of the resulting fragments are analyzed by gel electrophoresis.

There are three crucial things to remember in interpreting RFLP analysis. (*a*) In general, the base change detected by the restriction enzyme that leads to an RFLP is not in itself responsible for *disease*, but is a neutral change with no functional consequences. It can still be used, however, to mark a specific chromosome and follow its inheritance. Rarely will a restriction enzyme digest detect a disease-causing mutation unless the enzyme was specifically chosen for that purpose (as in the example in Figure 5.13). (*b*) The inheritance of RFLP alleles strictly follows Mendelian expectation. Thus, for example, the offspring of an AA individual and a BB individual would all be AB. (*c*) In using RFLPs to follow the inheritance of a chromosome in a family, the most useful RFLPs (also called markers) will be those for which most individuals are heterozygous. While the reasons for this will not become fully clear until we consider some examples, it may be intuitively apparent that one cannot follow the inheritance of the two specific chromosomes from a homozygous AA individual.

The RFLPs we have considered so far are simple single nucleotide changes that create or destroy a restriction site. A rarer but very useful type of polymorphism is diagrammed in Figure 5.19. These polymorphisms,

Figure 5.19. A variable number of tandem repeat (VNTR) polymorphism. The *boxed area* is a long array of a short tandemly repeated sequence. The number of the repeated elements varies from chromosome to chromosome, but is heritable. The different lengths can be visualized on a Southern blot, almost regardless of what restriction enzyme is used. An example of the results of analyzing three individuals with *Eco*RI and *Bam*HI using probe 1 demonstrates that all three are heterozygous, which is the major advantage of this sort of polymorphism. Probe 2, corresponding to the tandemly repeated region, detects a number of related VNTRs, in addition to the unique VNTR detected by probe 1, and thus gives rise to a much more complex and highly variable pattern.

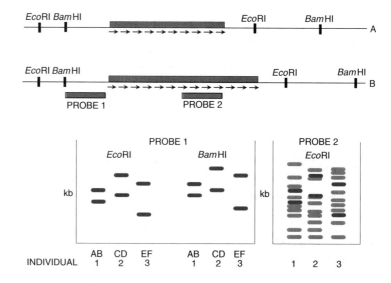

called length polymorphisms, minisatellites, or "variable number of tandem repeats" (**VNTRs**), are created by the presence of short sequences arranged in a head-to-tail fashion and repeated multiple times in a tandem array. The function of such sequences, if any, remains unknown, but the number of repeated units within such an element (and hence, the total length of the element) frequently varies from one homologous chromosome to another. In this setting, any restriction enzyme that cuts outside the tandem repeat will generate a fragment whose length will reflect the size of the VNTR. The feature that makes these polymorphisms particularly useful is that a large number of alleles are possible because the total length of the repeat may be highly variable from chromosome to chromosome. In Figure 5.19 is shown an example of such a VNTR polymorphism. Probe 1 corresponds to a segment of DNA unique to this particular VNTR polymorphism and thus detects only this single locus on a Southern blot. All three of the individuals shown are heterozygous at this locus. Probe 2 matches the tandem repeat of the VNTR polymorphism itself. Since the same tandem repeat is shared between a number of different VNTR polymorphisms scattered throughout the genome, probe 2 will detect multiple bands on a Southern blot from these multiple different polymorphisms. The complex pattern detected by a repeated probe like probe 2 simultaneously displays multiple polymorphic loci and is thus very rarely the same between two individuals. This pattern is often referred to as a "DNA fingerprint," an example of which is shown in Figure 5.20. This type of DNA identity analysis has found widespread use in paternity testing and forensic medicine. However, in practice, these analyses are now generally done with unique probes similar to probe 1 in Figure 5.19, which each detect a single, highly polymorphic VNTR. For such VNTRs with very large numbers of alleles, the chance of any two unrelated individuals carrying the same two alleles is very low, often less than 1%. By analyzing four or more such independent polymorphisms, the chance of any two unrelated individuals sharing the exact same pair of alleles at all of the loci becomes extremely small, unless they are monozygotic twins. An example of forensic DNA analysis is shown in Figure 5.21.

Since the repeated region in most VNTRs can be several thousand base pairs in length, a size that is difficult to amplify by standard PCR techniques, VNTRs must generally be analyzed by Southern blot analysis. However, another class of highly polymorphic markers has recently been developed that can be analyzed by PCR and thus is much more amenable to large-scale DNA typing. Though this class of polymorphisms also contains tandemly repeated sequences, the basic repeating unit is much shorter, generally only 2, 3, or 4 base pairs (di, tri, and tetranucleotide repeats, respectively). This class of polymorphisms is often referred to as "microsatellites" or simple sequence repeats (**SSRs**) (Fig. 5.22). As will be discussed in chapter 9, the identification of more than 10,000 markers of this type over the past few years has greatly facilitated mapping and linkage studies in humans, as well as a number of other species, dramatically speeding up the identification of disease genes purely on the basis of their position (positional cloning). Recently, unstable variations in the length of specific triplet repeats located within several genes have been identified as an important new mechanism for human disease mutation (see chapters 3 and 8).

The usefulness of DNA sequence polymorphisms may be clearer with the consideration of an example. As will be described in chapter 7, hemophilia A is an X-linked recessive disorder caused by mutations in the gene

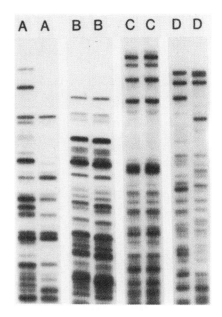

Figure 5.20. DNA fingerprint analysis using a single probe that detects a large number of VNTR polymorphisms located in widely scattered regions of the genome. Each pair of samples represents DNA from twins. Note the perfect match in B and C indicates that these are identical twins, whereas A and D are fraternal. Note that the fraternal twins share about half of the variable bands, as expected for first-degree relatives.

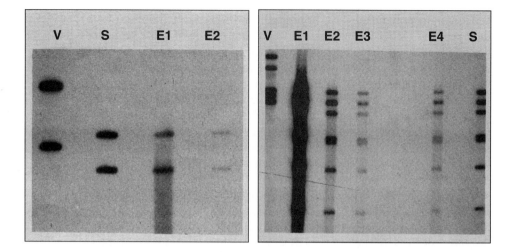

Figure 5.21.   VNTR polymorphisms and forensic DNA analysis.   The Southern blot at the left illustrates a single VNTR locus detected by a unique DNA probe, similar to probe 1 in Figure 5.19. Different bands are seen in DNA obtained from the victim (V) and the suspect (S). DNA prepared from evidence (E), collected at the crime scene matches the suspect's pattern. The probability of a chance match to the suspect can be estimated knowing the frequencies of the various VNTR alleles in the general population. By performing a similar analysis with multiple different VNTR polymorphisms, the probability of a chance match can be made extremely low. The Southern blot at the right was performed with a cocktail of 4 different single locus VNTR probes. There is a perfect match between the evidence and the suspect. Current forensic analysis generally employs at least four independent, highly polymorphic VNTR markers. (Reprinted with permission from DNA Fingerprinting[SM] and DNA Profiling. Germantown, MD: Cellmark Diagnostics. © 1989 by ICI Americas Inc.)

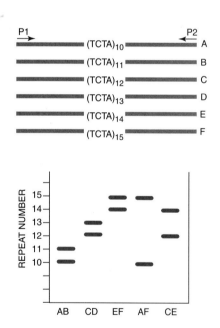

Figure 5.22.   A simple sequence repeat (SSR) polymorphism.   Each of the alleles for this polymorphism carries a different number of copies for the simple repeated sequence, TCTA. When this locus is amplified using primers P1 and P2, the products of the various alleles differ in length by multiples of the 4 base-pair repeat unit. These different sizes can easily be resolved by gel analysis.

for factor VIII. Defective factor VIII leads to an inability to form proper blood clots. The factor VIII gene has been cloned and is a very large gene approximately 200,000 bp in length (see Fig. 5.14). As illustrated in Figures 5.12 and 5.13, large deletions within the gene and point mutations leading to a change in a restriction site can occasionally be detected in hemophilia A patients by Southern blotting. As discussed in chapter 7, a unique rearrangement in the factor VIII gene leading to hemophilia A has recently been detected by Southern blot analysis in a large group of patients. However, about 1/2 of the mutations in the factor VIII gene that lead to hemophilia A are missense or nonsense mutations that are not easily detected by routine Southern blot analysis. Screening of the large factor VIII gene for each new mutation is not yet practical, outside of the research laboratory. In Figure 5.23 is shown a typical family in which hemophilia A is occurring. Note that there are affected males in generations IV and V. Inspection of the pedigree indicates that III-2, III-4, and III-5 are obligate heterozygotes for hemophilia A. Individual IV-4, whose risk of being a carrier is 50% based on the pedigree, wishes to be more sure of this risk before beginning a family. In general, carriers of hemophilia A are found to have approximately half the normal protein levels of factor VIII in the blood, so this can sometimes be used to distinguish carriers from homozygous normal females. However, there is considerable overlap between the carrier and normal ranges, so that an unequivocal distinction is often not possible based on protein measurement. In a family such as this, a more accurate way to determine whether IV-4 is a carrier is to use a DNA sequence polymorphism as a marker of the chromosome carrying the mutant allele. In Figure 5.23 is shown a restric-

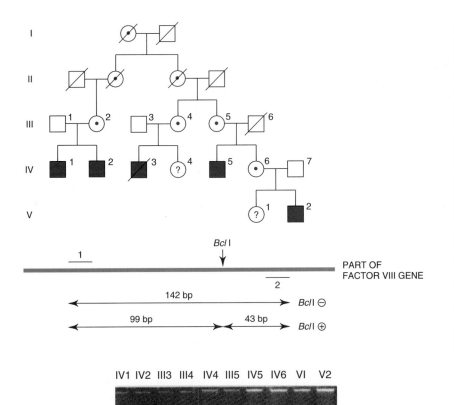

Figure 5.23. Analysis in a hemophilia A family using a DNA sequence polymorphism. Below the pedigree is a diagram of the region to be analyzed by PCR, showing the location of the primers and of the polymorphic *Bcl* I site. PCR with primers 1 and 2 gives a product of 142 bp, which when digested with *Bcl* I will give a 99-bp and a 43-bp product if the *Bcl* I site is present. The photograph shows the actual results of the analysis; the *numbers* above each lane correspond to the individual in the pedigree. A constant band at 67 bp is of unknown origin and can be ignored for the purposes of this analysis. The hemophilia A gene is associated with the presence of the 142-bp band (i.e., lacking the *Bcl* I site) in all of the affected males. Careful inspection reveals that individual IV-4 must be a hemophilia carrier. The status of individual V-1 cannot be determined because her mother is a homozygote for the polymorphism. (Reprinted with permission from Kogan SC, Doherty M, Gitschier J. An improved method for prenatal diagnosis of genetic diseases by analysis of amplified DNA sequences. Application to hemophilia A. N Engl J Med 1987;317:985–990.)

tion map of a region of an intron in the factor VIII gene that contains a polymorphism for the enzyme *Bcl*I.

PCR primers 1 and 2 flanking the polymorphic restriction site are used to amplify the target region, the amplified DNA is cut with *Bcl*I, and the fragments are directly run on a gel to determine whether the site is present. If the *Bcl*I site is present, digestion with this enzyme cuts the 142-bp product into bands of 99 and 43 bp, whereas if it is absent the full 142-bp length is seen. All of the males with hemophilia have the 142-bp band, indicating that the X chromosome carrying the hemophilia mutation lacks the *Bcl*I site. Individual IV-4 has inherited the *Bcl*I– allele from her mother, III-4, and is thus a hemophilia carrier. This example illustrates an important point noted above; the *Bcl*I RFLP itself (in an intron) is *not* the hemophilia mutation, but simply serves to mark the chromosome; other chromosomes with this same allele do not carry the hemophilia gene, as demonstrated by the normal allele in individual IV-6. While in this example we have considered an X-linked recessive disease, this type of analysis can also be used very successfully for autosomal dominant and autosomal recessive diseases, and we shall encounter many examples of this in later chapters. In addition, this PCR-based analysis is very rapid, with the results available in a few hours, and requires only a tiny amount of genomic DNA from each individual. PCR can be carried out, for example, using DNA prepared from saliva specimens (which contain enough epithelial cells to provide sufficient DNA for PCR) or even from archived blocks of paraffin-embedded tissue stored in surgical pathology laboratories from patients long since deceased.

OTHER METHODS FOR DETECTING DNA SEQUENCE DIFFERENCES

Since not all DNA sequence changes result in the convenient alteration of a restriction enzyme recognition site, other more general methods have been developed to screen for any known sequence difference. The ability to use PCR to generate an essentially pure sample of a single DNA fragment makes it possible to carry out precise hybridization experiments that allow the detection of single nucleotide differences. Figure 5.24 illustrates a method for doing this, applied to the detection of the mutation causing sickle cell anemia (see chapter 6). In addition to the oligonucleotides synthesized to carry out PCR, one also generates **allele-specific oligonucleotides** (ASOs) for the internal part of the fragment, located over the site of the DNA sequence difference. The ASOs are usually 15–19 bp in length; careful hybridization experiments (primarily by controlling the temperature and salt concentration) will allow the "perfect match" ASO to hybridize efficiently to its target, whereas the ASO with a single nucleotide mismatch will not hybridize. In general, one synthesizes ASOs for both of the possible sequences of a given region and separately tests each probe on PCR-amplified material, labeling the ASO so that it is possible to tell whether it hybridized or not to the PCR-amplified DNA.

An example, applied to the same hemophilia family of Figure 5.23, is shown in Figure 5.25. One ASO has been synthesized to be a perfect match for the chromosome containing the *Bcl*I site (TGATCA is the recognition site for *Bcl*I). The other ASO matches the chromosome that does not have the *Bcl*I site, which has TGAACA instead. Genomic DNA from the family has been amplified by PCR, and then small amounts of this DNA have been applied to nitrocellulose in elliptical slots. The upper strip has been hybridized with the labeled *Bcl*I+ ASO, and the lower strip with the labeled *Bcl*I− ASO. After washing off the excess ASO probes, the filter is placed against x-ray film. The results agree completely with the gel analysis shown in Figure 5.17. Note, however, that this ASO method did not depend on the presence of a restriction site at the location of the nucleotide difference between the chromosomes, but could have been applied to detect *any* difference. Also, one must know sequence information about a particular region to carry out the analysis, since the oligonucleotide PCR primers and the ASOs depend on this information. Many other PCR-based methods have been developed to rapidly detect known sequence differences. Several of these approaches are particularly amenable to automation and will likely form the basis for widespread DNA-based testing in the clinical laboratory of the future.

For cases in which the precise mutations are unknown, methods have also been developed to scan large segments of a target gene for possible sequence differences. Even for genes as large as factor VIII (Fig. 5.14), it is now possible to amplify all of the coding exons by PCR and efficiently screen through this sequence to identify unique mutations within a given patient's DNA. Several of these approaches are illustrated schematically in Figure 5.26. **Denaturing gradient gel electrophoresis** (DGGE) takes advantage

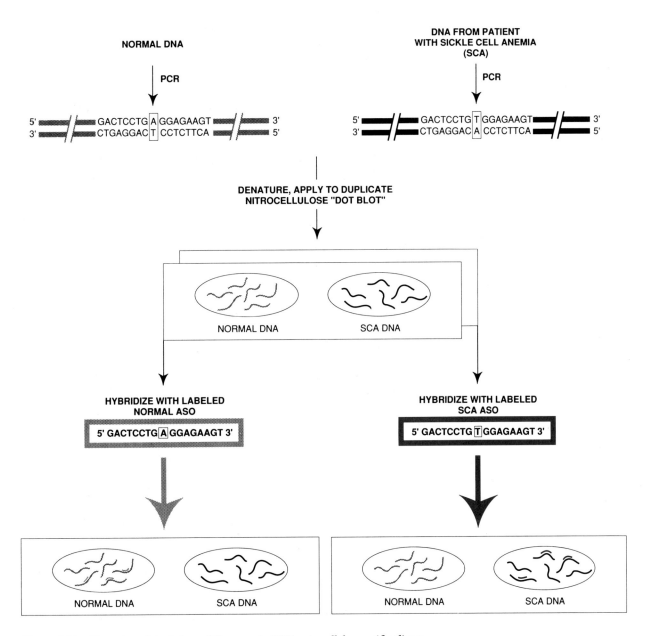

Figure 5.24. Detection of single base differences in DNA using allele-specific oligonucleotides (ASOs). In this example, the ASOs are designed to detect the difference between normal DNA and DNA containing the mutation causing sickle cell anemia. This disease is caused by an A to T change in the β-globin gene (see chapter 6). Under careful hybridization conditions, the labeled "perfect-match" ASO will stick to the target DNA, but a single-mismatch ASO will not; this allows a clear distinction of the two DNA samples.

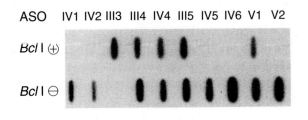

Figure 5.25. Analysis of the pedigree in Figure 5.23 using ASO testing of PCR-amplified DNA. The results of this analysis are consistent with the gel analysis in Figure 5.23. (Reprinted with permission from Kogan SC, Doherty M, Gitschier J. An improved method for prenatal diagnosis of genetic diseases by analysis of amplified DNA sequences. Application to hemophilia A. New Engl J Med 1987;317:985–990.)

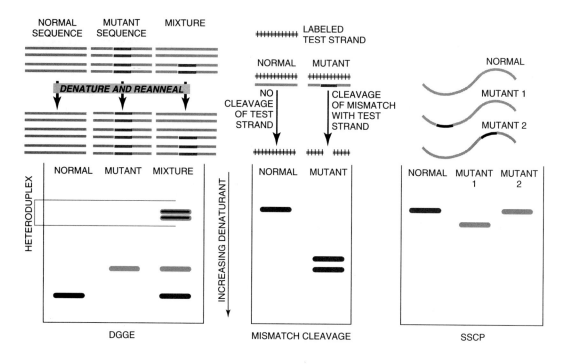

Figure 5.26.   Screening methods for mutation detection.   Several methods for screening a DNA sequence to identify new mutations are illustrated schematically. Denaturing gradient gel electrophoresis (DGGE) takes advantage of small differences in the melting behavior of two complementary strands of DNA based on their precise DNA sequence. The gel provides a gradient of denaturing conditions with the highest stringency toward the bottom of the gel. As a double-stranded DNA fragment makes its way through the gel, it will suddenly slow in mobility at the position where the strands begin to come apart. A single base-pair difference in sequence between the normal and mutant will result in slightly different melting behaviors and thus different mobilities in the gel. Heteroduplexes of a normal and mutant strand will contain one mismatched position that will markedly alter mobility by causing melting to occur at a lower denaturant condition. When the conditions are designed to detect mutations as heteroduplexes, nearly 100% can be detected. Mismatch cleavage methods form a heteroduplex between a labeled test DNA or RNA strand and a control normal sequence. The presence of a mutation will result in a mismatch at the corresponding position. A variety of chemical and enzymatic methods can then be used to cleave the heteroduplex at the position of mismatch. The labeled cleaved or uncleaved test strand is then visualized on a denaturing gel. The presence of smaller fragments adding up to the full size of the test strand will indicate the presence of a mutation. In addition, the size of the bands provides information about the location of the corresponding mutation. Chemical mismatch cleavage methods have been developed that detect nearly 100% of mutations. Single-strand conformational polymorphism (SSCP) analysis separates single-stranded DNA from the region of interest in a nondenaturing gel. The conformation of each single strand will vary slightly depending on its precise sequence content and these differences in conformation may be reflected in difference in gel mobility. However, not all sequence changes result in a significant difference in mobility, and thus, only a subset of mutations are detected by this approach.

Figure 5.27.   Generation of transgenic mice.   For the generation of transgenic mice by pronuclear injection, oocytes are obtained surgically just after fertilization, before the male and female pronuclei have fused. The cloned DNA to be transferred to the mouse genome is injected into the male pronucleus; the pronuclei then fuse, and in a proportion of eggs the injected DNA will be covalently integrated into a random site in the mouse genome. The oocytes are then reimplanted surgically into a foster mother whose uterus has been primed suitably by hormonal treatment. After delivery, the animals can be checked for the presence of the injected DNA by a Southern blot or PCR of a small amount of DNA, most conveniently prepared from a tail tip. Transcription of this sequence can be assessed by Northern blotting. In this example, animals *A* and *C* have incorporated the injected DNA, whereas *B* and *D* are negative. *C* has more DNA copies than *A* (commonly 1–200 copies occur) and also expresses the gene, whereas *A* does not. The transgene ordinarily is transmitted to offspring in a Mendelian fashion. The embryonic stem cell approach is shown on the right. ES cells are selected in culture for the desired DNA alteration. These cells are injected into an early stage of the embryo called a

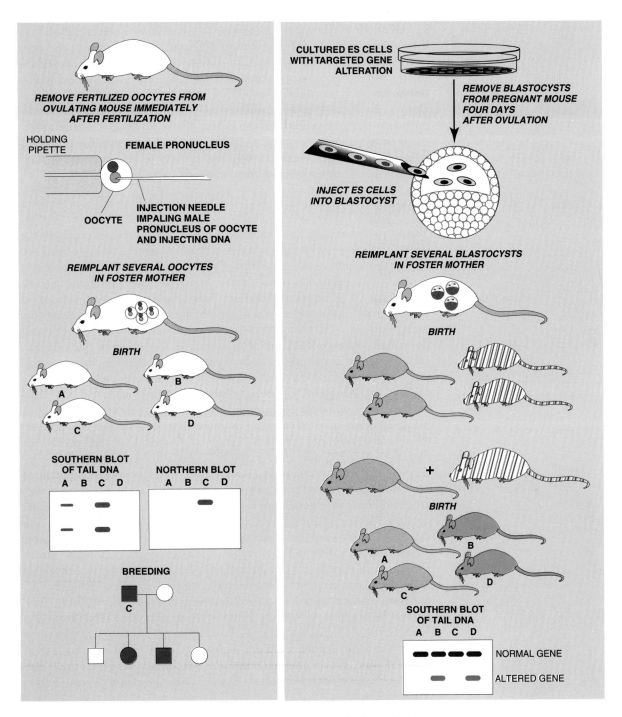

Figure 5.27. (*continued*) blastocyst, obtained from a pregnant donor. The injected blasto-cysts are reimplanted into a foster mother. The offspring mice are chimeric, with some cells derived from the original blastocyst and some from the ES cell. When this chimeric animal is bred with another mouse, it will contribute a germ cell either of ES or non-ES cell origin. ES-derived animals will carry the same genetic alteration as the original ES cell culture and can now be bred to establish a stable line of successfully engineered mice. The presence of the al-tered gene can be detected by Southern blotting or PCR.

of the altered mobility in a particular type of gel for DNA fragments carry-ing normal or mutant sequences. An even simpler approach, **single-strand conformational polymorphism** (SSCP) analysis generates single-stranded DNAs from PCR-amplified material that are then separated on the basis of differences in gel mobility owing to the single nucleotide mutation. Finally, several methods take advantage of specific enzymes or chemical procedures that efficiently cleave DNA at sites of mismatch between mutant and normal sequence. The cleaved fragments can then be detected in the gel, identifying both the presence of a mutation and its approximate location within the fragment. Under optimal conditions, the SSCP approach can detect as many as 70–80% of sequence differences, whereas DGGE and some of the mismatch cleavage procedures can detect nearly 100% of sequence differences within a given segment of DNA. Improvements in these mutation-scanning approaches may eventually lead to more widespread routine diagnosis of specific mutations in human genetic disease.

GENE TRANSFER

The sequence of a gene is extremely useful, as it predicts precisely the amino acid sequence of the resulting protein. However, it is not possible to look at the sequence of a gene or its flanking regions and predict how that gene will be regulated or in what tissues it will be expressed. To obtain this information, it is highly desirable to have a system for gene transfer, in which a gene can be sequenced, altered in any way desirable by removing certain sequences or changing others, and then placed back into cells and its expression into mRNA and protein studied. Genes can be put back into cells that grow in culture flasks by a variety of methods including simple precipitation of the DNA with calcium phosphate onto the surface of the cells, or stimulation of DNA uptake by the cells using electric shock (**electroporation**), or incubation with lipids (**lipofection**). By these approaches, many different types of cells can be induced to take up the DNA, which then finds its way into the nucleus and is expressed. In a small proportion of such transfected cells, the foreign DNA actually becomes covalently integrated into a chromosome at a random site. A number of recombinant viral vectors including retroviruses and adenoviruses can also be used to very efficiently introduce genes into cells. These methods are discussed in more detail in chapter 13. Introduction of recombinant genes into foreign cells can be used to manufacture recombinant proteins with normal or altered amino acid sequences and to study the DNA sequences responsible for the regulation of gene expression. In human genetics, these methods are used to produce large amounts of recombinant proteins for the treatment of patients with genetic deficiencies, such as the use of recombinant factor VIII to treat hemophilia A. Analysis of the function of mutant DNA sequences is also critical to distinguishing authentic disease mutations from neutral changes in DNA sequence and for understanding the molecular pathogenesis of disease. Finally, the introduction of an exogenous gene into human cells for the treatment of disease is the aim of the new field of gene therapy (chapter 13).

    Transgenic mouse technology provides a powerful set of tools for manipulating genes in the whole animal. In the standard approach, genes are transfected into mouse oocytes just after fertilization, using a very fine pipette to inject the purified DNA under direct vision. The oocyte is then reimplanted into a different mouse and normal embryogenesis of the injected egg proceeds. About 10–30% of the mouse progeny are found to have covalently integrated several copies of the injected DNA into their germline DNA, so that these sequences are transmitted in a Mendelian fashion to future offspring. In many instances, the injected gene is also transcribed by the mouse. This provides an excellent way of studying what sequences are necessary to direct proper developmental and tissue-specific expression of a given gene. The process is diagrammed in Figure 5.27.

Figure 5.28 shows a picture of a mouse that was derived from such an experiment, in which the injected gene was a growth hormone gene engineered in such a way as to produce large quantities of the hormone. The resulting increase in size of the mouse relative to its normal littermate is apparent.

An exciting recent development has been the ability to perform more precise targeted manipulations of the mouse genome. For these methods, DNA is introduced into embryonic stem cells (ES cells) grown in tissue culture (Fig. 5.27). ES cells can be modified in tissue culture and even after several passages, maintain their potency for contributing to the genetic makeup of a developing mouse embryo. Thus, when ES cells have been successfully engineered by sophisticated in vitro techniques to delete or subtly alter part of the sequence for a specific gene, mice derived from these ES cells will also carry this gene defect. ES cells carrying the desired change are injected into an early form of the mouse embryo called a blastocyst and reimplanted into a foster mother. A mouse derived from such an injected blastocyst will be a mixture composed of cells derived from the original blastocyst cells and those derived from the ES cells. A mouse composed of cells of mixed origin is termed a **chimera.** Germ cells (egg or sperm) in the chimeric mouse derived from the ES cells will stably carry the genetic alteration originally introduced into those cells, permitting a stable mouse line to be constructed. If a specific gene was disrupted in the ES cells, then matings between offspring of the chimeric mouse can eventually produce mice homozygous for the gene defect. Mice in which a specific gene has been disrupted in this way are often referred to as "**knockout**" mice. Using these approaches, it has now become possible to engineer transgenic mice carrying virtually any desired alteration of the genome, even including single-point mutations introduced into a specific gene target. In this way, powerful animal models can now be constructed for many human diseases for which the responsible gene is known. These animals can be used to study the pathogenesis of the human disease as well as to test new therapies.

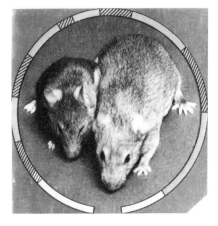

Figure 5.28. Mouse and supermouse. The smaller mouse on the *left* is a normal (nontransgenic) animal, whereas the larger mouse is transgenic for a rat growth hormone gene, which was constructed in such a way that growth hormone is overproduced. The transgenic mouse has attained a weight two to three times normal as a result of this intervention. (Reprinted with permission from Palmiter RD, Norstedt G, Gelinas RE, Hammer RE, Brinster RL. Metallothionein-human GH fusion genes stimulate growth of mice. Science 1983;222:809–814.)

Conclusion

We have reviewed the gross and detailed structure of genes and gene families and the powerful methods of recombinant DNA technology that have made possible such a remarkable understanding of human molecular biology. Armed with this background about normal structure and function, we are now ready to move forward into an analysis of the molecular basis of human disease, which will occupy us for the next two chapters.

SUGGESTED READINGS

Beaudet AL, Scriver CR, Sly WS, Valle D. Genetics, biochemistry, and molecular basis of variant human phenotypes. In: Scriver CR, Beaudet AL, Sly WS, Valle D, eds. The metabolic basis of inherited disease. 7th ed. New York: McGraw-Hill, 1995:53–118. *A general overview of recombinant DNA technology.*

Bronson SK, Smithies O. Altering mice by homologous recombination using embryonic stem cells. J Biol Chem 1994;269:27155–27158. *A discussion of the techniques for generating knockout mice by gene targeting.*

Grompe M. The rapid detection of unknown mutations in nucleic acids. Nat Genet 1993;5:111–116. *A summary of methods of screening for mutations.*

Lewin B. Genes V. New York: Oxford University Press, 1994. *An excellent textbook of basic molecular biology.*

Tjian R. Molecular machines that control genes. Sci Am 1995;272:54–61. *A review of transcription factors and the regulation of gene expression.*

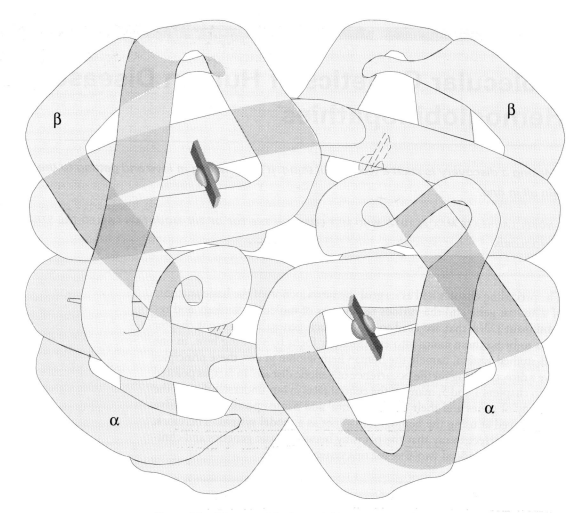

Figure 6.1.   Diagram of the hemoglobin tetramer.   The two α and two β chains, each of which binds a molecule of heme (the planar structure in the center of each subunit), are shown. (Reprinted with permission from Dickerson RE, Geis I. Hemoglobin: structure, function, evolution, and pathology. Menlo Park, CA: Benjamin/Cummings, 1983. © W Irving Geis.)

The Hemoglobin Genes

A scale drawing of the α- and β-globin gene regions of humans is shown in Figure 5.2. Both the α and β genes actually are part of gene clusters, with the β-globin cluster on chromosome 11 and the α-globin cluster on chromosome 16. These clusters contain, in addition to the major adult genes, α and β, other expressed sequences, which are used at different points in development. In both clusters, the genes are arranged so that their 5′ to 3′ direction of transcription is the same for all genes, and the genes used earliest in development are at the 5′ end of the cluster, and those used last, at the 3′ end. As noted in chapter 5, both clusters contain pseudogenes, remnants of once functioning genes, which have undergone mutations rendering them no longer capable of producing a protein. In both clusters, the majority of the DNA is located in intergenic regions of unknown and possibly dispensable function.

Figure 6.2 shows the pattern of expression of the functional genes in both of these clusters, plotted as a function of developmental age. In the first few weeks of life, hemoglobin synthesis occurs in the yolk sac. The major hemoglobin at that time is a tetramer of two ζ chains (encoded within the α cluster), and two ε chains transcribed from the β cluster. Very soon, how-

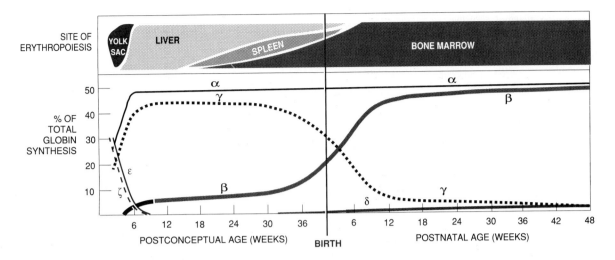

Figure 6.2.   Developmental pattern of expression of human hemoglobin.   The time course of production of the various globin chains is shown. At the *top* of the figure is diagrammed the primary site of hematopoiesis during these various stages. (Reprinted with permission from Weatherall DJ, Clegg JB. The thalassemia syndromes. 3rd ed. Oxford: Blackwell Scientific Publications, 1981.)

ever, production of these two globin chains rapidly diminishes and the α-globin cluster begins to transcribe α as its major product. There are actually two α genes, $\alpha 2$ and $\alpha 1$, but these are identical in their coding regions and therefore produce a single protein. The α genes then stay on for the remainder of the life of the individual.

The β-globin cluster, however, contains an additional set of genes, the fetal hemoglobin genes. This consists of a pair of genes, $^G\gamma$ and $^A\gamma$, which differ in their coding region by only one amino acid, which is glycine for $^G\gamma$ and alanine for $^A\gamma$ at position 136. As shown in Figure 6.2, the γ genes turn on as the embryonic genes are turning off, and during fetal life the major products from the β-globin cluster are $^G\gamma$ and $^A\gamma$. Beginning somewhat before birth and continuing for several months after birth, there is a smooth and carefully regulated switch from γ production to β production, so that at all times the sum of the two is kept approximately constant. This development switch cannot be attributed to the change in environment that occurs at birth because the switch is already underway by that time. It also cannot be attributed to a change in the site of hemoglobin production, although red cell production does switch at about the same time from the fetal liver to the bone marrow (Fig. 6.2). If one looks in the bone marrow at the time of birth, however, both γ and β are being produced at that site; thus, the switch occurs on a cell-by-cell basis.

Figure 6.3 shows the possible hemoglobin tetramers during this developmental pattern. All of these have been identified and have been given somewhat anachronistic names before an understanding of their molecular basis. In embryonic life, the major hemoglobin is hemoglobin Gower I. Hemoglobin Gower II and hemoglobin Portland are seen transiently during the time when the embryonic genes are turning off and the fetal genes are turning on. During fetal life the major hemoglobin is hemoglobin F, which includes both $\alpha_2{}^G\gamma_2$ and $\alpha_2{}^A\gamma_2$. In adult life, the major globin is hemoglobin A, which is a tetramer of two α and two β chains. There is also a minor adult globin called hemoglobin A_2, which is a tetramer consisting of two α chains and two δ chains. The δ gene has developmental timing similar to β, but it has acquired a number of alterations in its promoter, particularly in the CCAAT box region, which render it relatively inefficient. At least partly for this reason, the amount of δ mRNA is considerably lower than that of β mRNA. The net re-

Figure 6.3. A matrix diagram showing the possible tetrameric products of the α-globin cluster on chromosome 16 and the β-globin cluster on chromosome 11, together with their historical names.

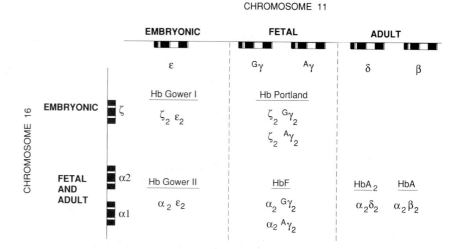

Figure 6.3. A matrix diagram showing the possible tetrameric products of the α-globin cluster on chromosome 16 and the β-globin cluster on chromosome 11, together with their historical names.

sult is that a normal adult individual has approximately 97.5% hemoglobin A, about 2% hemoglobin A_2, and about 0.5% hemoglobin F.

The expression of the γ genes in a fetal developmental program is a relatively recent evolutionary event, having appeared only in primates. It is speculated that this additional hemoglobin had advantages because of the longer gestation time in these species, which requires a more efficient means of ensuring adequate oxygen delivery to the growing fetus over an extended period of time. Fetal hemoglobin has a somewhat higher oxygen affinity than adult hemoglobin and thus is capable of extracting oxygen more efficiently across the placenta from the maternal circulation.

Normal Anatomy and Expression of the β-Globin Gene

Many of the general features of eukaryotic genes discussed in chapter 5 were first defined through study of the human β-globin gene, which is diagrammed in Figure 6.4. The promoter region of the β-globin gene contains a TATA box, but in this instance the sequence is actually just ATA. There is also a CCAAT box, and somewhat further upstream a sequence, CACCC, which is repeated once and is present in many other globin genes. Human β globin is exquisitely tissue-specific, being expressed in significant levels only in red blood cells and their precursors. Considerable progress has been made over the past few years toward understanding the molecular basis for this highly regulated expression. A number of sequence motifs within the β-globin promoter serve as targets for binding by tissue-specific transcription factors. An important example of such a factor is GATA-1. The GATA genes are a family of transcription factors that bind to DNA of the sequence (T/A) GATA (A/G). The binding motif for GATA-1 is found in multiple copies in the β-globin gene promoter as well as in the promoters of many other erythroid-specific genes, including all the hemoglobin genes. Transgenic mice that have been engineered to be deficient in GATA-1 by gene targeting in embryonic stem cells (see chapter 5) are unable to form red blood cells. The transcription factor EKLF binds to the CACCC motif and also contributes to the control of β-globin gene expression. A mutation in that CACCC sequence preventing binding of the EKLF transcription factor results in β-thalassemia (see below). Complex interactions between multiple other transcription factors and the β-globin gene promoter are also required for proper expression. Recently another critical regulator has been identified, quite a distance from the β-globin gene. This region is referred to as the **locus control region** (LCR), since

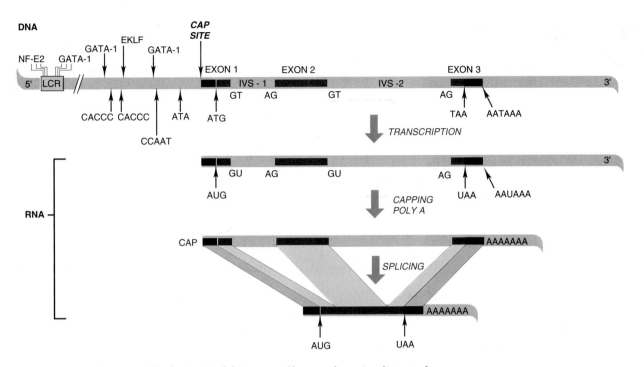

Figure 6.4.   A schematic of the human β-globin gene.   Shown at the *top* is a diagram of the genomic DNA, with important flanking regulatory sequences also indicated. Critical sequence motifs in the promoter are shown below the bar with several of the important transcription factors known to bind in this region indicated above the bar. The locus control region (LCR) required for efficient expression of all genes in the β-globin complex is also shown. It is located more than 50 kb upstream of the β-globin gene itself. The introns and their junctions with exons are also noted, as is the polyadenylation (AATAAA) site. The transcription of this gene into RNA is depicted, as is the processing of that RNA into a mature cytoplasmic message.

it is important for regulation of all of the genes within the β-globin cluster. The LCR is located 6–20 kb upstream of the ε-globin gene (see Figs. 5.2 and 6.4) and thus approximately 60 kb away from the β-globin gene. The LCR contains binding motifs for a number of erythroid-specific transcription factors including GATA-1 and NF-E2. The complex way in which interactions between the LCR and the promoters for each of the globin genes in the β cluster precisely regulate the switch from embryonic, to fetal, and eventually to adult globin (Fig. 6.3) is still a subject of intense investigation. As we shall see, manipulation of this developmental program could offer an important approach to therapy for a number of genetic disorders of the β-globin genes.

The β-globin gene consists of three exons and two introns, with the second intron considerably larger than the first. As shown in Figure 6.4, there are short 5′ and 3′ untranslated regions, and capping, polyadenylation, and splicing all proceed in the usual fashion. The resultant mRNA is then transported to the cytoplasm and its complete sequence is shown in Figure 6.5. Note the presence of the 7-methyl guanosine at the cap site, followed by a short stretch of untranslated RNA. The first AUG codon is surrounded by a box and denotes the start of translation of this RNA. This initial methionine is subsequently cleaved off of the polypeptide, so that the first amino acid of the mature protein is valine, which is coded for by GUG. There are a total of 146 amino acids in the mature polypeptide, and translation is terminated upon encountering the UAA stop codon. The remainder of the 3′ portion of the RNA represents untranslated sequence. The AAUAAA sequence, which is used in the nucleus as a signal for polyadenylation, is boxed, and a string of adenosine residues is attached 19 nucleotides to the 3′ side of this.

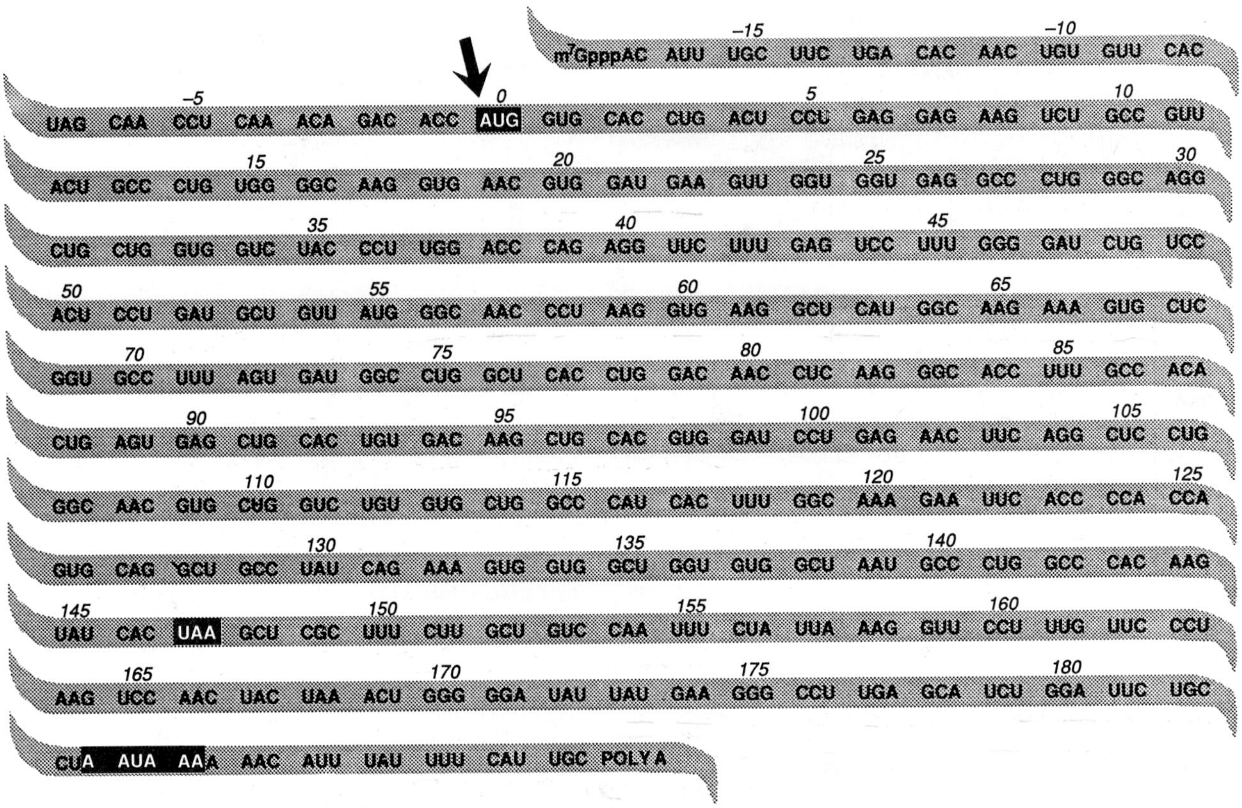

Figure 6.5.   The nucleotide sequence of human β-globin messenger RNA.   The AUG initiation codon is *boxed*, marked with an *arrow*, and numbered as *0*. The termination codon UAA (codon 147) is also marked. The polyadenylation signal near the 3' end of the message is also *boxed* and is followed 19 nucleotides later by a string of A residues.

We are now ready to take a look at the wide variety of mutations that have been described in the globin genes. These mutations can be divided into those causing qualitative abnormalities (such as sickle cell anemia) and those causing quantitative abnormalities (the thalassemias). Together, this whole group of disorders is referred to as the **hemoglobinopathies.**

Mutations Causing Qualitative Abnormalities in Globin

MISSENSE MUTATIONS

As described in chapter 2, a missense mutation results from a nucleotide change that alters the amino acid encoded by a particular 3-base codon. Because of the intense scrutiny to which the α- and β-globin genes have been subjected, a very large number of missense mutations have been described. Many of these do not cause any phenotypic abnormalities. As can be seen in Figure 6.6, most of the amino acids in both the α- and the β-globin genes have had missense mutations identified. Correlation of the phenotypes of these mutations with functional abnormalities seen in some of the mutations has led to a much better understanding of the functional domains of the hemoglobin tetramer, which are responsible for its properties. The general strategy of correlating the effect of mutations at specific locations in a molecule with the functional properties of that molecule is a powerful one with far-reaching implications.

The most common missense mutation in the β-globin gene leads to sickle cell anemia in the homozygote. The incidence of this disease in the

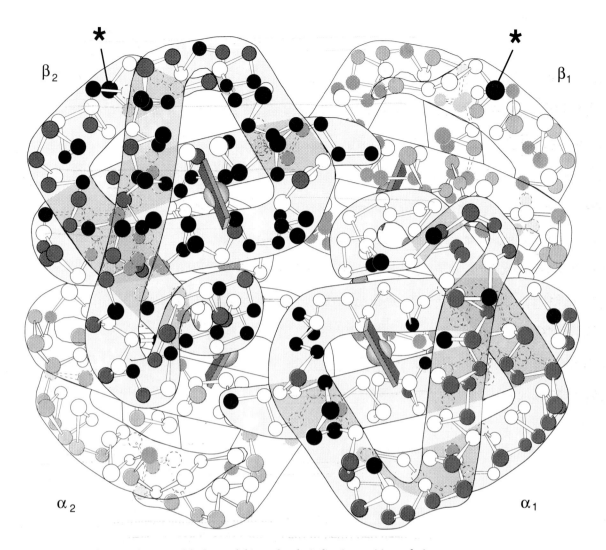

Figure 6.6. Schematic drawing of the hemoglobin molecule, indicating positions of missense mutations in the α and β subunits. This figure is based on all the reported hemoglobin mutations as of 1982. The very large number of abnormal hemoglobins already known at that time is evident, involving 170 of the 287 total amino acid positions in the α and β chains. *Shaded circles* indicate positions where altered amino acids had been observed, and mutations leading to abnormal hemoglobin function are indicated in *dark red* in the two closest subunits, α₁ and β₂. The β6 location of the sickle mutation is indicated with an *asterisk*. As of 1996, a total of 586 α and β chain variants have been identified, involving 238 of the 287 possible amino acid positions. (Reprinted with permission from Dickerson RE, Geis I. Hemoglobin: structure, function, evolution, and pathology. Menlo Park, CA: Benjamin/Cummings, 1983.)

black population is approximately 1 in 500 births, and the disease causes significant morbidity and mortality. The disorder is recessive, but carriers are easily detected. Using the Hardy-Weinberg law, described in chapter 4, one can predict that, if the incidence of the disease (q^2) is 1 in 500, the carrier frequency ($2pq$) is approximately 8%, and carrier screening confirms this result. Given that homozygous sickle cell anemia causes severe disease with shortening of life and decrease in reproductive potential, it may seem remarkable that this gene has reached such a high frequency in the black population. As described in chapter 4, however, there appears to be a clear-cut explanation for this occurrence. Specifically, heterozygotes for sickle cell anemia are moderately protected from the most severe and lethal consequences of infection with the malarial parasite, which apparently has led to

DNA

	codon 5	6	7
β^A	...CCT	GAG	GAG ...
β^S	...CCT	G**T**G	GAG ...
β^C	...CCT	**A**AG	GAG ...

PROTEIN

	5	6	7
β^A	...Pro	Glu	Glu ...
β^S	...Pro	**Val**	Glu ...
β^C	...Pro	**Lys**	Glu ...

Figure 6.7. The DNA and protein abnormalities in codon 6, which lead to sickle hemoglobin (β^S) and hemoglobin C (β^C).

selection for this gene over the long term. Thus, even though the homozygotes (1 in 500) are selected against, the moderate selection for heterozygotes (1 in 12) has allowed the gene to reach its high frequency in areas of the world where malaria has been endemic.

Sickle cell anemia is the first human disease to be successfully understood at the molecular level. The basic abnormality in sickle cell anemia was first postulated by Linus Pauling in 1949. Using careful analysis of the hemoglobin protein, Vernon Ingram subsequently demonstrated that the sickle cell β-globin gene differed by a single amino acid at position 6. The normal residue at this position is glutamic acid, whereas in sickle cell anemia valine is present instead. Subsequently, cloning and sequencing the respective genes has revealed the expected change in the DNA sequence, namely that the sequence for codon 6 is changed from GAG in the normal gene to GTG in sickle cell disease. Interestingly, another relatively common β-globin chain missense mutation, called hemoglobin C, also results from an alteration at codon 6, changing GAG to AAG and resulting in a lysine at this position (Fig. 6.7).

It is remarkable indeed that a single nucleotide change of the 3 billion nucleotides in the haploid human genome results in the wide array of severe clinical problems experienced by individuals with sickle cell anemia. The basis of these problems is diagrammed in Figure 6.8. The underlying problem is that the valine for glutamic acid replacement results in hemoglobin tetramers that, when deoxygenated, can aggregate into arrays rather than remaining soluble. As shown in Figure 6.8, these arrays can become almost crystalline in their structure. Thus, every time a red cell carrying sickle hemoglobin travels through the circulation and becomes deoxygenated, the hemoglobin within it aggregates. This in turn deforms the red cell, making it relatively inflexible and rendering it unable to traverse the fine capillary beds, which have diameters smaller than the red cell itself. After repeated cycles of deoxygenation and reoxygenation, some cells become irreversibly sickled. The result of all this is plugging of the microcirculation, particularly in areas of low oxygen tension. Bones are particularly affected, leading to the frequent and severe bone pain experienced in a sickle cell "crisis." Over the long term, this recurrent plugging of the circulation leads to significant damage to internal organs, especially the heart, lungs, and kidneys. Cerebrovascular accidents are another serious complication. Because of the destruction of red cells containing hemoglobin crystals, sickle cell patients are chronically anemic, and that contributes to the cardiac stress.

Despite remarkable progress in our understanding of the molecular pathology of sickle cell anemia, advances in treatment have been disappointing. The slow progress in improving therapy for this very common and life-threatening disorder serves as a sobering reminder for modern molecular medicine that rapid progress in basic research may prove difficult to directly translate into clinical benefit. Despite many decades of frustration in the treatments of patients with sickle cell anemia, recent results offer some promise. Selected patients with severe disease have recently been treated with a mild form of chemotherapy (hydroxyurea) that causes an increase in fetal hemoglobin production and improvement of red blood cell function. In addition, a number of patients have now been cured by bone marrow transplantation, though the major risk associated with this procedure restricts its use at present to only the most severely affected patients.

The diagnosis of sickle cell anemia usually can be readily made by examination of the blood smear (Fig. 6.8) in the presence of a typical clinical

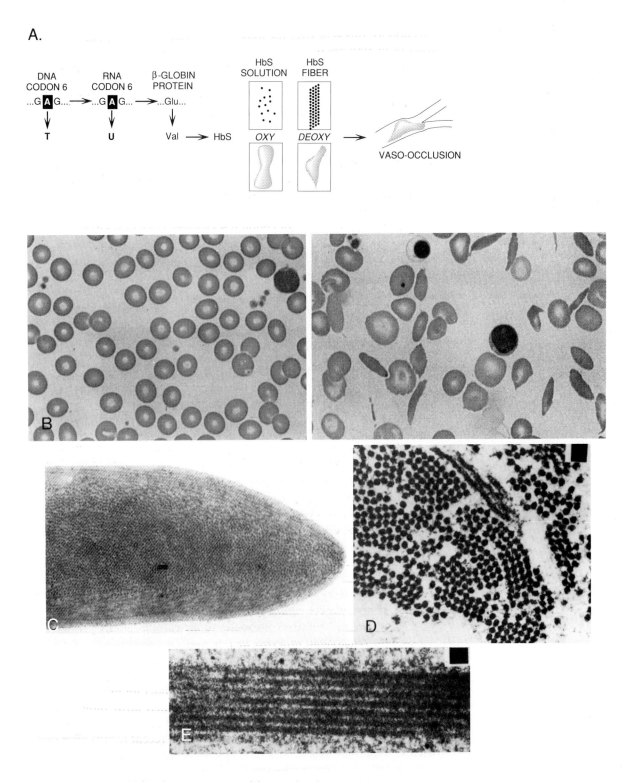

Figure 6.8.   Molecular pathogenesis of sickle cell anemia.   A. Deoxygenated sickle hemoglobin crystallizes within the red cells leading to rigidity and inability to traverse small capillaries. **B.** The sickled cells are visible in a blood smear on the *right*, with a normal blood smear on the *left* for comparison. **C.** Electron micrographs of deoxygenated sickle cells reveal fibers of hemoglobin, seen at higher magnification in both transverse **(D)** and longitudinal **(E)** orientation. (Reprinted with permission from Bunn HF, Forget B. Hemoglobin: molecular, genetic, and clinical aspects. Philadelphia: WB Saunders, 1986.)

Figure 6.9.   Hemoglobin electrophoresis. Hemoglobin samples are loaded at the position marked *origin* and then placed under an electric field; the distance traveled reflects total charge of the molecule. This allows separation of hemoglobins A, S, C, and A_2 (C and A_2 travel very close together). A normal individual (AA, *lane 3*) has primarily hemoglobin A with a small amount of hemoglobin A_2. A sickle homozygote (SS, *lane 2*) has only hemoglobin S and A_2. Hemoglobin samples from AC (*lane 4*) and SC (*lane 1*) individuals are also shown. (Reprinted with permission from Weatherall DJ, Clegg JB. The thalassemia syndromes. 3rd ed. Oxford: Blackwell Scientific Publications, 1981.)

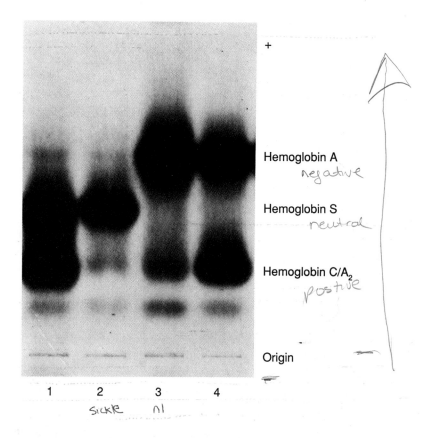

syndrome. Carriers can be diagnosed by exposing their red blood cells to very low oxygen tension, under which circumstances even blood from a heterozygote can be made to sickle. It is important to note, however, that heterozygotes (often referred to as having sickle trait) are not symptomatic, with the possible exception of very low oxygen tension environments such as high altitude unpressurized flight.

To be certain of the diagnosis, however, hemoglobin electrophoresis is usually carried out. As shown in Figure 6.9, hemoglobins that differ in charge can be separated by their migration in an electric field. Because the sickle mutation alters a negatively charged amino acid (glutamic acid) to a neutral one (valine), the result is a significant alteration in the migration of the protein on a gel in an electric field. Such gels can also detect the small amount of hemoglobin F and hemoglobin A_2 in the blood; these appear in a different position than hemoglobin A. Hemoglobin C, which, as noted above, represents a two-charge difference from hemoglobin A because of the mutation of a negatively charged amino acid to a positively charged amino acid (lysine) at codon 6, results in a band on the gel that migrates even more slowly than hemoglobin S toward the positive electrode and travels very close to the position of hemoglobin A_2. Many of the other missense mutations shown in Figure 6.6 were initially detected by the presence of an abnormal band in hemoglobin electrophoresis.

When red blood cells are available, electrophoresis of the hemoglobin itself may be the most direct way to diagnose these abnormalities. However, in some situations such as prenatal diagnosis, it is risky or impossible to obtain a pure blood sample from the individual to be tested. Since the DNA encoding the β-globin gene is represented in all cells of the organism, it is possible to diagnose the presence of the sickle mutation by directly analyzing the DNA from any available source of cells. As will be described in a later chapter, such cells can be obtained by amniocentesis or chorionic villus biopsy far more easily than one could obtain a fetal blood sample.

One method by which one can diagnose the presence of the sickle mutation in a DNA sample is diagrammed in Figure 6.10. The enzyme *Mst*II recognizes the sequence CCTNAGG, where N is any nucleotide. Thus, the sequence of codons 5 and 6 and the first base of codon 7 normally constitute a restriction site for this enzyme. The sickle mutation, however, abolishes this *Mst*II site because the mutation of A to T makes this region no longer a match for the restriction enzyme. This is a somewhat fortuitous occurrence. Restriction enzyme recognition sites do not comprise an infinite set; only a subset of single base changes that cause disease in humans alter a restriction site and can thus be detected by this direct approach. Since the sickle mutation does destroy a restriction site, heterozygotes and homozygotes can be identified by cutting their DNA with *Mst*II and analyzing the results with a Southern blot, as shown in Figure 6.10. The normal β-globin allele, which contains the *Mst*II site at codon 6, leads to a 1.15-kb band when probed with a sequence from the 5'-flanking region of the gene. This fragment is 1.35 kb, however, in the sickle allele because the site at codon 6 is lost, and the next adjacent site is located 200 bp further to the 3' side (within the β-globin gene). Homozygous normal individuals, heterozygotes, and homozygous affected individuals can then be distinguished using this approach. In practice, this type of analysis is currently most often performed by PCR. PCR primers matching the sequences on either side of this codon 6 mutation will amplify a DNA fragment, which can subsequently be digested with *Mst*II and analyzed directly on a gel, as described in chapter 5. In addition, with the power of PCR, it is no longer necessary to identify a restriction enzyme that can distinguish between the normal and mutant alleles, since many other methods can also be applied. An example using the polymerase chain reaction (PCR) and allele-specific oligonucleotides (ASOs) was given in Figure 5.24.

Sickle cell anemia is one of the few genetic diseases in which this direct approach to DNA diagnosis can be applied. This is possible because *(a)* the

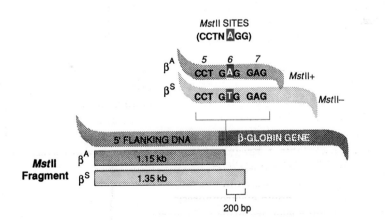

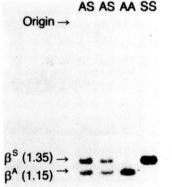

Figure 6.10.   Diagnosis of the sickle mutation using Southern blotting analysis.   The abolition of the normal *Mst*II site in codons 5, 6, and 7 by the sickle mutation is shown. On the *right* is the result of a Southern blot of DNA from individuals who are homozygous A (AA), homozygous S (SS), or AS heterozygotes. The probe is a genomic fragment from 5' flanking DNA. (Reprinted with permission from Bunn HF, Forget BG. Hemoglobin: molecular, genetic, and clinical aspects. Philadelphia: WB Saunders, 1986.)

mutation is known at the DNA level; and *(b)* all individuals with the disease have the same mutation, i.e., there is no allelic heterogeneity. For most other genetic diseases, such as the thalassemia syndromes discussed later in this chapter, multiple different mutations can all produce the same disease phenotype. In these cases, one of the screening methods described in chapter 5 must generally be applied. This process is considerably more complicated, with the possibility of missing a subset of mutations or identifying amino acid substitutions that may or may not represent the actual disease causing mutation.

FRAMESHIFT MUTATIONS

As described in chapter 2, frameshift mutations occur when there is an insertion or deletion of a small number of nucleotides that are not a multiple of three. When the RNA from such a mutant gene is translated, the amino acid sequence beyond the point of the frameshift is completely garbled. There are several possible effects of this. If the frameshift occurs near the 5′ end of the coding region, the protein may bear little resemblance to its normal counterpart or may be rapidly degraded and impossible to identify. The net result of this is a virtual absence of a recognizable protein product, which falls in the thalassemia category we will consider shortly. However, if the frameshift mutation is near the end of the protein, the result can be a qualitative abnormality in which the carboxy-terminal end of the polypeptide has acquired an entirely new stretch of amino acids. An example of this, shown in Figure 6.11, is hemoglobin Cranston. (Abnormal hemoglobins are often

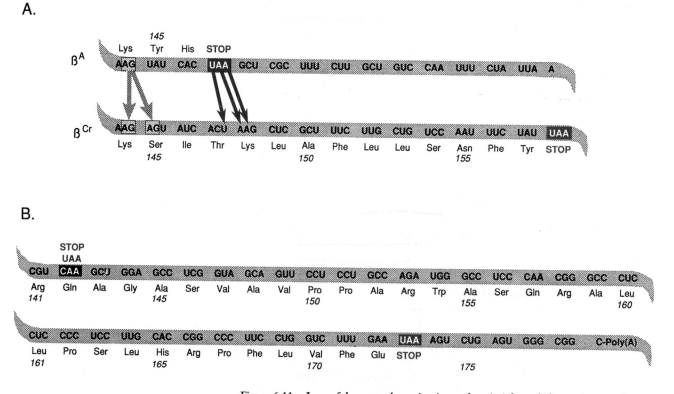

Figure 6.11. Loss of the normal termination codon. A. A frameshift mutation near the end of the β-globin gene, leading to hemoglobin Cranston (β^{Cr}). **B.** Mutation of the normal α-globin termination codon 142 to result in hemoglobin Constant Spring, containing an extra 31 amino acids at the carboxy terminus.

named by the geographic location where the patient in whom the abnormality was first described resided.) Here a 2-nucleotide insertion has occurred between codons 144 and 145 of the β-globin gene, almost at the end of the coding region. The result of this is that the normal termination codon 6 nucleotides further along is shifted out of frame and is therefore not read as stop. Thus, translation proceeds obliviously into the normally 3′-untranslated region, and a protein consisting of 157 amino acids is produced before the next fortuitous termination codon is encountered.

A similar situation occurs in hemoglobin Constant Spring, which is an analogous mutation of an α-globin gene. In this situation the normal termination codon, UAA, is mutated to CAA, which codes for glutamine instead of stop. Therefore, this is not truly a frameshift but can be thought of as the opposite of a nonsense mutation. The result is that translation continues to read into the normally 3′-untranslated region of the α-globin RNA, continuing for an additional 31 amino acids until encountering an in-frame stop at codon 173 (Fig. 6.11). Thus, the resulting α-globin chain is entirely normal for the first 141 amino acids but contains this unusual carboxy-terminal tail. As it turns out, this renders the α-globin protein somewhat unstable, so that the result is a combined qualitative and quantitative abnormality in α-globin production.

Another interesting and important source of mutation is a phenomenon called **unequal crossing over.** As described in chapter 2, homologous chromosomes line up during meiosis I based on their similar sequence over the entire length of a chromosome; at this time crossing over between homologous chromosomes occurs. If a stretch of duplicated nucleotide sequences exists, it is possible for the lining up process to occur improperly. Should a crossover occur between chromosomes that are misaligned, the net result will be a deletion or duplication. An example is shown in Figure 6.12. A nearly perfect duplication of the sequence GCTGCACGTG is found in codons 91–94 and in codons 96–98 of the β-globin gene. If the first copy of this sequence lines up with the second (rather than with itself), and a crossover occurs within this region, the result is the deletion or duplication of amino acids 91–95. This deletion has in fact been observed and is denoted as hemoglobin Gun Hill. This deletion of 15 nucleotides keeps the reading

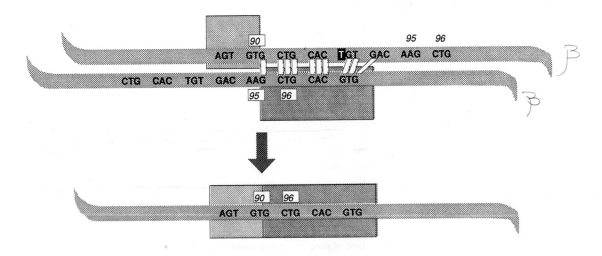

Figure 6.12. Generation of hemoglobin Gun Hill by unequal crossing over between homologous regions during meiosis.

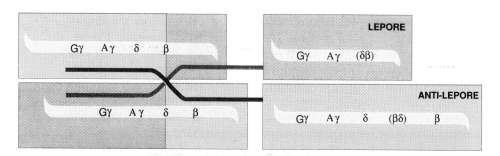

Figure 6.13. Unequal crossing over between the δ and β genes to generate hemoglobins Lepore (a hybrid δβ gene) and anti-Lepore (a hybrid βδ gene).

frame intact, so that the amino acids from 96 on are still correct in the translated protein.

A much larger deletion can occur if the δ- and β-globin genes, which are approximately 90% homologous to each other, happen to line up improperly during meiosis and participate in a crossover. This event is diagrammed in Figure 6.13. The chromosome resulting from a crossover (indicated by the *gray line*) would thus be a hybrid adult globin gene consisting of the 5′ end of the δ gene and the 3′ end of the β gene. Several such variants have been observed, depending upon the precise localization of the point of crossover; all are called Lepore hemoglobins. Since, as noted above, the promoter of the δ-globin gene has sustained a number of mutations, which render it relatively inefficient, the Lepore hemoglobin is produced at reduced amounts. Thus, this is another example of a combined quantitative and qualitative abnormality.

Note that this sort of unequal crossover has an alternative outcome. As shown by the *red line* in Figure 6.13, the result will be a chromosome with intact δ and β genes, with a hybrid β-δ gene inserted between them. In this situation the hybrid gene has the 5′ sequences of β and the 3′ sequences of δ. This is known as an "anti-Lepore" hemoglobin. Individuals with this chromosome will make relatively normal amounts of δ and β, but in addition will produce the novel anti-Lepore hemoglobin.

Globin Chain Imbalance: The Thalassemias

Until this point we have been considering primarily qualitative abnormalities of δ- and β-globin chains that result from alterations in the coding region of these genes. The thalassemias, on the other hand, are hereditary abnormalities of hemoglobin production in which the primary difficulty is a *quantitative* deficiency of either β-globin, leading to β-thalassemia, or α-globin, leading to α-thalassemia. Thalassemia derives from the Greek word thalassa, which means "sea." This name was applied because of the relatively high frequency of these disorders in individuals living around the Mediterranean Sea. In fact, the thalassemias are common not only in the Mediterranean area but also in parts of Africa and Southeast Asia. As in sickle cell anemia, the distribution of the thalassemias coincides with the frequency of malaria, and the high frequency of thalassemia alleles in these areas is felt to be a reflection of the advantage that a heterozygote for one of these conditions has when infected with the malarial parasite.

The pathogenesis of the thalassemias is diagrammed in Figure 6.14. In the normal situation, equal amounts of α- and β-globin chains are produced, so that they are able to combine stoichiometrically to generate appropriate hemoglobin tetramers. As a result, red blood cells in a normal adult are

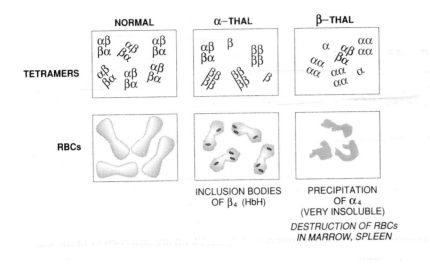

Figure 6.14. Schematic diagram of the pathogenesis of the thalassemias. *RBCs*, red blood cells.

loaded with a high concentration of hemoglobin and have a mean cell volume of about 90 mm^3. α-Thalassemia is characterized by a relative deficiency of α-globin chains but normal production of β-globin chains. If some α chains are still being made, a small amount of normal tetramers will form, but there will be a large excess of β chains. Under these circumstances, β is capable of forming homotetramers (β$_4$). This hemoglobin, which is called **hemoglobin H** (HbH), can be visualized as inclusion bodies within the red cells of individuals with α-thalassemia. HbH has markedly reduced ability to function as an oxygen carrier. The result of this β-chain excess and α-chain deficiency is that the red cells are reduced in size (50–80 mm^3, depending on the severity of the disease), and in number, resulting in anemia.

In β-thalassemia, it is the β-globin chains that are deficient. Under these circumstances, α-globin is in excess and is also capable of forming homotetramers. These tetramers, however, are *very* insoluble and precipitate within red blood cells, leading to their premature destruction in the bone marrow and marked trapping in the spleen. Again, red cells from individuals with β-thalassemia are reduced in size (50–80 mm^3), as well as in number.

α-THALASSEMIA

The genetics of α-thalassemia were initially puzzling, since individuals with this disorder seemed to have a wide range of α-globin production, extending from none at all (leading to stillbirth) to very near normal levels. Much of this confusion was clarified by the realization that each chromosome 16 carries two functioning α-globin genes, leading to a total of four genes in the normal situation. The α-thalassemias generally involve inactivation of anywhere from one to all four of these genes, and therefore the wide range of severity has a reasonable explanation. The possible outcomes of inactivating α-globin genes are diagrammed in Figure 6.15. If three of the four genes are functioning, the clinical abnormalities are extremely subtle and such individuals are completely asymptomatic. This is denoted as the "silent carrier" state; it is also anachronistically called α-thalassemia 2. A somewhat more transparent designation for this genotype is αα/α- or α-/αα (Fig. 6.15). If two of the four α-globin genes have been inactivated, this is denoted as "α-thalassemia trait" or α-thalassemia 1. There are two possible ways in which this could occur; in one situation, commonly seen as the cause of α-thalassemia 1 in Southeast Asia, both α-globin genes on one chromosome are defective, whereas both α-globin genes on the other chromosome are

Figure 6.15.   Gradation and severity of α-thalassemia, ranging from the normal situation in which all four genes are functioning to the lethal hydrops fetalis, in which no α-globin production occurs.

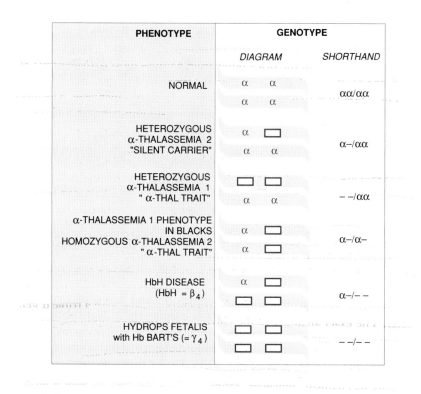

PHENOTYPE	GENOTYPE	
	DIAGRAM	SHORTHAND
NORMAL	α α α α	αα/αα
HETEROZYGOUS α-THALASSEMIA 2 "SILENT CARRIER"	α ☐ α α	α–/αα
HETEROZYGOUS α-THALASSEMIA 1 " α-THAL TRAIT"	☐ ☐ α α	– –/αα
α-THALASSEMIA 1 PHENOTYPE IN BLACKS HOMOZYGOUS α-THALASSEMIA 2 " α-THAL TRAIT"	α ☐ α ☐	α–/α–
HbH DISEASE (HbH = β₄)	α ☐ ☐ ☐	α–/– –
HYDROPS FETALIS with Hb BART'S (= γ₄)	☐ ☐ ☐ ☐	– –/– –

normal (αα/——). Blacks with α-thalassemia 1, however, usually have the alternative arrangement in which one α-globin gene on each chromosome is functioning normally (α-/α-). Therefore, these individuals are homozygous for an α-thalassemia 2 chromosome. The α-thalassemia 1 phenotype is also relatively benign; the mean cell volume is reduced, but these individuals are relatively asymptomatic.

A more severe situation occurs if only one of the four α genes is functioning. This could arise, for example, if one parent (α-/αα) carried an α-thalassemia 2 chromosome and the other parent carried the Southeast Asian variety of α-thalassemia 1 (αα/——). If both parents passed along their thalassemia chromosomes to a child, then the child (α-/——) would be markedly deficient in α-globin production. The net result of this would be a 4 to 1 predominance of β-globin chains leading to quite detectable levels of β_4 tetramers. In fact, the presence of significant amounts of β_4 has led to the designation of this situation as hemoglobin H disease. These individuals have moderate to marked anemia, which is present at birth. Their mean cell volume is quite low (about 50). This is not, however, a lethal condition.

The most severe situation, in which there are no functioning α-globin genes (——/——), leads to stillbirth or early neonatal death. In this situation, the predominant fetal hemoglobin is a tetramer of γ chains known as **hemoglobin Bart's.** This hemoglobin has virtually no oxygen-carrying capacity, so that the fetal tissues are deprived of oxygen, except for the small amount that is dissolved in the blood. In addition, there is a profound anemia. Heart failure results because of the efforts of an unoxygenated heart to pump the small amount of dissolved oxygen in the blood to oxygen-starved tissues. As the heart fails, marked edema (hydrops fetalis) occurs, and this condition is generally incompatible with life. This genotype can only arise when each parent carries a ——/ chromosome. Most commonly, this results from both parents having the Southeast Asian variety of α-thalassemia 1 (αα/——), although occasionally one parent carries hemoglobin H disease (α-/—). Hydrops fetalis is most commonly seen in individuals of Southeast Asian origin and is relatively rare in the black population because most α-thalassemia alleles in the black population are of the α-/ type.

The causes of α-thalassemia are diverse at the molecular level. The most common abnormality, leading to loss of one α-globin gene on a chromosome, is unequal crossing over. As shown in Figure 6.16, there is a high degree of homology of the nucleotide sequence including and surrounding the α2 and α1 globin genes. The X and Y blocks shown in the figure represent regions that are greater than 90% identical to each other, and the Z block is greater than 99% identical. This is an ideal setup, therefore, for unequal crossing over. If the two homologous chromosomes align incorrectly, with the Z block of the α1 gene lined up with the Z block of the other α2 gene, a crossover in this interval can have two outcomes. In one situation, as shown at the top of the figure, a deletion occurs with the 5′ end of the resulting single α gene deriving from α2, and the 3′ end deriving from α1. In fact, most α-thalassemia 2 alleles have arisen by this mechanism. Alternatively, the other outcome of such an event leads to a chromosome with a triple α gene cluster. The exact anatomy of the chromosome depends upon the point of crossover, which can occur in the X and Y blocks as well as the Z. In support of this hypothesis, the triple α-globin gene chromosome is also seen at reasonably high frequency in most populations.

This mechanism, however, cannot explain the loss of *both* α-globin genes on one chromosome (—/). Such chromosomes also are usually found to harbor deletions; in this instance the deletions are large, remove both α-globin genes, and cannot be easily explained by unequal crossing over. Finally, in a few situations, loss of function of an α-globin gene has been shown to arise from more subtle mutations such as nonsense or frameshift abnormalities, but in contrast to β-thalassemia (see below), these mutations are in the minority.

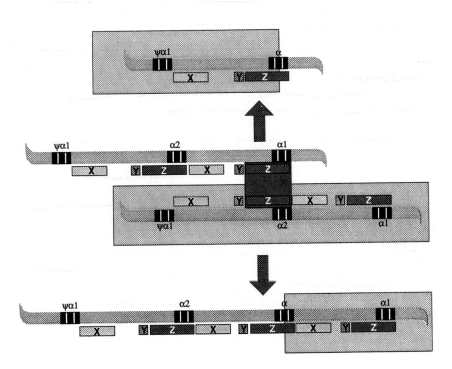

Figure 6.16. Misalignment of the α-globin cluster during meiosis leading to α-thalassemia. In the *middle* of the figure are shown two chromosomes that have lined up incorrectly so that α1 from one chromosome is matched with α2 from the homologous chromosome. If a crossover occurs in the Z box region, the outcome can be either a chromosome with only a single α gene (shown above), or a chromosome with three α genes (shown below).

PHENOTYPE	β— GENE GENOTYPE

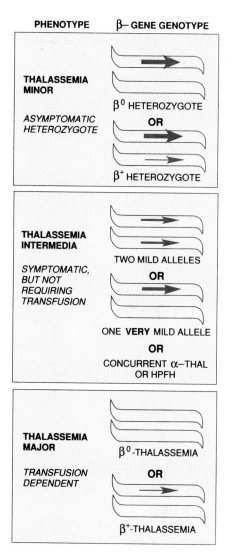

THALASSEMIA MINOR

ASYMPTOMATIC HETEROZYGOTE

β⁰ HETEROZYGOTE

OR

β⁺ HETEROZYGOTE

THALASSEMIA INTERMEDIA

SYMPTOMATIC, BUT NOT REQUIRING TRANSFUSION

TWO MILD ALLELES

OR

ONE **VERY** MILD ALLELE

OR

CONCURRENT α—THAL OR HPFH

THALASSEMIA MAJOR

TRANSFUSION DEPENDENT

β⁰-THALASSEMIA

OR

β⁺-THALASSEMIA

Figure 6.17. Possible genotypes that can give rise to phenotypes of β-thalassemia minor, β-thalassemia major, or β-thalassemia intermedia.   The thickness of the *arrow* indicates the level of transcription from each β-globin gene. Note that concurrent α-thalassemia can lead to less severity of disease because of an improvement in balance of chain synthesis (Fig. 6.14). Hereditary persistence of fetal hemoglobin (*HPFH*) is also beneficial in β-thalassemia because the increased γ chains can partially make up for the deficiency in β.

β-THALASSEMIA

In β-thalassemia it is the β-globin chains that are deficient. Since there is only one β-globin gene per chromosome 11, the potential for unequal crossing over is much reduced. When this does occur between δ and β, it results in hemoglobin Lepore as noted above; because the homology between δ and β is considerably less than the two α-globin genes, this is a relatively rare event. Loss or decreased function of the β-globin gene, therefore, is in general found to be caused by other mechanisms.

The genetics of β-thalassemia are complicated by the large number of mutations that can result in decreased or absent function of a β-globin gene. The disease is inherited in an autosomal recessive fashion. Carriers are detectable, however, by the fact that their red cells have reduced volume, and they have characteristic mild increases in hemoglobin A_2 and hemoglobin F by hemoglobin electrophoresis. As in α-thalassemia, the genetic analysis is somewhat complicated by the large number of possible mutations and by the historical terminology that developed before the molecular basis of β-thalassemia was understood.

Figure 6.17 shows the possible phenotypes arising from mutations at the β-globin locus and the genotypes that can underlie them. Beginning at the most severe, β-thalassemia major represents the homozygous state in which both β-globin genes contain mutations that prevent them from producing normal amounts of β-globin protein. If both β genes are completely nonfunctional, there will be no hemoglobin A whatsoever; this is denoted as $β^0$-thalassemia. If one or both of the mutations still allows the production of small amounts of β-globin, then this is denoted as $β^+$-thalassemia. Individuals with β-thalassemia major are transfusion-dependent and experience a variety of major medical problems, which will be described below.

Heterozygotes for β-thalassemia are said to have "thalassemia minor" and are asymptomatic. In general, they carry one normal β-globin gene and one that has a mutation that reduces or destroys its function. It is usually impossible to tell by looking at the level of β-globin in such an individual whether the thalassemia allele carried is a $β^+$ or a $β^0$ mutation because the normal chromosome is producing the vast majority of β-globin in both situations.

A somewhat confusing term is the designation "thalassemia intermedia," which has been used clinically to designate individuals who are significantly anemic and symptomatic but do not require transfusion. Such individuals have abnormalities in both of their β-globin genes, but one or both of these mutations is relatively mild so that a significant amount of β-globin production still occurs. An alternative mechanism for thalassemia intermedia is for an individual to have α-thalassemia along with $β^+$-thalassemia. As can be appreciated from Figure 6.14, if *both* α- and β-globin production are reduced, the phenotype will be milder because of a lack of the destructive $α_4$ precipitates within red cells.

Whereas α-thalassemias are primarily caused by deletions, β-thalassemia is usually the result of more subtle mutations. Intense work over the past decade has demonstrated a dizzying array of mutational events that can give rise to this phenotype. There are now more than 100 different mutations that have been shown to cause β-thalassemia, so this disorder is a prime example of allelic heterogeneity. Because of this wide diversity of mutations, most individuals with β-thalassemia major are in fact compound heterozygotes, having inherited a different mutation from each parent.

A diagram of some of the β-thalassemia mutations is shown in Figure 6.18. The mutations in the β-globin gene are scattered throughout the length of the gene, including the 5′-flanking region where the promoter lies. One

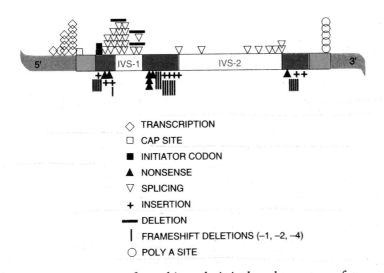

Figure 6.18. Schematic diagram of some of the mutations that have been shown to cause β-thalassemia. (Adapted from Kazazian HH Jr. The thalassemia syndrome: molecular basis and prenatal diagnosis in 1990. Sem Hematol 1990;27:209–228.)

◇ TRANSCRIPTION

☐ CAP SITE

■ INITIATOR CODON

▲ NONSENSE

▽ SPLICING

+ INSERTION

━ DELETION

| FRAMESHIFT DELETIONS (–1, –2, –4)

○ POLY A SITE

of the points to carry away from this analysis is that almost every feature of the gene has been a target for thalassemia mutations. Thus, this is an example of "Murphy's Law of the Genome"—anything that can go wrong, will.

It is not important to absorb all of the details of this array of mutational events, but it is useful to consider some of the categories in a bit more detail. One interesting category consists of individuals with point mutations in the promoter of the gene, as shown in Figure 6.19. Six different mutational events that have occurred in the ATA box are shown, as well as six mutations in the CACCC sequence, which was previously described as being a consistent feature of β-globin genes. Individuals with any one of these mutations do make β-globin mRNA from the mutated gene, but at approximately 10% of the normal amount. This represents the ultimate proof that these sequences are crucial for efficient transcription of the β-globin gene. Thus far, no mutations in the CCAAT box have been identified. A single mutation has been identified at the cap site (the first nucleotide in the mRNA, Figure 6.18). This mutation may affect the efficiency of transcription or interfere with the capping process, which is required for mRNA stability.

A number of mutations interfere with the efficient translation of the β-globin mRNA into protein, including mutations in the translation initiation codon itself (Fig. 6.18). Chain terminator mutations, in which translation is stopped prematurely, can result from nonsense mutations or frameshift mutations. In most of these situations in Figure 6.18, the abnormality occurs early enough in the coding region that the resulting protein is missing one-half or more of its structure and is totally nonfunctional. This contrasts with hemoglobin Cranston and hemoglobin Constant Spring described above, in which the abnormality occurs very near the end of the protein, and therefore function is still maintained. Chain terminator mutations early in the coding region usually lead to a product that is very unstable and is rapidly degraded within the cell. Thus, homozygotes for these mutations have β⁰-thalassemia.

An interesting array of abnormalities occurs in the splicing signals, and these mutations have added considerably to our understanding of the normal

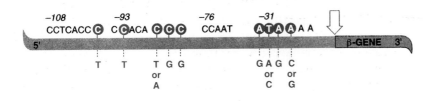

Figure 6.19. Mutations in the β-globin promoter that have been found to give rise to β⁺-thalassemia.

splicing process. Some of these splicing abnormalities are relatively easy to understand, as they alter the invariant GT sequence at the beginning of an intron or the AG at the end. Since these sequences are absolutely required for normal splicing, it is not surprising that these lead to β^0-thalassemia. Somewhat more subtle, however, are mutations that do not occur in the invariant nucleotides but affect the consensus region of the donor or the acceptor. In Figure 6.20, for example, mutations in the donor sequence of the first intron are shown. Those that alter the first nucleotide, abolishing the normal GT sequence, lead to β^0-thalassemia, but mutations at positions 5 and 6 within the intron lead to reduced ability of this RNA to splice correctly yet still result in detectable amounts of normal β-globin. Thus, these mutations in the homozygous state lead to β^+-thalassemia.

A particularly instructive mutation, and the most common cause of β^+-thalassemia in the Mediterranean region, is a mutation within intron 1 that does not actually affect the sequence of the normal donor or acceptor site. This mutation, shown in Figure 6.21, is a simple point mutation of a G to an A at position 110 of intron 1 and occurs 21 nucleotides upstream of the normal splice acceptor site. The result of this mutation is the creation of an AG sequence, which previously did not exist at that location. This AG sequence is preceded by a long run of pyrimidines, and although the sequence is not an ideal fit for the consensus acceptor sequence, it functions extremely well. As shown in Figure 6.21, when this mutation is present, 90% of the splicing events use the new AG as the acceptor site, and only 10% splice into the correct site. The abnormally spliced RNA contains an additional 19 nucleotides in the mature RNA, which normally would have been removed during splicing. Because this is not a multiple of 3, the result is a frameshift mutation in all subsequent coding regions. Therefore, the abnormally spliced RNA does not give rise to useful protein, and only the 10% of the RNA that is normally spliced is useful. The phenotype is thus β^+-thalassemia in a homozygote.

An even more bizarre mutation is represented by hemoglobin E, a very common variant carried by up to 30% of the population in some parts of Southeast Asia. This hemoglobinopathy represents a puzzling combination of a qualitative and quantitative abnormality. As shown in Figure 6.22, hemoglobin E arises from a point mutation in codon 26 in which the normal GAG codon is mutated to an AAG, resulting in a change from glutamic acid to lysine. One would predict that this would lead to a hemoglobin with abnormal electrophoretic mobility; this is, in fact, observed.

Figure 6.20. Five mutations that have been described in the beginning of the first intron of the β-globin gene.

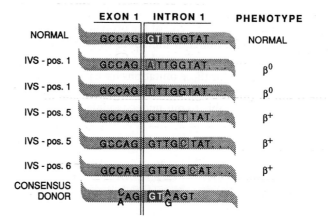

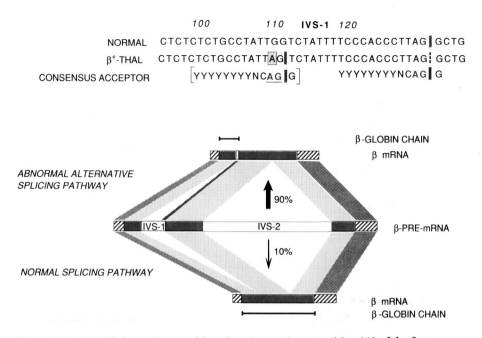

	100	110	**IVS-1**	120

NORMAL   CTCTCTCTGCCTATTGGTCTATTTTCCCACCCTTAG┆GCTG

β⁺-THAL   CTCTCTCTGCCTATT[AG]┆TCTATTTTCCCACCCTTAG┆GCTG

CONSENSUS ACCEPTOR   [YYYYYYYYYNC<u>AG</u>┆G]   YYYYYYYYYNCAG┆G

Figure 6.21.   β⁺-Thalassemia caused by a G to A mutation at position 110 of the first intron.   This leads to creation of an abnormal splice acceptor site, as the new sequence contains an AG. As shown in the lower part of the diagram, this abnormal splicing pathway is used about 90% of the time. Only 10% of the message is spliced properly and can give rise to normal β-globin chains. Y = C or T; N = any nucleotide. The invariant AG in the consensus acceptor is *underlined. Vertical lines* indicate location of splice.

However, individuals with this mutation produce only about 60% of the normal amount of β-globin from this mutant allele, and the reduction cannot be explained on the basis of protein stability. The reason for this additional quantitative reduction in protein production became clear when the pattern of splicing of the mutant gene was investigated. As shown in Figure 6.22, the sequence of codons 24–27 is actually a rather good fit for the consensus donor signal for splicing. In the normal situation, of course, this potential donor signal is not used at all. The nucleotide immediately following the GT in an ideal intron donor can be either A or G, but A is preferred, occurring about twice as often as G in this position. Apparently, the β^E mutation, which converts a G in this position to an A, activates this "cryptic" splice site so that it begins to function in a rather efficient way. The result of this event is that about 40% of the splices remove the sequence from codon 25 to the end of exon 1, or a total of 16 nucleotides. Again, because this is not a multiple of 3, the abnormally spliced message is out of frame in exon 2, resulting in termination at an out-of-frame stop codon. Thus, the 40% abnormally spliced RNA does not give rise to any detectable β-globin protein. The normally spliced RNA contains the β^E mutation. Thus, the result of this is a combined quantitative and qualitative abnormality from a single mutation.

A final interesting mutation shown in Figure 6.18 is a point mutation in the signal for polyadenylation, in which the AATAAA is converted to an AACAAA. Although transcription occurs normally, the cleavage and addition of A residues, which is required for normal processing and transport to the cytoplasm, is impaired, with the net outcome being a β⁺-thalassemia phenotype.

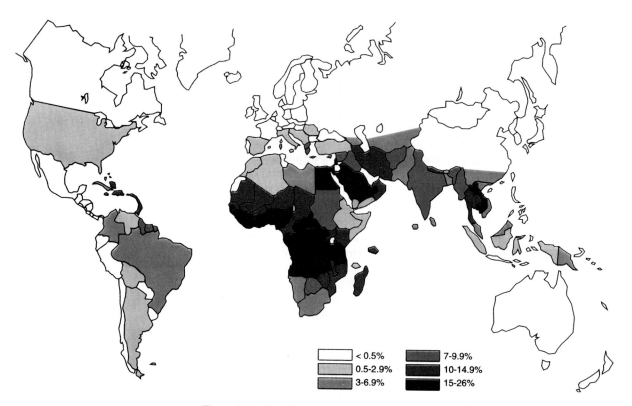

< 0.5%		7-9.9%	
0.5-2.9%		10-14.9%	
3-6.9%		15-26%	

Figure 7.5. World distribution of G6PD deficiency showing approximate population frequency. (Redrawn from Luzzatto L, Mehta A. Glucose-6-phosphate dehydrogenase deficiency. In: Scriver CR, Beaudet AL, Sly WS, Valle D, eds. The metabolic and molecular bases of inherited disease. 7th ed. New York: McGraw-Hill, 1995:3367–3398.)

G6PD deficiency is a paradigm of pharmacogenetics, the study of the genetic basis for differences in response to drugs. Several other polymorphisms have been described that specifically affect drug metabolizing enzymes and may account for differences in therapeutic efficiency of drugs as well as for idiosyncratic reactions to drugs among different individuals. Genetic differences in drug metabolizing enzymes among different races may account for observed racial differences in therapeutic efficiency of drugs (for example, differences in β-blocker effects between Orientals and Caucasians) and for the greater susceptibility of Orientals to alcohol-induced facial flushing and palpitations. Garrod's concept of chemical individuality also suggested that there might be genetic differences in response to exogenous pathogenic agents that might account for differences in susceptibility to disease. α_1-Antitrypsin deficiency provides an excellent example of just such a situation.

α_1-Antitrypsin Deficiency

The serine proteases are a group of closely related proteolytic enzymes with serine in their active site, which play a key role in coagulation and fibrinolysis and in kinin and complement activation. The activities of these enzymes are controlled at least in part by specific inhibitors known collectively as serine protease inhibitors, or serpins. The serine protease inhibitor found in highest concentration in plasma is α_1-antitrypsin, a 52-kDa glycoprotein, which accounts for 90% of the total α_1-globulin in plasma. Despite its name, the major function of α_1-antitrypsin is to inhibit the activity of elastase generated by neutrophils in the lung. The major phenotype of α_1-antitrypsin

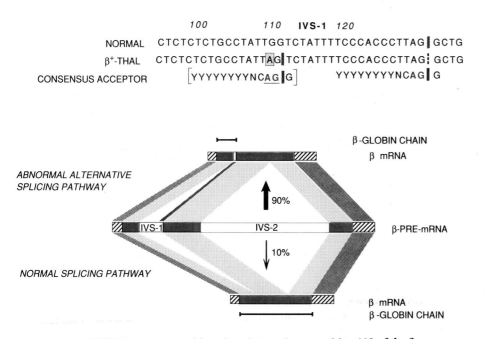

Figure 6.21. β⁺-Thalassemia caused by a G to A mutation at position 110 of the first intron. This leads to creation of an abnormal splice acceptor site, as the new sequence contains an AG. As shown in the lower part of the diagram, this abnormal splicing pathway is used about 90% of the time. Only 10% of the message is spliced properly and can give rise to normal β-globin chains. Y = C or T; N = any nucleotide. The invariant AG in the consensus acceptor is *underlined*. *Vertical lines* indicate location of splice.

However, individuals with this mutation produce only about 60% of the normal amount of β-globin from this mutant allele, and the reduction cannot be explained on the basis of protein stability. The reason for this additional quantitative reduction in protein production became clear when the pattern of splicing of the mutant gene was investigated. As shown in Figure 6.22, the sequence of codons 24–27 is actually a rather good fit for the consensus donor signal for splicing. In the normal situation, of course, this potential donor signal is not used at all. The nucleotide immediately following the GT in an ideal intron donor can be either A or G, but A is preferred, occurring about twice as often as G in this position. Apparently, the β^E mutation, which converts a G in this position to an A, activates this "cryptic" splice site so that it begins to function in a rather efficient way. The result of this event is that about 40% of the splices remove the sequence from codon 25 to the end of exon 1, or a total of 16 nucleotides. Again, because this is not a multiple of 3, the abnormally spliced message is out of frame in exon 2, resulting in termination at an out-of-frame stop codon. Thus, the 40% abnormally spliced RNA does not give rise to any detectable β-globin protein. The normally spliced RNA contains the β^E mutation. Thus, the result of this is a combined quantitative and qualitative abnormality from a single mutation.

A final interesting mutation shown in Figure 6.18 is a point mutation in the signal for polyadenylation, in which the AATAAA is converted to an AACAAA. Although transcription occurs normally, the cleavage and addition of A residues, which is required for normal processing and transport to the cytoplasm, is impaired, with the net outcome being a β⁺-thalassemia phenotype.

Figure 6.22. The mutation in hemoglobin E. This mutation gives rise to both a quantitative abnormality, owing to activation of a cryptic splice donor site, and a qualitative abnormality, because the properly spliced message will contain a lysine instead of glutamic acid at codon 26.

The A in codon 26 is apparently enough to activate this otherwise cryptic splice donor site, which is then used in 40% of the splicing events.

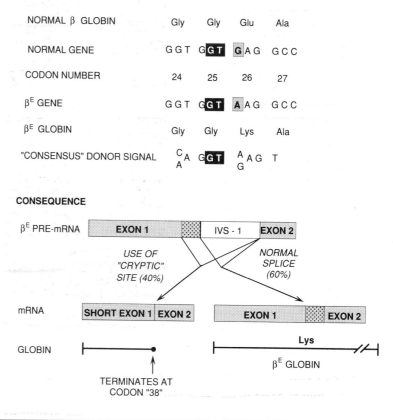

MECHANISM

NORMAL β GLOBIN	Gly	Gly	Glu	Ala
NORMAL GENE	G G T	G **GT** **G** A G	G C C	
CODON NUMBER	24	25	26	27
β^E GENE	G G T	G **GT** **A** A G	G C C	
β^E GLOBIN	Gly	Gly	Lys	Ala
"CONSENSUS" DONOR SIGNAL	^C A	G **GT** ^A A G	T	

CONSEQUENCE

β^E PRE-mRNA   EXON 1   IVS-1   EXON 2

USE OF "CRYPTIC" SITE (40%)   NORMAL SPLICE (60%)

mRNA   SHORT EXON 1 EXON 2   EXON 1   EXON 2

GLOBIN   Lys

TERMINATES AT CODON "38"   β^E GLOBIN

Clinical Aspects of β-Thalassemia Major

Thalassemia major, also called Cooley's anemia after Dr. Thomas Cooley who first described this disorder, is usually not apparent at birth because the switch of fetal to adult hemoglobin is still incomplete and the deficiency of β-globin chains is not yet of consequence. However, during the first year of life, as fetal globin production progressively drops, symptoms of severe anemia become apparent. Because of this anemia, the bone marrow, within which the majority of red blood cells are destroyed before ever being released into the circulation, makes a massive effort at blood production. The cortex of the bones becomes thinned, which can lead to pathologic fractures as well as distortion of the bones of the face and the skull. The liver and spleen are also markedly enlarged and act as additional sites of red blood cell production (Fig. 6.23). If not treated, death usually occurs in the first decade of life owing to severe anemia, debilitation, and infection.

These symptoms can be effectively alleviated by blood transfusion, since this supplies normal red blood cells and suppresses the overactive bone marrow. However, in the long run, transfusion is a two-edged sword. The reason for this relates to the mechanism of iron metabolism. Normally the total amount of iron in the body is regulated completely at the level of absorption. No efficient mechanism exists for increasing iron excretion when body stores accumulate. In the process of transfusion, total body levels of iron rise continuously, and with no means of excretion, the iron deposits in the heart, liver, pancreas, and other organs. This leads to a gradual failure of these organs, particularly the heart, and an inexorable downhill course. In Figure 6.24 is shown a survival curve for individuals with thalassemia major treated with transfusion. Although survival is relatively nor-

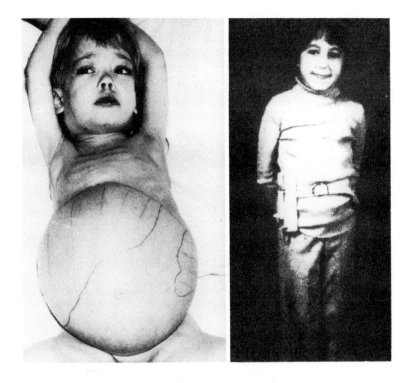

Figure 6.23.   The clinical picture of thalassemia major.   The individual on the *left* is 18 months old and has received no treatment. She shows marked enlargement of the liver and spleen (the borders of which have been marked on her abdomen), which are attempting to increase blood production. The individual on the *right* has been treated with a transfusion program and has a normal appearance. She is wearing an infusion pump that subcutaneously administers desferrioxamine to handle the iron overload, which is an otherwise eventually fatal complication of transfusion therapy. (Reprinted with permission from Weatherall DJ, Clegg JB. The thalassemia syndromes. 3rd ed. Oxford: Blackwell Scientific Publications, 1981.)

mal in the first decade of life, the effects of iron overload become apparent after this, leading to death in the teens and twenties.

Some hope has been provided for this situation by the availability of drugs that chelate iron and lead to its excretion in the urine. The most commonly used drug, desferrioxamine, appears to be capable of chelating enough iron to keep up with chronic transfusions, but only if given continuously and subcutaneously through an infusion pump (Fig. 6.23). Chelation therapy has been shown to significantly reduce the complications of iron overload, including cardiac disease (Fig. 6.24). However, the current methods of administration are inconvenient and painful, and an effective iron chelator that could be given orally is badly needed.

As for sickle cell anemia, bone marrow transplantation is potentially curative, though this procedure carries the potential for significant morbidity and mortality. Nonetheless, this approach has found more widespread use in thalassemia, given the uniformly poor prognosis in untreated patients with the severe form of the disease and the limitations of current chelation therapy. In the most recent studies, more than 80% of severe β-thalassemia patients appear to be cured by this treatment. Large-scale population screening and prenatal diagnosis has also had a dramatic impact on the incidence of β-thalassemia major in selected high-risk populations. Figure 6.25 shows the birthrate of β-thalassemia homozygotes on the island of Sardinia. Currently, only 4–5 cases per year arise compared with approximately 100 per year in 1975.

A final group of mutations to be considered in this chapter is that in which the developmental timing of globin production is altered. Individuals with hereditary persistence of fetal hemoglobin (HPFH) continue to produce increased amounts of hemoglobin F (greater than 1% of total) as adults, in the absence of other causes. In some instances these individuals may even pro-

Hereditary Persistence of Fetal Hemoglobin

Figure 6.24. Transfusion and iron chelation therapy for thalassemia. The top graph shows the survival curve for individuals with thalassemia major treated with transfusion but without iron chelation therapy. (Redrawn from Weatherall DJ, Clegg JB. The thalassemia syndromes. 3rd ed. Oxford: Blackwell Scientific Publications, 1981.)

Survival has been improved over this curve by the introduction of agents that stimulate iron excretion. Treatment with desferrioxamine to remove excess iron results in reduction of the complications of iron overload, including cardiac disease as shown in the bottom graph. The black line indicates the cardiac disease-free survival among patients with the most effective chelation therapy (< 33% of serum ferritin measurements > 2500 mg/L; ferritin is a laboratory measure of total body iron stores). The red line shows survival in patients with frequent elevated ferritin measurements (33–67% of ferritin measurements > 2500 mg/L), and the gray line, survival among patients for whom most ferritin measurements are markedly elevated (67% > 2500 mg/L). (Redrawn from Olivieri NF, Nathan DG, MacMillan JH, Wayne AS, Liu PP, McGee A, Martin M, Koren G, Cohen AR. Survival in medically treated patients with homozygous β-thalassemia. N Engl J Med 1994;331:574–578.)

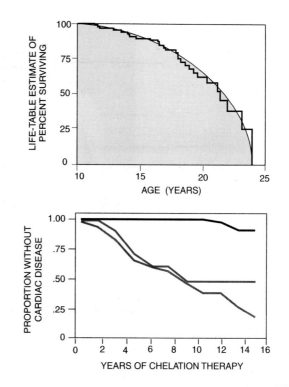

duce 100% fetal hemoglobin. Somewhat surprisingly, this is a benign condition, and such individuals are usually unaware of the hemoglobin abnormality. One might expect that fetal hemoglobin, with its somewhat increased oxygen affinity, might lead to symptoms if its production continued throughout adult life, but these are sufficiently subtle that they do not cause overt clinical disease.

The significance of HPFH is twofold. In the first place, mutations in developmental timing may provide clues to the general control of gene expression, which would advance our understanding in this area. Secondly, an ability to understand the control of fetal globin gene expression might allow manipulation of this situation in individuals with sickle cell anemia or β-thalassemia, in which turning the fetal globin genes back on would probably be curative.

The molecular basis of HPFH turns out to be heterogeneous (Fig. 6.26). Many such individuals have large deletions of the δ- and β-globin extending a considerable distance to the 3′ side. The fetal globin genes are not deleted, however, and by a poorly understood mechanism continue to be

Figure 6.25. Decrease in the birthrate of β-thalassemia homozygotes in Sardinia. (Redrawn from Cao A, et al. Clinical experience of management of thalassemia: the Sardinian experience. Sem Hematol 1996;33:66–75.)

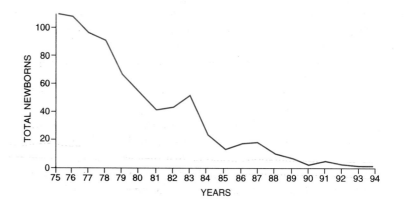

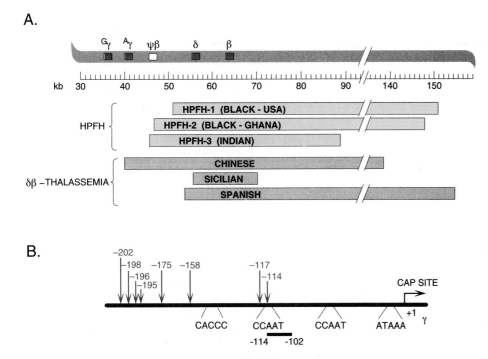

Figure 6.26.   Molecular mechanisms leading to HPFH.   In **(A)** are shown three HPFH deletions that remove large segments of DNA at the 3' end of the β-globin cluster including the adult genes. Not all such deletions lead to HPFH, however, as shown by the three δβ-thalassemia mutations also diagrammed. In **(B)** are shown the location of mutations (numbered relative to the cap site) in the promoter of either the Gγ or the Aγ fetal globin genes that have been found in individuals with HPFH (marked with *arrows* above the *line*). These positions presumably mark the location of important control sequences, but most do not involve the usual promoter elements (CACCC, CCAAT, or TATA). The bar beneath the sequence indicates the location of a small deletion in one patient that removes the second CCAAT box.

transcribed at high levels throughout life, rather than turning off at about the time of birth. Not all large deletions that remove the δ- and β-globin genes have this phenotype, however. Figure 6.26*A* also shows three mutations of the same type in which the fetal genes do turn off in their usual fashion. Since the δ and β genes are missing on the affected chromosome, the phenotype is therefore δβ-thalassemia. The reason why some deletions lead to HPFH and others to thalassemia is still not understood.

Other individuals with HPFH do not have major deletions in the β-globin cluster. In general, these individuals overproduce either Gγ or Aγ, but not both, and also continue to make substantial amounts of β-globin from their affected chromosome. Cloning and sequencing studies have demonstrated that these individuals carry point mutations in the promoter region of the overexpressed fetal globin gene, and the point mutations so far identified are shown in Figure 6.26*B*. As can be seen, these are scattered over a region 5' to the start of transcription of the gene and presumably identify sequences involved in the normal switching mechanism. One of these mutations, located 114 bp 5' to the start of transcription, occurs at the second C in one of the duplicated CCAAT boxes and a small deletion in another patient removes most of this sequence. Most of the other mutations fall in regions of the promoter not previously suspected to be important for control. One hypothesis for the mechanism of these mutations would be that they fall in a binding site for a repressor that is normally involved in shutting off fetal globin production but which cannot bind as well in the presence of a mutation. This hypothesis is under active study. What is learned from an analysis of HPFH mutations may well turn out to have clinical use in the attempt to develop effective treatments for sickle cell anemia and β-thalassemia.

Conclusion

In this chapter we have considered a wide variety of mutational events occurring in the human hemoglobin genes. Currently this system is the best studied of any set of loci in humans, and the rich array of mutational events is likely to foreshadow the findings with many other genes as our understanding of molecular genetics increases. For the student of genetics, the exact details of these mutations are not particularly critical; what is important, however, are the principles that emerge and the profound implications that an understanding of the mechanism of these mutations has for normal gene function. Truly, as Bateson advised some 70 years ago, "Treasure your exceptions."

SUGGESTED READINGS

General

Bunn HF, Forget BG. Hemoglobin: molecular, genetic, and clinical aspects. Philadelphia: WB Saunders, 1986. *A superb and thoroughly referenced work on human hemoglobin, from protein structure and function through molecular biology.*

Dickerson RE, Geis I. Hemoglobin: structure, function, evolution, and pathology. Menlo Park, CA: Benjamin/Cummings, 1983. *A beautifully illustrated short volume on the structure of the hemoglobin protein.*

Stamatoyannopoulos G, Nienhuis AW, Majerus PW, Varmus H. The molecular basis of blood disease. 2nd ed. Philadelphia: WB Saunders, 1994. *Also a superb reference text. Chapters on hemoglobin molecular biology and hemoglobin switching are particularly relevant.*

Weatherall DJ, Clegg JB. The thalassemia syndromes. 3rd ed. Oxford: Blackwell Scientific Publications, 1981. *Encyclopedic work on the clinical and laboratory aspects of thalassemia. Most of the information in the book predates the explosion of information made possible by recombinant DNA, however.*

Weatherall PJ, Clegg JB, Higgs DR, Wood WG. Hemoglobinopathies. In: Scriver CR, Beaudet AL, Sly WS, Valle D, eds. The metabolic and molecular bases of inherited disease. 7th ed. New York: McGraw-Hill, Inc., 1995. *An up-to-date review by one of the founders of the field.*

Classic References

Ingram VM. A specific chemical difference between the globins of normal human and sickle cell anemia hemoglobin. Nature 1956;178:792.

Pauling L, Itano H, Singer SJ, et al. Sickle cell anemia: a molecular disease. Science 1949; 110:543.

Biochemical and Molecular Genetics of Human Disease

"It is an old experience that through her errors, Nature often grants us unexpected insights into her secrets which are otherwise a closed domain."

—A. LOEWY AND C. NEUBERG (FROM ÜBER CYSTINURIE. HOPPE-SEYLER'S PHYSIOL CHEM 43:338–354, 1904)

"Whatever it is you're studying, you're better off if you have a mutant."

—ANONYMOUS

In the previous chapter, the detailed dissection of the molecular pathology of the human hemoglobin molecule illustrated the rich diversity of mutational mechanisms that cause human genetic disease and introduced the principles of molecular genetics of human disease. In this chapter, we will consider several other genetic diseases that are also well understood at a biochemical and molecular level. The examples chosen are not intended to be exhaustive; rather the specific diseases have been chosen because they illustrate specific principles of medical genetics. Sir Archibald Garrod's pioneering studies on alkaptonuria established the field of biochemical genetics and introduced the concept of the "inborn errors of metabolism." His insights into the principles of biochemical genetics, based on careful studies of human patients, are a paradigm of clinical investigation. The fortuitous observation of drug-induced anemia and the characterization of glucose-6-phosphate dehydrogenase deficiency defined the field of pharmacogenetics. α_1-Antitrypsin deficiency illustrates how a single mutation in a nonenzymatic protein, a protease inhibitor, can predispose to a common serious disease, emphysema, by interacting with an all-too-common environmental toxin, cigarette smoke. The brilliant investigations of familial hypercholesterolemia illustrate beautifully the dynamic interface between basic genetics and clinical medicine, clarifying on the one hand the normal cellular process of receptor-mediated endocytosis and, on the other hand, a major cause of coronary artery disease. Studies on hemophilia provide important insights into the basic molecular mechanisms of human mutation. Finally, molecular analysis of collagen disorders is increasing our understanding of "protein suicide" and the mechanisms by which dominantly inherited disorders of structural proteins cause disease.

In 1908, Archibald Garrod delivered the prestigious Croonian lectures to the Royal College of Physicians of London on the topic of "The Inborn Errors of Metabolism." He presented the results of his studies on four rare disorders in humans: alkaptonuria, pentosuria, cystinuria, and albinism. Alkaptonuria is characterized by black urine and degenerative arthritis of the

Inborn Errors of Metabolism

spine and large joints. The urine is actually colorless when passed, but quickly turns black when exposed to air, secondary to the oxidation of the large amounts of homogentisic acid present in it. The deposition of endogenous homogentisic acid autooxidation products in cartilage and collagenous tissues accounts for the blue- or black-pigmented palate, black deposits in the sclerae of the eyes, and the degenerative changes in the large joints and in the intervertebral discs of the spine (Fig. 7.1). The ochre color of these cartilaginous deposits, when viewed under the light microscope, gave rise to the term ochronosis to describe this form of arthritis.

Garrod found that when homogentisic acid was fed to alkaptonuric subjects, it was excreted quantitatively in the urine; none was excreted by normal subjects. Furthermore, the amount of endogenous homogentisic acid excreted by alkaptonuric patients was increased by feeding them a high-protein diet and specifically by feeding the amino acids phenylalanine and tyrosine. Normal individuals fed these amino acids did not excrete any measurable homogentisic acid. Garrod interpreted these observations to indicate that homogentisic acid was a normal metabolic product of phenylalanine and tyrosine metabolism and that it was immediately converted to another metabolite and did not accumulate; however, in individuals with alkaptonuria, its further metabolism was blocked, and it accumulated and was excreted in the urine in large amounts. His hypothesis was proven 50 years later by the demonstration that the livers of alkaptonuric patients had no detectable homogentisic acid oxidase, the enzyme responsible for the further metabolism of homogentisic acid (Fig. 7.2). Garrod generalized from his studies on alkaptonuria that individual steps in metabolism were the work of unique enzymes. He wrote in 1908:

Figure 7.1. Deposition of homogentisic acid oxidation products in tissue. A. Pigmentation of the hard palate in a patient with alkaptonuria. **B.** Deeply pigmented costal cartilage in a patient with alkaptonuria. (Reproduced with permission from McKusick VA. Heritable disorders of connective tissue. 4th ed. St. Louis: Mosby, 1972.)

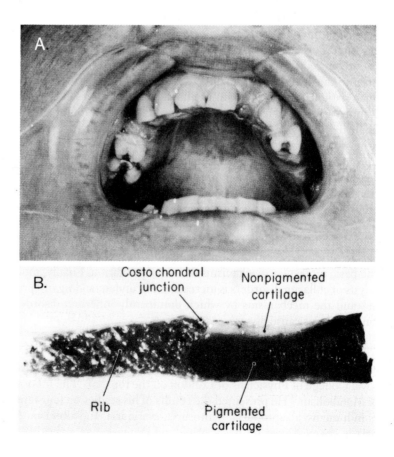

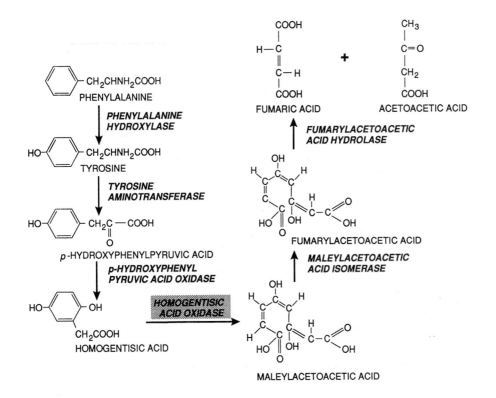

Figure 7.2.   Enzymatic steps in the catabolism of phenylalanine and tyrosine to aceto-acetic acid.

"The conception of metabolism in block is giving place to that of metabolism in compartments. The view is daily gaining ground that each successive step in the building up and breaking down . . . of individual fractions of proteins and of individual sugars is the work of special enzymes set apart for each particular purpose."

Garrod was also struck by the familial distribution of alkaptonuria. He noted that the abnormality is:

" . . . apt to occur in several brothers and sisters whose parents do not exhibit the anomaly and direct transmission from parent to child is very rare."

In 8 of 17 families with alkaptonuria, the parents were first cousins. Garrod consulted his friend, the distinguished English biologist William Bateson (who coined the term "genetics"). Bateson interpreted this familial pattern in light of the newly rediscovered laws of Mendel, pointing out that the mating of first cousins gives exactly the conditions most likely to enable a rare, recessive character to show itself. Alkaptonuria was thus the first autosomal recessive human disease recognized. The implication of this insight was that the normal allele was in some way necessary for the production of a specific enzyme in the unaffected individual. This was the first clue that genes may exert their effects by coding for enzymes. Garrod's work presaged the concept of one gene-one enzyme, which was established in the 1940s and 1950s by the pioneering work of George Beadle and Edward Tatum. Beadle and Tatum, studying the mold *Neurospora*, used UV light and x-rays to create nutritional, or auxotrophic, mutants, which lacked the ability to catalyze specific metabolic steps. They showed that individual metabolic steps in *Neurospora* were controlled by individual enzymes and that single mutations altered single functions. Beadle and Tatum had done their work in ignorance of Garrod's observations; however, Beadle paid tribute to Garrod in his Nobel Prize acceptance speech in 1958:

" . . . we had rediscovered what Garrod had seen so clearly so many years before. By now we knew of his work and were aware that we had added little if anything new in principle."

Finally, Garrod recognized the concept of biochemical and genetic individuality:

"The existence of chemical individuality follows of necessity from that of chemical specificity. Even those idiosyncrasies with regard to drugs and articles of food which are summed up in the proverbial saying that what is one man's meat is another man's poison presumably have a chemical (and genetic) basis."

Thus, Garrod laid the groundwork for the study of pharmacogenetics, discussed below, as well as the conceptual framework for the genetic basis of susceptibility to disease caused in part by exogenous agents discussed in chapter 4.

Garrod's views were well ahead of his time. Despite his dominant position in English medicine (he succeeded Sir William Osler as the Regius Professor of Medicine at Oxford), his work on the inborn errors of metabolism had little immediate impact on clinical medicine or genetics. Garrod predicted that many more inborn errors would be found, suggesting that there was an "almost countless variety of such sports." In fact, few additional inborn errors of metabolism were discovered for many years, most likely because serious inborn errors caused death early in infancy and went unrecognized at a time when infectious diseases were a major cause of infant mortality.

The explosion in knowledge about inborn errors of metabolism had to wait until the introduction of antibiotics, which dramatically reduced the frequency of death in infancy from infectious causes, and the improvement in nutrition and control of such disorders as infant diarrhea. In addition, certain technical advances were also very important. These included the development of paper chromatography to separate amino acids and other metabolites from each other in urine and blood, the development of human cell culture techniques, which allowed investigators to study tissue from patients without requiring constant access to the patients, and subsequently the development of molecular techniques, which allowed a much more sophisticated approach to human biochemical disorders.

During the Korean War, when United States soldiers were given the drug primaquine for antimalarial prophylaxis, approximately 10% of black servicemen developed an acute but self-limited anemia secondary to the intravascular breakdown of red blood cells (hemolysis). A smaller number of white soldiers, usually of Mediterranean origin, developed a similar but often more severe hemolytic anemia. The basis for the drug-induced hemolytic anemia was found to be a genetically determined deficiency of the enzyme glucose-6-phosphate dehydrogenase (G6PD), which catalyzes the first step in the hexose monophosphate shunt pathway. One important function of this pathway of glucose metabolism is the generation of NADPH, which is required to maintain the level of glutathione and reduced sulfhydryl groups to protect cellular proteins against oxidative damage (Fig. 7.3).

Approximately 10% of black men were found to have a G6PD that was altered in electrophoretic mobility and had only 15% of normal enzymatic activity. These men were clinically entirely normal unless they were exposed to certain drugs such as the antimalarial primaquine, or sulfonamide or nitrofurantoin antibiotics, or to certain infections such as viral hepatitis or bacterial pneumonias. Under these circumstances, they developed an acute hemolytic anemia. Young red blood cells from affected individuals were found to be more resistant to oxidant damage and to have higher levels of G6PD activity than did older red blood cells. It was subsequently found that the abnormal G6PD, designated A-, had decreased stability in vivo with a reduction in half-life from 62 to 13 days. Although the same defect was found in other cell types, the clinical phenotype was limited to anemia. This is because mature red blood cells lack both a nucleus and ribosomes and thus are unable to synthesize new mRNA and proteins to replace proteins that are degraded. Therefore, an oxidant stress would selectively hemolyze old red cells with diminished G6PD activity. In an otherwise healthy individual, the bone marrow is able to respond to this stress with increased production of red blood cells. These young red blood cells, because of their normal levels of G6PD, would be resistant to the oxidant stress. Therefore, as long as the bone marrow was able to increase red cell production, the hemolytic anemia was self-limited even in the continued presence of the offending drug.

In some Mediterranean G6PD-deficient individuals, especially children, ingestion of fava beans (the common broad bean in the Mediterranean region) causes a dramatically severe acute hemolytic crisis (favism), often requiring blood transfusion. As early as the 5th century BC, the Greek historian Herodotus had described an unusual response of some Greeks to the ingestion of fava beans. Thus, G6PD deficiency is a striking confirmation of Garrod's prediction that idiosyncratic reactions to drugs and articles of food could be the result of inborn errors of metabolism.

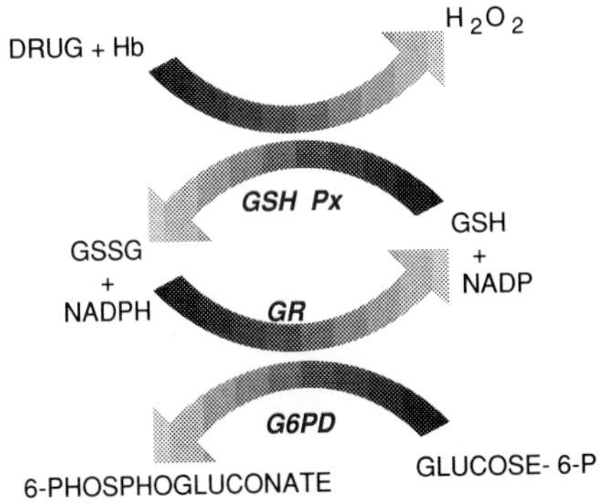

Family studies indicated that G6PD was encoded by a gene on the X chromosome, and the gene was subsequently mapped to the end of the long arm of the X chromosome, between the hemophilia A locus (discussed below), and that for color vision. The G6PD gene spans some 19 kb, contains 13 exons, and encodes a protein of 514 amino acids.

G6PD variants were initially described by differences in electrophoretic mobility on starch gels. G6PD B is the wild-type found in most populations. G6PD A, so named because of its more rapid electrophoretic mobility, is a common variant in the black population (10% of African-American males); it has full enzymatic activity. G6PD A-, discussed above, migrates like A, but has only 15% of the enzymatic activity of G6PD A or B.

Recent studies have defined the molecular defect in these and other G6PD variants (Fig. 7.4). An A → G change at nucleotide 376 in exon 5 re-

Pharmacogenetics

Figure 7.3. **Role of G6PD in the generation of NADPH used to protect the red blood cell against oxidative damage.** NADPH is necessary for the glutathione reductase (GR)-catalyzed reduction of oxidized glutathione (GSSG) to reduced glutathione (GSH). The latter is oxidized by glutathione peroxidase (GSH Px) in the presence of peroxides.

GAOHE 32 His → Arg

1

2

SUNDERLAND Δ Ile 35

3

METAPONTO 58 Asp → Asn

AURES 48 Ile → Thr

4

SWANSEA 75 Leu → Pro

68 Val → Met

LAGOSANTO 81 Arg → His

KONAN* 81 Arg → Cys

A—*

5

CHINESE-4 131 Gly → Val

A 126 Asn → Asp

ILESHA 156 Glu → Lys

SANTA MARIA

MAHIDOL 163 Gly → Ser

PLYMOUTH 163 Gly → Asp

CHINESE-3 165 Asn → Asp

A—*

COIMBRA 198 Arg → Cys

181 Asp → Val

6

SIBARI 212 Met → Val

MEDITERRANEAN* 188 Ser → Phe

MINNESOTA 213 Val → Leu

7

SANTIAGO 198 Arg → Pro

HARILAOU 216 Phe → Leu

227 Arg → Leu

STONYBROOK 242,3 Δ Gly Thr

MEXICO CITY 227 Arg → Gln

WAYNE 257 Arg → Gly

8

SEATTLE* 282 Asp → His

CHINESE-1 279 Thr → Ser

MONTALBANO 285 Arg → His

VIANGCHAN* 291 Val → Met

CHINESE-5 342 Leu → Phe

KALYAN* 317 Glu → Lys

9

IERAPETRA 353 Pro → Ser

323 Leu → Pro

MT. SINAI

LOMA LINDA 363 Asn → Lys

CHATHAM 335 Ala → Thr

10

BEVERLY HILLS* 387 Arg → His

TOMAH 385 Cys → Arg

NASHVILLE* 393 Arg → His

IOWA* 386 Lys → Glu

PUERTO LIMON 398 Glu → Lys

GUADALAJARA 387 Arg → Cys

RIVERSIDE 410 Gly → Cys

ALHAMBRA 394 Val → Leu

TOKYO 416 Glu → Lys

JAPAN 410 Gly → Asp

ATLANTA-1 428 Tyr → Stop

PAWNEE 439 Arg → Pro

MAEWO* 454 Arg → Cys

TELTI 440 Leu → Phe

CANTON* 459 Arg → Leu

SANTIAGO DE CUBA 447 Gly → Arg

KAIPING* 463 Arg → His

CASSANO 449 Gln → His

ANDALUS 454 Arg → His

13

COSENZA 459 Arg → Pro

CAMPINAS 488 Gly → Val

sults in a substitution of aspartic acid for asparagine at amino acid position 126; the substitution of the acidic amino acid aspartic acid for the basic amino acid asparagine presumably accounts for the more rapid electrophoretic mobility of the A and A- variants relative to the B, or wild-type, G6PD. A second mutation in G6PD A-, a G → A change in nucleotide 202 in exon 4, results in a substitution of methionine for valine at amino acid 68 and presumably accounts for the decreased stability of the variant.

In the Mediterranean variant of G6PD, the activity of the enzyme is barely detectable and there is a greater risk of hemolytic anemia. A C → T transition at nucleotide 563 in exon 6 results in the substitution of phenylalanine for serine at amino acid 188 and presumably accounts for the decreased catalytic activity and stability of this variant enzyme.

More than 60 independent mutations had been described at the DNA level, spanning almost the entire coding region (Fig. 7.4). Surprisingly, almost all of these are missense mutations, and the majority of these are transition mutations involving a C → T change where the C residue is in a CpG dinucleotide on either the coding or noncoding strand. CpG dinucleotides are thought to represent mutational "hot spots" because the cytosine is often methylated and 5-methylcytosine can undergo spontaneous deamination to thymidine. The phenotype of these mutations is highly variable; most are asymptomatic, but some can cause a chronic hemolytic anemia, even in the absence of triggering infections or drugs, and others cause severe neonatal jaundice and kernicterus (brain damage secondary to deposition of bilirubin). These more severe mutations appear to cluster in exon 10 near the NADP binding domain.

More than 400 allelic variants have been described at the protein level, many of which occur at polymorphic frequencies. Most mutant alleles are named after the geographic area in which they were first described and cover the alphabet from Aachen in West Germany to Zhitomir in the Ukraine.

G6PD deficiency is common, affecting approximately 400 million people worldwide (Fig. 7.5). It is found in high frequency in African, Mediterranean, and Asiatic populations in which malaria has been endemic, leading to the view that resistance to falciparum malaria may account for this balanced polymorphism. The incidence of G6PD deficiency is greater than 60% in some Kurdish Jewish groups, more than 30% in some villages in Sardinia, 13% among Saudis, and greater than 10% among African-American males. Multiple different mutant alleles account for G6PD deficiency in different parts of the world suggesting convergent evolution, rather than spreading of a favorable mutation by migration of populations. Although there appears to be no benefit to the G6PD-deficient hemizygote, women heterozygous for the mutant G6PD A- have been found to have lower parasite counts and are relatively resistant to severe malaria.

Figure 7.4   Mutations of the human G6PD gene.   The amino acid substitutions found in the different named variants are shown on a sketch of the G6PD gene. Exons are shown as numbered black boxes. The red shaded variants are those associated with chronic hemolytic anemia. Asterisks indicate that other named variants have been found to have the same mutation. Two mutations are found in G6PD Mount Sinai and in the three different types of G6PD A-. (Reprinted with permission from Vulliamy T, Beutler E, Luzzatto L. Variants of glucose-6-phosphate dehydrogenase are due to missense mutations spread throughout the coding region of the gene. Hum Mutat 1993;2:159–167.)

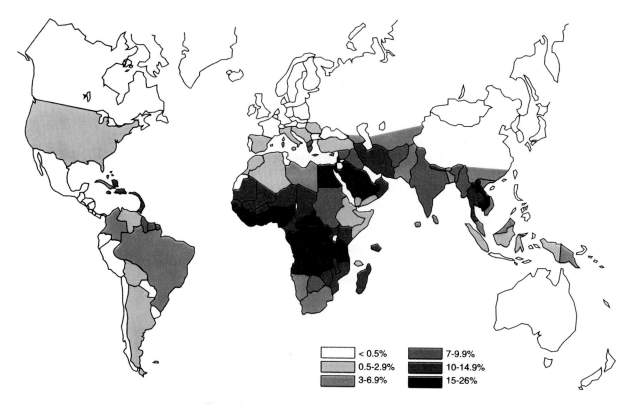

Figure 7.5.   World distribution of G6PD deficiency showing approximate population frequency.   (Redrawn from Luzzatto L, Mehta A. Glucose-6-phosphate dehydrogenase deficiency. In: Scriver CR, Beaudet AL, Sly WS, Valle D, eds. The metabolic and molecular bases of inherited disease. 7th ed. New York: McGraw-Hill, 1995:3367–3398.)

G6PD deficiency is a paradigm of pharmacogenetics, the study of the genetic basis for differences in response to drugs. Several other polymorphisms have been described that specifically affect drug metabolizing enzymes and may account for differences in therapeutic efficiency of drugs as well as for idiosyncratic reactions to drugs among different individuals. Genetic differences in drug metabolizing enzymes among different races may account for observed racial differences in therapeutic efficiency of drugs (for example, differences in β-blocker effects between Orientals and Caucasians) and for the greater susceptibility of Orientals to alcohol-induced facial flushing and palpitations. Garrod's concept of chemical individuality also suggested that there might be genetic differences in response to exogenous pathogenic agents that might account for differences in susceptibility to disease. α_1-Antitrypsin deficiency provides an excellent example of just such a situation.

α_1-Antitrypsin Deficiency

The serine proteases are a group of closely related proteolytic enzymes with serine in their active site, which play a key role in coagulation and fibrinolysis and in kinin and complement activation. The activities of these enzymes are controlled at least in part by specific inhibitors known collectively as serine protease inhibitors, or serpins. The serine protease inhibitor found in highest concentration in plasma is α_1-antitrypsin, a 52-kDa glycoprotein, which accounts for 90% of the total α_1-globulin in plasma. Despite its name, the major function of α_1-antitrypsin is to inhibit the activity of elastase generated by neutrophils in the lung. The major phenotype of α_1-antitrypsin deficiency is destruction of pulmonary alveoli resulting in chronic obstructive pulmonary disease or emphysema.

The gene for α_1-antitrypsin is highly polymorphic, with more than 75 different alleles described in the European population. The different forms of α_1-antitrypsin, frequently designated as Pi for proteinase inhibitor, are commonly distinguished by differences in electrophoretic mobility upon isoelectric focusing gels. Variants are assigned a letter based on their migration toward the anode. The most common allele in the European population is Pi^M (actually four distinct alleles differing by a single amino acid but with the same electrophoretic mobility), with an allele frequency of 0.95; 90% of white Europeans have the MM genotype. Two mutant alleles, S and Z, account for most of the disease associated with α_1-antitrypsin deficiency. The frequency of the important Pi genotypes and the activity associated with each is indicated in Table 7.1. Pi^{ZZ} is associated with 10–15% of normal activity and is found in approximately 1 in 2500 whites of Northern European descent. This mutant accounts for most of the illness associated with α_1-antitrypsin deficiency. Homozygous Pi^{SS} reduces α_1-antitrypsin activity by only 50–60% and does not cause disease. However, heterozygous Pi^{SZ} individuals have 30–35% of normal activity and may develop emphysema. In addition, more than a dozen rare alleles have been described that cause severe deficiency or absence ("null alleles") of detectable α_1-antitrypsin.

Individuals with α_1-antitrypsin deficiency have at least a 20-fold increased risk of developing emphysema; 80–90% of deficient individuals eventually develop this condition. Activated neutrophils elaborate elastase that, if unchecked by the proteinase inhibitor, can cause destruction of lung tissue. Furthermore, they release oxygen radicals and chlorinated oxidants that can oxidize the methionine at the active site of α_1-antitrypsin. Such oxidation decreases the rate of association of the inhibitor with neutrophil elastase 2000-fold, markedly reducing its ability to inhibit elastase activity. The unopposed elastase activity is thought to cause destruction of the lung.

Clinical and epidemiologic studies indicate that α_1-antitrypsin deficiency causes much more severe disease in cigarette smokers than in nonsmokers. The basis for this is probably the effect of smoking on the elaboration of oxygen radicals by neutrophils and macrophages. Thus, the interaction of an environmental agent, cigarette smoke, with a genetic predisposition, deficiency of α_1-antitrypsin, results in severe lung disease. Nonsmokers with α_1-antitrypsin deficiency also develop emphysema, but they tend to do so later in life than smokers, and although life expectancy is decreased relative to unaffected individuals, it is not nearly so severely decreased as it is in deficient subjects who are cigarette smokers (Fig. 7.6).

Individuals with Pi^{ZZ} also develop liver disease, thought to be the result of accumulation of aggregates of the mutant protein in the rough endoplasmic reticulum of hepatocytes. Approximately 10–15% of affected patients develop a neonatal cholestatic hepatitis and approximately 20% of those children develop juvenile cirrhosis. Approximately 20% of adults with α_1-

Table 7.1.   Clinically Important Pi Genotypes

	Pi Genotype				
	MM	MZ	SS	SZ	Z
Frequency	0.90	0.038	0.001	0.0012 (1/800)	0.0004 (1/2500)
Activity (% control)	100	60	50–60	30–35	10–15

Figure 7.6. Cumulative probability of survival, given that 20 years of age is reached, in smoking and nonsmoking Pi^{ZZ} individuals compared with all Swedish individuals. (Reprinted with permission from Larsson C. Natural history and life expectancy in severe α_1-antitrypsin deficiency, Pi Z. Acta Med Scand 1987;204:345–351.)

■ SMOKING Pi^{ZZ} MALES AND FEMALES
□ NONSMOKING Pi^{ZZ} MALES AND FEMALES
△ ALL SWEDISH FEMALES
▲ ALL SWEDISH MALES

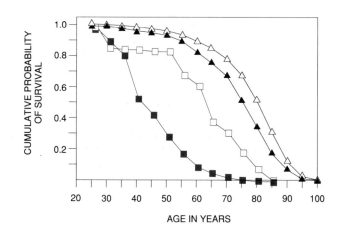

antitrypsin deficiency also develop cirrhosis of the liver and with it an increased risk of primary carcinoma of the liver.

The gene for α_1-antitrypsin occupies approximately 12 kb on chromosome 14, and encodes a 1.4-kb mRNA transcript that encodes a 394-amino acid protein. The Pi^S variant results from a GAA to GTA mutation in exon 3 causing the substitution of valine for glutamic acid at position 264. This results in the production of an inhibitor with decreased stability. The Pi^Z variant results from a mutation in exon 5 changing GAG, encoding glutamic acid at position 342, to AAG, encoding lysine. This mutation modifies the three-dimensional structure of the protein causing it to aggregate within the rough endoplasmic reticulum. As a consequence, only 15% of the mutant protein is secreted by the hepatocyte. In addition, the altered protein appears to be less effective as an inhibitor of neutrophil elastase than is the normal form. The rare "null" mutations, in which little or no immunoreactive protein is detectable in serum, are caused by small insertions or deletions that lead to a frame shift and premature termination of translation.

Although more than 20 mutations cause deficiency of α_1-antitrypsin, only two mutations, Z and S, cause the great majority of disease associated with a deficiency of this protease inhibitor. Therefore, it is feasible to offer prenatal DNA diagnosis for this condition, for example, by using allele-specific oligonucleotide probes (Fig. 7.7), a technique discussed in chapter 5. Therapy of α_1-antitrypsin deficiency has been attempted by administration of human inhibitor purified from plasma or made by recombinant DNA technology. Studies in a series of patients with already established pulmonary disease have indicated that weekly or monthly injections of purified inhibitor can restore α_1-antitrypsin levels in blood and alveolar fluid to levels that ought to be protective against neutrophil elastase activity. Obviously, patients with α_1-antitrypsin deficiency, even more than unaffected individuals, must be strongly encouraged not to smoke cigarettes. Future prospects for replacement therapy include the delivery of inhibitor directly to the lungs by aerosol and by the development of alternative synthetic inhibitors of elastase. Lung transplantation has been used successfully in some patients with end-stage emphysema.

Gene therapy is also being explored (see chapter 12). Mouse fibroblasts have been transfected with human α_1-antitrypsin cDNA and found to synthesize the inhibitor both in vitro and after implantation of the cells into the peritoneal cavity of immunodeficient nude mice. Other strategies involve modifying adenovirus to carry the gene directly to epithelial cells lining the lung. Unfortunately, replacement either with purified inhibitors or by somatic cell gene therapy will not prevent the liver disease associated

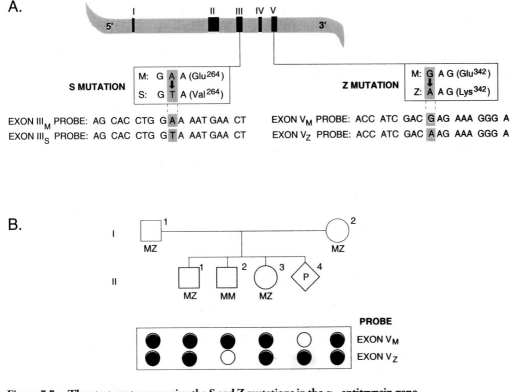

Figure 7.7.   The strategy to recognize the S and Z mutations in the α₁-antitrypsin gene using synthetic allele-specific oligonucleotide probes.   A. The structure of the α₁-antitrypsin gene is shown with its five exons (*solid boxes* labeled I-V). The *boxes* below the gene structure indicate the mutations encoding the S and Z forms of α₁-antitrypsin. The pairs of 19-mer oligonucleotide probes used to detect these two mutations are shown at the *bottom* of the figure. (Modified with permission from Nukiwa T, Brantly M, Garver R, Paul L, Courtney M, LeCrocq J-P, Crystal RG. Evaluation of "at-risk" α₁-antitrypsin genotype SZ with synthetic oligonucleotide gene probes. J Clin Invest 1986;77:528–537. Modified with permission of the American Society for Clinical Investigation.) **B.** Prenatal diagnosis of a fetus with Pi^ZZ α₁-antitrypsin deficiency using synthetic allele-specific oligonucleotide probes. Genomic DNA was obtained from the individuals shown in the pedigree, including the fetus at risk, and amplified using the polymerase chain reaction. Amplified DNA was applied to nylon filter membranes as "dot blots" and hybridized with labeled oligonucleotide probes specific for the Z and M sequences. Radioactivity was detected by autoradiography. Pi typing in the parents and siblings of the fetus at risk was carried out by standard electrophoretic techniques. DNA from I-1 and I-2 and II-1 and II-3 hybridized with both probes confirming heterozygosity for Pi MZ; DNA from II-2 hybridizes only with the M-specific probe. DNA from the fetus hybridized only with the Z-specific probe, indicating homozygosity for the mutant allele.

with the ZZ genotype unless endogenous mutant gene expression can be turned off.

α₁-Antitrypsin deficiency is a very common autosomal recessive disorder in the Caucasian population (it is rare in blacks and Asians). Although many individuals with this condition appear to be asymptomatic until late in life when they develop pulmonary emphysema or cirrhosis of the liver, they are at high risk if exposed to a specific environmental agent, cigarette smoke. Thus, α₁-antitrypsin is a paradigm of an "ecogenetic" disorder, resulting from the interaction of an unfortunately common environmental factor with a specific genetic predisposition to disease. Biochemical and molecular investigations have determined the nature of the two common mutations that cause disease associated with α₁-antitrypsin deficiency, have provided techniques for highly accurate prenatal diagnosis of this disease, and have facilitated the development of replacement therapy and the beginnings of somatic gene therapy.

Familial Hypercholesterolemia

Familial hypercholesterolemia (FH) is an autosomal dominant disease affecting 1 in 500 individuals and is found in approximately 5% of myocardial infarction patients younger than 60 years of age. The disease is characterized by elevated serum cholesterol (300–600 mg/dL, normal less than 230) and a low-density lipoprotein (LDL) cholesterol of greater than 200 mg/dL. Approximately 50% of affected adults manifest deposits of cholesterol (xanthomas) in extensor tendons, typically an irregular thickening of the Achilles tendons, and xanthelasmata, yellowish fatty deposits of the eyelids. Most significantly, patients with familial hypercholesterolemia have early onset of atherosclerotic cardiovascular disease. The medical and family history of W. H. presented in chapter 3 (Fig. 3.3) is typical for this condition. It is important to emphasize that, given the autosomal dominant inheritance, diagnosis of an affected individual immediately identifies a population at high risk of hypercholesterolemia and premature atherosclerotic heart disease. All first-degree relatives have a 50% chance of being affected and should be tested for this condition. Hypercholesterolemia is present in childhood so the condition can be detected early and dietary and drug intervention begun before atherosclerotic heart disease develops. Because the disease is relatively common, mating between heterozygotes occasionally occurs (1/500 × 1/500 = 1/250,000) and homozygous affected offspring occur with a frequency of approximately 1 in 1 million. Homozygous affected individuals have very high blood cholesterol levels (600–1200 mg/dL), frequently suffer heart attacks in childhood, and often die of coronary artery disease in the second or third decade of life. Familial hypercholesterolemia is important not only because it is common, serious, and treatable, but because the elegant investigations of Michael Brown and Joseph Goldstein, for which they were awarded the Nobel Prize in 1985, beautifully illustrate the dynamic interface between medicine and genetics.

THE CELLULAR DEFECT IN FAMILIAL HYPERCHOLESTEROLEMIA

Brown and Goldstein astutely selected cultured skin fibroblasts from homozygous affected individuals as their model system. They demonstrated that fibroblasts from such patients had high levels of β-hydroxy-β-methylglutaryl-CoA reductase (HMG-CoA reductase), the rate-limiting enzyme in cholesterol biosynthesis, and that the enzyme activity was not normally repressed by incubation in the presence of LDL. The defect, however, was not in the regulation of HMG-CoA reductase per se, and thus not in cholesterol biosynthesis, but rather in the delivery of the regulatory signal, cholesterol. Using radioiodinated LDL, they demonstrated specific, saturable binding of LDL to the surface of normal cells. Electron microscopic studies indicated that the LDL receptor was not distributed randomly on the cell surface but rather was located in specialized structures called coated pits that contain a specific protein, clathrin. Binding of LDL particles to LDL receptors in coated pits resulted in their subsequent internalization and in the degradation of the apoprotein to amino acids and the cholesterol esters in the LDL particle to free cholesterol. Free intracellular cholesterol, in the form of oxygenated derivatives such as 25-hydroxycholesterol, triggered three important regulatory events: a marked decrease in the synthesis of HMG-CoA reductase, resulting in decreased endogenous synthesis of cholesterol; increased activity of acyl-CoA:cholesterol acyltransferase (ACAT), resulting in increased cholesterol esterification and storage; and importantly, decreased synthesis of LDL receptors, resulting in a decrease in cellular uptake of exogenous cholesterol (Fig. 7.8).

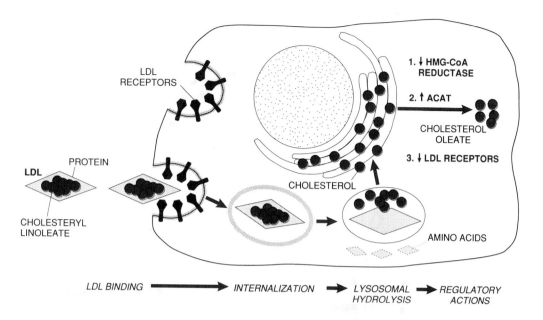

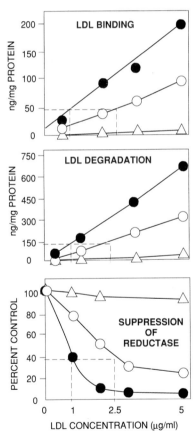

Figure 7.8. Sequential steps in the LDL receptor pathway in cultured mammalian cells. *HMG-CoA reductase* denotes β-hydroxy-β-methylglutaryl coenzyme A reductase; *ACAT* denotes acyl-CoA:cholesterol acyltransferase; *vertical arrows* indicate the directions of regulatory effects. (Reprinted with permission from Brown MS, Goldstein JL. Receptor-mediated endocytosis: insights from the lipoprotein receptor system. Proc Natl Acad Sci USA 1979;76:3330–3337.)

Fibroblasts from patients homozygous for familial hypercholesterolemia failed to bind and internalize LDL and thus to repress HMG-CoA reductase. Therefore, the defect in familial hypercholesterolemia appeared to be a deficiency of functional LDL receptors. Patients with the more common partial deficiency of LDL receptors, i.e., those heterozygous for familial hypercholesterolemia who have one normal allele encoding a normal LDL receptor, show an intermediate defect. Cultured fibroblasts from heterozygotes show normal regulation of HMG-CoA reductase by LDL but only at higher concentrations of ambient LDL than are necessary in normal fibroblasts (Fig. 7.9). Thus, normal regulation occurs at the expense of an increased LDL cholesterol level. These studies, in addition to defining the molecular defect in FH, also elucidated a very important normal cellular process, namely, receptor-mediated endocytosis, a process by which cells specifically bind and internalize a variety of important ligands including hormones, growth factors, enzymes, and nutritional signals.

THE LDL RECEPTOR

Purification of the LDL receptor and cloning of its cDNA and gene indicated that the receptor is synthesized on the endoplasmic reticulum, glycosylated during its passage through the Golgi complex, and is inserted into the membrane as an integral membrane protein of approximately 160 kDa apparent molecular mass. The domain structure of the LDL receptor was defined by analysis of its amino acid sequence as well as study of specific mutations (Fig. 7.10). The N-terminal end of the molecule contains the ligand binding domain that has a strongly negative charge and is composed of seven repeated units of 40 amino acids, each containing 6 cysteines. This domain is followed by a domain that resembles the precursor to epidermal growth factor (EGF). A short stretch containing O-linked sugars is followed by a membrane-spanning region and a 50-amino acid cytoplasmic tail at the car-

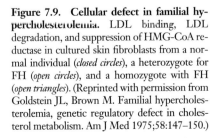

Figure 7.9. Cellular defect in familial hypercholesterolemia. LDL binding, LDL degradation, and suppression of HMG-CoA reductase in cultured skin fibroblasts from a normal individual (*closed circles*), a heterozygote for FH (*open circles*), and a homozygote with FH (*open triangles*). (Reprinted with permission from Goldstein JL, Brown M. Familial hypercholesterolemia, genetic regulatory defect in cholesterol metabolism. Am J Med 1975;58:147–150.)

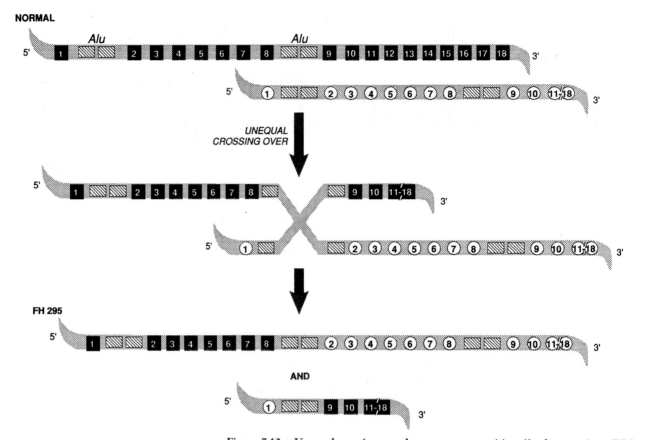

Figure 7.12.   Unequal crossing over between two repetitive *Alu* elements in an LDL receptor gene from an FH homozygote.   Two copies of the normal receptor gene, one with exons indicated by *bold rectangles*, and the other with exons indicated by *light circles*, are aligned to illustrate the point of unequal crossing over in FH 295. The crossing over involved *Alu* elements in both genes that paired with each other. The recombination event is predicted to yield one gene with two copies of exons 2–8 and a hypothetical gene in which exons 2–8 are deleted. The exons are denoted by *numbered boxes;* exons and introns are not drawn to scale. (Redrawn from Lehrman LE, Goldstein JL, Russell DW, Brown MS. Duplication of seven exons in the LDL receptor gene caused by Alu-Alu recombination in a subject with familial hypercholesterolemia. Cell 1987;48:827–835. © Cell Press.)

generation of deletion and insertion mutations in this and other genes (see chapter 6).

The various mutations affecting the LDL receptor gene have been grouped into five functional classes (Fig. 7.13). Class 1 alleles, accounting for approximately 20% of the total, produce virtually no detectable LDL receptor protein (null alleles). These mutations, most frequently nonsense or frameshift mutations, are distributed randomly among the exons of the gene. The absence of truncated protein may reflect the instability and rapid degradation of the mutant mRNA (as observed in some forms of β-thalassemia caused by nonsense mutations) or of the abnormal protein. Class 1 mutations may also occur in the promoter region; in this case, no mRNA or protein is produced. Class 2 mutations block the transport of the nascent LDL receptor protein from the endoplasmic reticulum to the Golgi apparatus. More than half of FH "homozygotes" (compound heterozygotes) have at least one allele of this type. Two-thirds of these mutations are in the ligand binding domain, with a striking preponderance in repeat number 5; most are missense mutations of highly conserved residues. Other class 2 mutations are found in the EGF precursor homology domain, the most highly con-

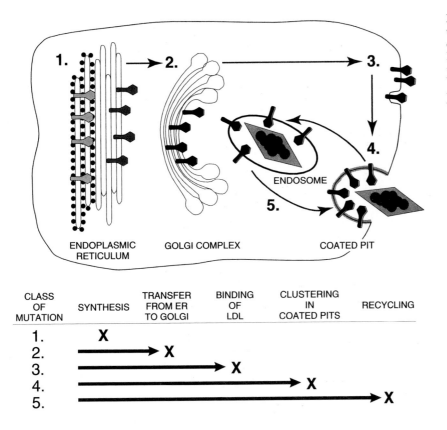

Figure 7.13.   Five classes of mutations at the LDL receptor locus.   See text for discussion. (Redrawn from Goldstein JL, Hobbs HH, Brown MS: Familial hypercholesterolemia. In Scriver CR, Beaudet AL, Sly WS, Valle D, eds. The metabolic and molecular bases of inherited disease. 7th ed. New York: McGraw-Hill, 1995:1981–2030.)

CLASS OF MUTATION	SYNTHESIS	TRANSFER FROM ER TO GOLGI	BINDING OF LDL	CLUSTERING IN COATED PITS	RECYCLING
1.	X				
2.		X			
3.			X		
4.				X	
5.					X

served region in the LDL receptor. Mutations that interfere with intracellular transport of nascent proteins have also been found to be a frequent cause of other genetic diseases involving membrane or secretory proteins. The Pi^Z mutation causing α_1-antitrypsin, discussed earlier, is a case in point.

Class 3 mutations encode a receptor that reaches the cell surface, but fails to bind ligand normally. Virtually all are the result of in-frame insertions or deletions in the ligand binding domain or the EGF precursor homology domains. Deletion of any of the cysteine-rich repeats results in decreased binding of LDL, which binds receptor via its single apoB-100 apoprotein, but generally not of intermediate-density lipoproteins (IDL, discussed below), which bind via multiple copies of apoE. The exceptions are deletions of repeat 5, which diminish both LDL and IDL binding, and often have a more severe phenotype.

Class 4 mutations encode receptors that reach the cell surface and bind LDL normally, but are not localized to clathrin-coated pits and fail to internalize bound LDL. These mutations, which include missense, nonsense, and frameshift mutations as well as deletions, may involve the cytoplasmic domain alone, or this domain and the membrane-spanning region.

The first receptor mislocation mutation was discovered because cultured fibroblasts from a boy with the clinical picture of homozygous familial hypercholesterolemia showed near normal binding of LDL but deficient internalization and, hence, deficient regulation of HMG-CoA reductase. Analysis of fibroblasts from his parents indicated that no functional LDL receptor was encoded by his mother's mutant allele, whereas the LDL receptor encoded by his father's mutant allele was not found in coated pits but was inserted in the cell membrane at random; this LDL receptor was able to bind LDL but not to internalize it. In this mutation, a TAT encoding tyrosine at position 807 was changed to TGT encoding cysteine (Fig. 7.14). Proof that this mutation

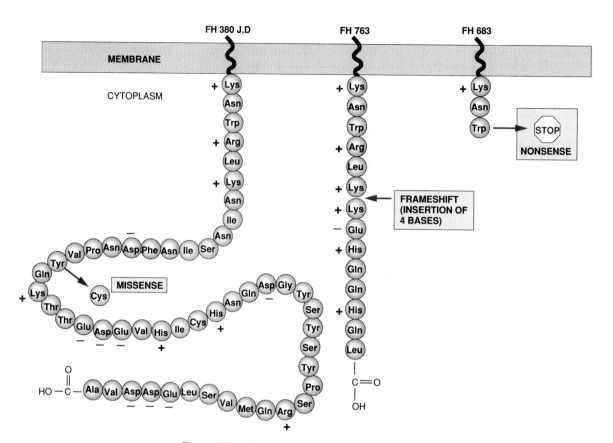

Figure 7.14. Mutations affecting the cytoplasmic domain of the LDL receptor in three FH homozygotes with the internalization-defective form of FH. (Reprinted with permission from Brown MS, Goldstein JL. A receptor-mediated pathway for cholesterol homeostasis. Science 1986;232:34–47. © The Nobel Foundation, 1986.)

caused the receptor mislocation phenotype was obtained by using oligonucleotide site-directed mutagenesis to mutate the normal LDL receptor cDNA so as to mimic the mutation in this patient. The mutated cDNA was transfected into a variant line of Chinese hamster ovary cells lacking LDL receptor. The transfected cells expressed LDL receptor randomly on the membrane but not in coated pits. Other mutations affecting the C-terminal end of the LDL receptor, such as the 7.8-kb deletion discussed above, result in a failure to anchor the receptor in the membrane and in secretion out of the cell of more than 90% of the newly synthesized receptor.

Finally, class 5 mutations encode receptors that bind and internalize LDL receptor in coated pits, but fail to release the ligand in endosomes and fail to recycle back to the cell surface (called recycling-defective mutants). These mutations, found in approximately 20% of FH "homozygotes," are most often missense mutations in the 5'-end of the EGF precursor homology domain. Conserved regions within this domain are apparently essential for normal receptor recycling. If ligand is not released from the receptor, the receptor-ligand complex is degraded.

Thus, the analysis and functional classification of a variety of mutations causing FH has resulted in a better understanding of the domain structure of this important receptor and the functional properties of each structural domain. This analysis has also allowed correlation of specific mutations with certain cellular and clinical phenotypes. Patients with mutations that diminish but do not eliminate LDL receptor function tend to have lower plasma levels of LDL-cholesterol, less severe atherosclerotic cardiovascular disease, and better response to therapy (see below) than patients whose mutations encode totally dysfunctional receptors. Nevertheless, the plasma LDL concentration and clinical phenotype can vary considerably among affected individuals within the same family who have the same mutation. This variability could reflect the modifying effects of other genes and/or environmental factors. In one instructive family, one-third of individuals heterozygous for an LDL-receptor mutation, documented at the cellular or molecular level, had normal plasma LDL. In this family there was evidence for an autosomal dominant gene, unlinked to the LDL receptor locus, that mollified the effect of the FH mutation.

It is now possible to screen for FH and provide prenatal diagnosis at the DNA level. In those populations in which there is a single, common mutation, this can be accomplished by direct detection of the mutation. However, in most populations such as that in North America, in which there are multiple mutations in the LDL receptor, molecular diagnosis is accomplished by linkage analysis using DNA polymorphisms, provided that affected family members are available. The availability of multiple DNA polymorphisms spanning the LDL receptor gene allows construction of haplotypes that can be used to follow the segregation of the mutant gene in families at risk.

PHYSIOLOGY OF THE LDL RECEPTOR PATHWAY

Although the cellular and molecular defect in familial hypercholesterolemia was defined in cultured skin fibroblasts, the major site of cholesterol biosynthesis and uptake is the liver. Subsequent studies showed that liver contains the same LDL receptor system defined in fibroblasts and that 70% of hepatic LDL uptake is mediated by LDL receptor-dependent pathways. The pathophysiologic role of LDL receptor deficiency in familial hypercholesterolemia was further defined by studies on an animal model, the Watanabe heritable hyperlipidemic (WHHL) rabbit. The homozygous mutant rabbit lacks LDL receptors and has markedly elevated cholesterol, closely mimicking human familial hypercholesterolemia. LDL cholesterol levels are elevated because of a combination of increased production of LDL from intermediate-density lipoproteins (IDL), which are normally taken up by hepatic LDL receptors, and reduced clearance of LDL secondary to the reduced number of LDL receptors. Further confirmation of the role of LDL receptors in atherosclerosis has come from studies in mice. Using homologous recombination in embryonic stem cells, mice homozygous for targeted disruption of the LDL receptor gene were produced. These mice had significantly elevated plasma LDL cholesterol, and when fed a high-fat diet, developed severe atherosclerosis associated with markedly increased LDL cholesterol. Wild-type mice on the same diet did not show these changes. Finally, administration of recombinant adenovirus encoding the human LDL receptor to the receptor-deficient mice restored hepatic LDL receptor activity and normal cholesterol metabolism.

THERAPEUTIC IMPLICATIONS OF THE LDL RECEPTOR MODEL

The studies of Brown and Goldstein predicted that one might be able to increase the number of hepatic LDL receptors in heterozygous deficient individuals by increasing hepatic demand for cholesterol. Decreasing exogenous cholesterol by decreasing dietary cholesterol and saturated fat does produce a modest and limited decrease in LDL cholesterol concentration in affected individuals. A more significant decrease in blood cholesterol is achieved by interfering with the enterohepatic circulation of bile acids using anion exchange resins such as cholestyramine (Fig. 7.15). Bile acids, con-

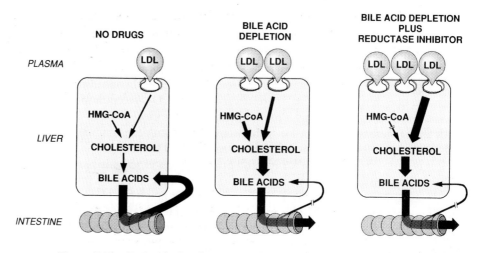

Figure 7.15. Rationale for the use of a bile acid-binding resin and an inhibitor of HMG-CoA reductase in the treatment of FH heterozygotes. (Reprinted with permission from Brown MS, Goldstein JL. A receptor-mediated pathway for cholesterol homeostasis. Science 1986;232:34–47. © The Nobel Foundation, 1986.)

taining significant amounts of cholesterol, are normally secreted into the bile and reabsorbed in the terminal ileum and returned to the liver. By interfering with the reabsorption of bile acids, cholesterol levels can be reduced by 25–30% in heterozygotes with familial hypercholesterolemia. This is presumably associated with an increased number of hepatic LDL receptors. Unfortunately, hepatocytes also respond to this decrease in cholesterol returning via the enterohepatic circulation by increasing the amount of HMG-CoA reductase and endogenous cholesterol biosynthesis. Endogenous cholesterol biosynthesis can be inhibited by a class of drugs called statins, which are potent competitive inhibitors of HMG-CoA reductase. Inhibition of endogenous HMG-CoA reductase results in an increase in LDL receptor number and, when used together with bile acid sequestering agents, can lower blood cholesterol to the normal range in heterozygotes with familial hypercholesterolemia. Under these conditions the amount of cholesterol available to the liver remains normal, but this is accomplished by increasing the number of LDL receptors in face of a decrease in blood LDL cholesterol concentration (Fig. 7.15). Thus, understanding the LDL receptor pathway has resulted in the development of rational and effective therapeutic approaches to this serious disease.

In homozygotes with familial hypercholesterolemia, LDL receptor number generally cannot be increased. Such patients have been helped by a liver transplant, often coupled with a heart transplant because of the serious damage caused by the premature atherosclerotic coronary artery disease. Somatic gene therapy for this disease is under active investigation and clinical trials are currently in progress (chapter 13).

The LDL receptor model also may be relevant to hypercholesterolemia and cholesterol regulation in the general population not affected with familial hypercholesterolemia. Studies on the LDL receptor in several species including humans have suggested that the receptor has evolved in humans to function at a much lower blood LDL cholesterol concentration than is generally found in Western populations. Thus, the receptor is saturated at the usual concentrations of LDL cholesterol found in "normal" individuals, and LDL receptor synthesis is suppressed. Lowering dietary intake of cholesterol and saturated fats might be expected to increase modestly the synthesis of new

LDL receptors. Treatment of patients with "non-familial" hypercholesterolemia with statins has now been shown to lower LDL cholesterol by 25 to 35%, and, importantly, to reduce the frequency of heart attacks by 25 to 30%.

The elucidation of the molecular pathology of familial hypercholesterolemia illustrates clearly the dynamic interface between medicine and genetics. Two medically trained investigators began by studying the problem of coronary artery disease, focusing their efforts on an inborn error of metabolism, an accident of nature, familial hypercholesterolemia. Astutely, they focused on a rare and (relatively) pure mutant, homozygous familial hypercholesterolemia. Applying a succession of appropriate and state-of-the-art methods ranging from those of cell biology, biochemistry, and immunology to those of molecular biology, they made major contributions to the understanding of normal and abnormal cholesterol metabolism; they discovered and defined the role of the LDL receptor and developed a rational and successful therapy for familial hypercholesterolemia, a common and serious disease. Along the way, they defined and characterized receptor-mediated endocytosis, a mechanism of universal importance and significance for eukaryotic cells, and made major contributions to understanding molecular mechanisms of mutation and the role of unequal crossing over in the evolution of genes. Finally, because the mevalonate synthesis pathway is involved in the production of various isoprenoid compounds, some of which are involved in cell growth regulation, understanding the regulation of cholesterol biosynthesis may lead to important insights into treating disorders of growth regulation such as cancers.

Hemophilia

According to the Talmud, as early as the second century AD, a rabbi exempted a male infant from circumcision because his mother's sister had three sons who had died of bleeding following circumcision. This apparent understanding of X-linked inheritance is one of the earliest recognitions of human genetic disease. This bleeding syndrome was rediscovered in the late 18th and early 19th century as classic hemophilia, and afflicted several of the royal houses of Europe (Fig. 7.16).

Blood coagulation is controlled by a complex regulatory circuit of enzymes, cofactors, and inhibitors as illustrated in Figure 7.17. Defects at a number of steps in this pathway can lead to similar bleeding symptoms. The various plasma proteins making up the clotting cascade were readily accessible to researchers and for this reason were a target of intense study in the early days of medical science. The existence of patients with defects in nearly all of these components also contributed significantly to progress in understanding blood clotting. The clinically most significant inherited bleeding disorder is hemophilia A, which results from deficiency in blood coagulation factor VIII. Factor VIII is a nonenzymatic cofactor for the serine protease, factor IX. Deficiencies of either factor VIII or factor IX result in a similar block to normal coagulation, leading to clinically indistinguishable bleeding disorders. Defects in factor IX are referred to as hemophilia B. Since factor VIII and factor IX are located on the X chromosome, hemophilia A and hemophilia B are both X-linked recessive in inheritance.

A wide range of severity is observed among hemophilia A patients that can be directly correlated with the residual amount of factor VIII activity in the blood. As with many diseases caused by abnormalities in enzyme function, minimal symptoms occur until factor VIII levels drop below 5% of normal and individuals with levels greater than 25% generally exhibit normal clotting function. Total absence of factor VIII activity ($< 1\%$ of normal),

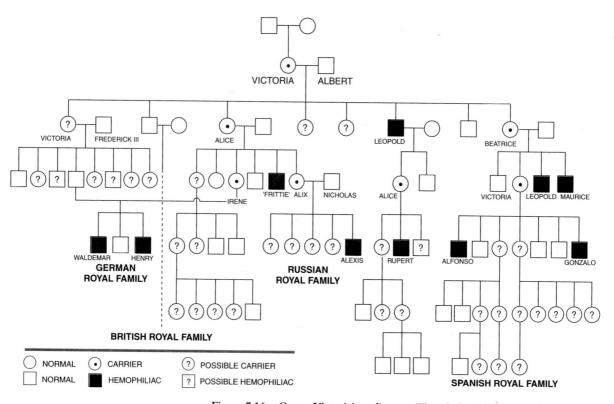

Figure 7.16.   Queen Victoria's pedigree.   Though the X-linked recessive inheritance pattern suggests a defect in either the factor VIII or factor IX gene, the distinction between these two disorders (hemophilia A and hemophilia B) was not known at the time. Queen Victoria, a carrier of hemophilia A, passed the hemophilia allele to her affected son Leopold and to her daughters, Alice and Beatrice, both of whom had affected sons and grandsons. The current British Royal family is descended from a normal male and thus unaffected. (Reprinted with permission from Kazazian HH, Tuddenham EGD, Antonarakis SE. Hemophilia A and parahemophilia. Deficiencies of coagulation factors VIII and V. In: Scriver CR, Beaudet AL, Sly WS, Valle D, eds. The metabolic and molecular bases of inherited disease. 7th ed. New York: McGraw-Hill, 1995:3241–3267.)

Figure 7.17.   The blood coagulation cascade.   It is currently believed that coagulation is initiated primarily through tissue factor, with the intrinsic pathway, including factor VIII and factor IX, functioning primarily as an amplification loop. The complex of coagulation factor IX and factor VIII activates factor X to Xa to form the prothrombinase complex, which in turn generates thrombin, leading to deposition of the fibrin blood clot. Deficiency of either factor IX or factor VIII results in a decrease in factor X activation, with a subsequent deficiency in clot formation leading to the bleeding phenotype of hemophilia.

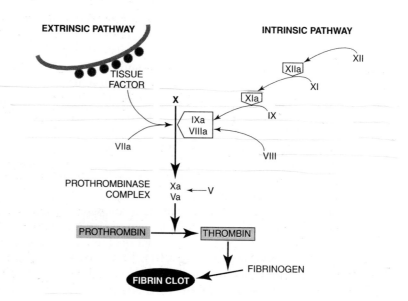

classified as severe hemophilia A, is observed in 70% of cases. Severe hemophilia patients suffer from frequent episodes of bleeding, often spontaneously or after minimal trauma. Bleeding into the joints (hemarthrosis) is a particularly common problem (Fig. 7.18). Repeated bleeding into the joint eventually leads to chronic damage often producing severe disability, sometimes requiring joint replacement. Bleeding can occur in many other organs, including the brain, a frequent cause of death in these patients. Treatment is replacement of the missing factor, first performed by whole blood transfusion and later with increasingly purified concentrates of factor VIII. These factor VIII concentrates are prepared from blood pooled from many thousands of donors. Unfortunately, the procedures used before the mid 1980s failed to inactivate common viral contaminants and, as a result, approximately 90% of patients treated with factor VIII concentrates between 1979 and 1985 were inadvertently infected with the HIV virus. Many of these patients have died of AIDS, and AIDS treatment has become an integral part of hemophilia clinical management. Donor screening for HIV along with improved procedures for factor VIII preparation have effectively eliminated the HIV risk for all patients who began treatment after 1985. Cloning of the factor VIII gene in 1984 by two biotechnology companies was driven in large part by the prospect of a safe recombinant factor VIII product, which was finally approved for human use in 1994. Analysis of the factor VIII gene also made possible the identification of numerous hemophilia A mutations, as described below.

The incidence of hemophilia A in males, although often stated to be 1/10,000, is more likely to be as high as 1/5000; thus, the mutant allele frequency (q) is also 1/5000. Heterozygous female carriers of hemophilia A (frequency of 1/2500) have approximately 50% levels of factor VIII and are completely asymptomatic. The incidence of clinical hemophilia A in women because of homozygosity for a mutant allele is predicted to be approximately

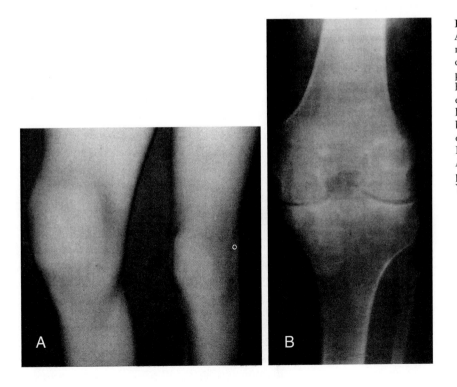

A   B

Figure 7.18.   Hemarthrosis in hemophilia A. **(A)** shows an acute hemarthrosis in the right knee. **(B)** is a radiograph showing the chronic destructive bony changes of hemophilic arthropathy resulting from repeated hemarthroses. There is rarefaction of bone, enlargement of the condyles, and loss of cartilage. (Reproduced by permission from Ginsburg D. Hemophilia and other inherited disorders of hemostasis and thrombosis. In: Rimoin DL, Connor JM, Pyeritz RE, Emery AEH. Emery and Rimoin's principles and practice of medical genetics. 3rd edition New York: Churchill Livingstone, 1996.)

1/25,000,000 (1/5000 × 1/5000, q²). Hemophilia A in females may also result from extreme skewing of X-inactivation or a translocation or other X chromosomal defect interfering with X inactivation (see chapter 8). In 1935, Haldane proposed that one-third of males with a lethal X-linked disorder should represent new mutations. This prediction, sometimes referred to as the Haldane hypothesis (see chapter 4), is based on the assumption that one-third of the mutant alleles on X chromosomes are carried in males and will be lost in each generation. Therefore, if the population remains in equilibrium with respect to disease incidence, these alleles must be replaced by an equal number of new mutations. Studies of factor VIII gene mutations have indeed borne out this prediction.

THE FACTOR VIII GENE

The factor VIII gene is located at the tip of the long arm of the X chromosome (Xq28) (Fig. 7.19). It is a large gene, containing 26 exons and spanning 186 kb, thus constituting 0.1% of the X chromosome. To date, a total of 78 large deletions and 223 point mutations or small insertions or deletions have been identified in the factor VIII gene. Given the high frequency of new mutations, unrelated families can generally be expected to carry different mutations. The large variety of resulting defects has provided a wealth of information about the structure and function of the factor VIII protein. Following the general paradigm described in chapter 5 for the hemoglobinopathies, nearly every type of defect has been observed. These include large deletions removing part or all of the factor VIII gene, and small insertions or deletions resulting in frameshift mutations. Numerous nonsense mutations have been identified throughout the molecule, resulting in premature truncation of the protein and loss of function. Finally, a large number of missense mutations that interfere with particular steps in the activation or function of factor VIII have been characterized. For example, a number of different amino acid substitutions have been observed replacing the arginine at codon 372, which is a thrombin cleavage site required for the activation of factor VIII. Loss of this activation site results in a hemophilia phenotype that varies from mild to severe depending, at least in part, on the specific amino acid substitution. A number of mutations have also been observed at another thrombin activation site, arginine 1689. Mutation of tyrosine 1680 to phenylalanine produces a moderately severe hemophilia phenotype, presumably because of loss of the posttranslation modification (sulfation) that normally occurs at this tyrosine. This sulfation is required for interaction of factor VIII with von Willebrand factor.

Approximately one-third of point mutations in the factor VIII occur at CpG dinucleotides, a "hot spot" for mutation in the human genome. Though by chance, only 1/16 of dinucleotides should be CpGs, approximately one-third of factor VIII point mutations occur at these sites. A high frequency of mutation at these positions has also been identified in other genes, such as G6PD, discussed earlier in this chapter.

Because of the large number of different possible mutations and large size of the factor VIII gene, it is often difficult to identify the specific defect in a given family. When multiple affected family members are available, analysis of DNA sequence polymorphisms within the factor VIII gene allows prenatal diagnosis and carrier detection to be performed by genetic linkage, as discussed in chapter 5. However, in families with only a single affected member, linkage analysis is not applicable. A number of screening methods have been developed, as discussed in chapter 5, to search for specific mutations. Using these approaches to screen all exons and intron/exon borders, mutations can be identified in nearly all patients who have an ab-

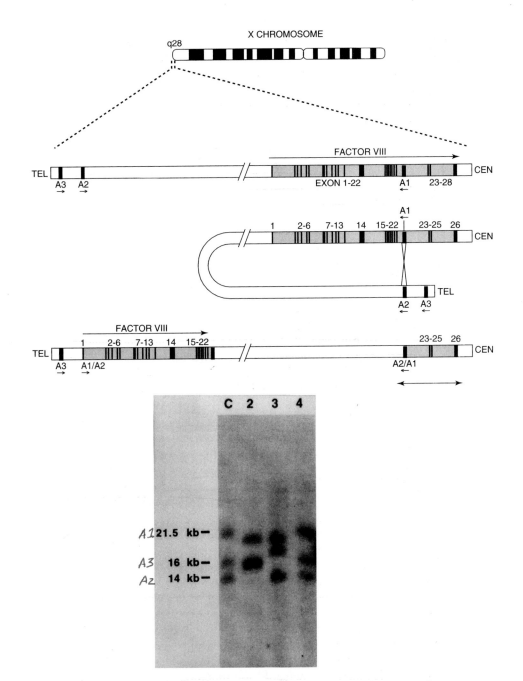

Figure 7.19. Diagram of the factor VIII gene and the mechanism for the common hemophilia gene inversion. The factor VIII gene is located near the tip of the long arm of the X chromosome. The A gene, whose function is still unknown, is present in 3 copies in this region of the X chromosome, one within factor VIII intron 22 (A1), and 2 more distal near the tip of the X chromosome (A2 and A3). Homologous recombination between the A1 gene and one of the two upstream copies (A2 or A3) results in inversion of a segment of the factor VIII gene including exons 1–22. This inversion results in complete loss of factor VIII function and severe hemophilia A. The recombination is shown here between A1 and A2, though either A2 or A3 can be involved. The Southern blot at the bottom of the figure shows the analysis of patients' DNA digested with the restriction enzyme *Bcl*I, using the A gene as probe. A control DNA sample is shown in lane C. The 21.5-kb band corresponds to A1, the 14-kb band to A2, and the 16 kb band to A3. The hemophiliac DNA in lane 2 carries the inversion resulting from recombination between A1 and A2. The DNA in lane 3 demonstrates recombination involving A1 and A3. Lane 4 is DNA from a hemophiliac who does not carry the inversion. In both types of inversion, the A1-specific band is altered in size, as is the band corresponding to the other copy of the A gene (A2 or A3) involved in the recombination. (Redrawn from Lakich D, Kazazian HH Jr, Antonarakis SE, Gitschier J. Inversions disrupting the factor VIII gene are a common cause of severe haemophilia A. Nat Genet 1993;5:236–241.)

normal factor VIII protein present in their plasma. Not surprisingly, these patients are almost invariably found to have missense mutations within the coding sequence, leading to a single amino acid substitution that results in loss of, or decreased amount of, factor VIII function.

A NOVEL MECHANISM FOR RECURRENT MUTATION

However, by the screening approaches described above, mutations can be identified in only about half of patients with *no detectable factor VIII* protein. Approximately 5% of these patients are found to have large deletions in the gene, detectable by Southern blot analyses, leaving 40–50% of severe hemophilia patients in whom no defect could be identified. Nearly all members of this large group of patients have now been shown to share the same defect, an inversion of a segment of the distal X chromosome leading to disruption of the factor VIII gene. The mechanism for this inversion is illustrated in Figure 7.19. The inversion occurs via homologous recombination between a small gene, called gene A, located within intron 22 of the factor VIII gene, and one of two additional copies of gene A located upstream of factor VIII, toward the tip of the X chromosome. The resulting inversion disrupts the factor VIII gene by removing the C-terminus of the protein encoded by exons 23–26. Remarkably, this same mutation occurs recurrently in unrelated patients. This unique molecular mechanism provides an approach to DNA diagnosis in this large group of patients. Southern blot analysis, which detects this inversion (Fig. 7.19), can now identify the defect in approximately 45% of severe hemophilia A patients.

This unique intrachromosomal homologous recombination event is unprecedented in other human diseases. It has recently been shown to occur only during male meiosis, presumably because of the requirement for an unpaired X chromosome. This observation has important clinical implications; the mother of a child carrying this defect can generally be assumed to be a carrier, even in the absence of a family history, with the recombination event often traceable to the maternal grandfather.

HEMOPHILIA B

Deficiency of factor IX results in hemophilia B. The prevalence of this disease is approximately one-tenth that of hemophilia A. The factor IX gene is located approximately 10 centimorgans from the factor VIII gene, is 34 kb in length and contains 8 exons. Similar to hemophilia A and factor VIII, hemophilia B is associated with a large number of mutations in the factor IX gene. Point mutations occur throughout the coding sequence, one-third at CpG dinucleotides. Again, as predicted by the Haldane hypothesis, approximately one-third of the mutations appear to have arisen *de novo*. However, unlike hemophilia A, no common recurrent mutation mechanism has been identified, making routine mutation detection difficult. A unique variant of hemophilia B, termed factor IX Leiden, has proved particularly instructive. These patients suffer from severe hemophilia that dramatically improves at puberty. Mutations have been identified in the factor IX promoter in these patients that appear to make the gene dependent on androgenic stimulation for high levels of gene expression. Thus, the level of factor IX is low in childhood, but increases at puberty.

Defects in a number of other clotting factors in the cascade shown in Figure 7.17 cause phenotypes similar to those encountered in hemophilia A and B patients. However, since the relevant genes are all located on autosomes (another example of locus heterogeneity), inheritance is autosomal recessive. Most of these disorders are rare.

Hemophilia is an example of an inherited disorder for which recent advances in molecular genetics have had a major impact. Identification of mutations leading to hemophilia A now provide powerful tools for DNA testing, including prenatal diagnosis. Cloning of the factor VIII gene has also led to the production of recombinant factor VIII, which provides an effective and safe replacement therapy for many patients. Finally, the hemophilias are an attractive target for long-term treatment by somatic gene therapy approaches. Simple replacement of the missing protein into the plasma compartment should result in complete resolution of bleeding symptoms, as has already been demonstrated with transfusion of factor VIII concentrates. In addition, precise regulation of gene expression, a difficult obstacle for current gene therapy strategies, is not required since even small increases of protein level could result in marked clinical improvement, and levels several times normal are unlikely to cause any significant complications. Early studies in experimental animals have demonstrated the feasibility of factor VIII and factor IX replacement by somatic gene therapy and it is conceivable that this approach may become a standard part of the treatment for hemophilia A in the future.

Collagen and its Disorders

The majority of inborn errors of metabolism, representing mutations in the genes for specific enzymes, are inherited in a recessive fashion. The quantity of most enzymes is sufficient that a reduction to 50%, as would occur in a heterozygote for an autosomal recessive condition, does not cause any phenotypic abnormality. In the example of familial hypercholesterolemia, however, in which the mutation is in a cell surface receptor gene, a reduction to 50% of the normal amount of receptor does lead to significant metabolic derangement. Mutations in nonenzymatic proteins including receptors, carrier proteins, and structural proteins are capable of creating disease in the heterozygous state and, hence, exhibiting a dominant inheritance pattern. In addition to the LDL receptor, among the best understood dominant genetic defects are the "heritable disorders of connective tissue," at least some of which arise from mutations in the genes for human collagen.

STRUCTURE OF COLLAGEN

Collagen is not only the most abundant structural protein, but also the most abundant protein of any sort in the human body. In some tissues such as bone, cartilage, tendons, and ligaments, collagens constitute 50 to 90% of the protein present. Although there are several types of collagen (see below), the basic structure common to all of them is a triple helix composed of three very long polypeptide chains. When initially assembled, this trimer includes globular domains at the amino and carboxy termini (Fig. 7.20), with the majority of the molecule being a tightly wound triple-helical domain. This precursor molecule, called procollagen, is then modified in the extracellular space by proteolytic cleavage of the globular domains and self-assembly of the triple-helical segments into an ordered array, which makes up a collagen fibril. Additional stability results from the covalent cross-linking of adjacent collagen molecules.

At least 18 different types of collagen have been identified in the human body, which differ in their structure and their tissue distribution. Table 7.2

PROCOLLAGEN MOLECULE

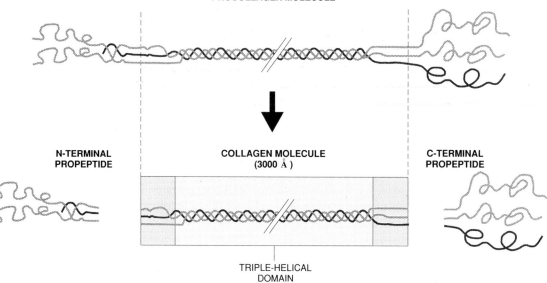

N-TERMINAL
PROPEPTIDE

COLLAGEN MOLECULE
(3000 Å)

C-TERMINAL
PROPEPTIDE

TRIPLE-HELICAL
DOMAIN

Figure 7.20.   Schematic representation of the structure of the procollagen and collagen molecules. Procollagen is formed by the assembly of three collagen polypeptide monomers. The *two light strands* are $\alpha_1(I)$, and the *one dark strand* is α_2. Once the molecule is secreted, cleavage of the N-terminal and C-terminal domains occurs, generating a 3000-Å long triple-helical collagen molecule.

provides information of the three most abundant and best characterized fibrillar collagens. Type I, which is ubiquitous but especially important in bones, tendons, and ligaments, is a heterotrimer made up of two $\alpha 1(I)$ chains and one $\alpha 2(I)$ chain. Type II collagen is a homotrimer of $\alpha 1(II)$ chains and accounts for over 50% of the dry weight of cartilage. Type III collagen, a homotrimer of $\alpha 1(III)$, is found in small amounts in many tissues in association with type I collagen, but is a major component of the walls of hollow organs of the gastrointestinal tract, of the uterus, and of large blood vessels, and plays a critical role in their structural integrity.

The 28 collagen genes are distributed throughout the human genome and are represented on 12 different chromosomes. These genes are large, ranging up to 40 kb in size, and contain as many as 52 exons.

The central triple-helical region of collagen is a remarkable protein structure. In this domain, each polypeptide chain of each of the different collagens consists of repeats of an amino acid sequence that can be written (Gly-X-Y)$_n$. In the fibrillar collagens (types I, II, III, V, and IX), there is an unbroken sequence of more than 300 of these triplets. The X position is frequently occupied by proline, and the Y position by the unusual amino acids hydroxyproline or hydroxylysine, which are generated by posttranslational modification of proline and lysine. Every third amino acid is in the

Table 7.2.   Major Types of Fibrillar Collagen

Collagen Type	Chains	Collagen Genes	Chromosomal Location	Procollagen Molecule	Tissue Distribution	Disease
I	$\alpha 1(I)$	COL1A1	17	$[\alpha 1(I)]_2\alpha 2(I)$	Bone, tendon, skin	Osteogenesis imperfecta
	$\alpha 2(I)$	COL1A2	7			
II	$\alpha 1(II)$	COL2A1	12	$[\alpha 1(II)]_3$	Cartilage, Vitreous	Chondrodysplasia
III	$\alpha 1(III)$	COL3A1	2	$[\alpha 1(III)]_3$	Skin, arteries, uterus, intestine	EDS IV

center of the triple helix in a restricted space that can only accommodate glycine, the smallest of the amino acids. The side chains of the amino acids in positions X and Y are on the surface of the triple helix. This repeating triplet of amino acids is critical for the normal assembly of collagen fibers and for the stability of the molecule. Mutations, especially of the glycine, tend to cause destabilization of the triple helix with a failure of collagen fibers to attain their normal configuration and strength.

INHERITED DISORDERS OF COLLAGEN

The molecular genetics of two disorders that fall in the category of "heritable disorders of connective tissue," namely osteogenesis imperfecta and the Ehlers-Danlos syndromes, have recently been defined. Understanding the basic pathogenesis of these diseases has clarified a novel molecular mechanism of disease, namely "protein suicide."

Osteogenesis Imperfecta

The term osteogenesis imperfecta (OI) is used to describe a clinically heterogenous group of disorders characterized by brittle bones. Type I OI, affecting approximately 1 in 15,000 individuals, is the most common, and is inherited in an autosomal dominant fashion. Affected individuals have a blue color to their sclerae that is apparent at birth, and are subject to frequent fractures that may begin in infancy, but tend to diminish after puberty. The long bones of the arms and legs, the ribs, and small bones of the hands and feet are most commonly fractured, but the fractures heal normally and usually without deformity. In about half the families with Type I OI, affected individuals have hearing loss beginning in the late teens, probably the result of fixation of the bones in the middle ear.

Biochemical analysis of cultured skin fibroblasts from Type I OI patients showed that they synthesized only half the usual amount of proα1(I) chains of Type I procollagen. At the molecular level, a variety of mutations have been discovered including multiple exon deletions or insertions and nonsense mutations, all of which result in the synthesis of only half the normal amounts of functional proα1(I) chains; products of the mutant allele are virtually absent from the cytoplasm of cultured fibroblasts. Since Type I collagen requires a 2:1 ratio of α1(I) to α2(I) protein chains for normal triple-helix formation, there is an excess of α2 chains that are degraded. Thus, as shown in Figure 7.21, only half of the normal amount of type I collagen is produced. This presumably accounts for the fragility of bones that characterizes this disorder. Thus, unlike the situation in which the protein product is an enzyme, a reduction in amount of a structural protein to 50% has significant phenotypic consequences.

Type II OI is a much more severe disorder, with innumerable fractures present at birth, and death usually occurring in the first few weeks or months of life. Figure 7.22 shows an x-ray of an affected individual, demonstrating the large number of congenital fractures and the telescoping of the long bones that occurs as a result of greatly reduced structural support. Here the collagen deficiency is much more marked. The mineralized bone, lacking the protein scaffolding, which functions in a similar fashion to steel rods in reinforced concrete, is easily crumpled by routine movements of the fetus in the womb. The molecular basis of type II OI turns out to be a bit of a surprise. Whereas the mutations that give rise to the milder type I disease are usually null mutations that completely inactivate one allele of the COL1A1

Figure 7.21.   The mechanism for collagen deficiency in type I and type II osteogenesis imperfecta. The molecular cause of these two disorders is heterogenous; shown here are typical examples. In type I OI, the example shown reflects an inactivation of one allele of the α_1(I) gene, resulting in only 50% of the normal amount of this polypeptide. The outcome is a 50% reduction in procollagen molecules, with degradation of the excess α_2 chains. In type II OI, however, typically there is a qualitative defect in one of the α chains, as in this example in which an amino acid substitution in the α_1(I) chain is indicated in *red*. If this substitution inhibits proper triple-helix formation, then three-quarters of the trimers will be abnormal and will undergo degradation, and only one-quarter will survive.

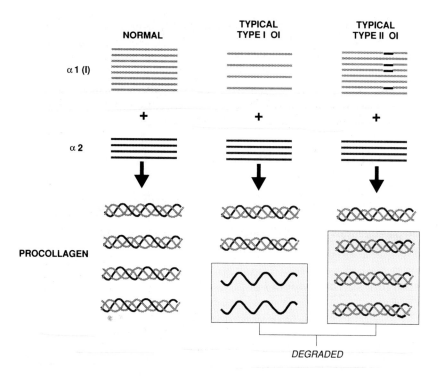

gene (which encodes α_1(I) collagen), the mutations in type II disease are much more subtle. Typically, these involve point mutations affecting glycine residues or rearrangements in the α_1(I) or α_2(I) genes (*COL1A1* and *COL1A2*), which are compatible with production of a relatively normal amount of qualitatively abnormal protein from the affected allele. The fact that such subtle mutations cause such severe disease presents a challenging paradox, but one that has now been resolved. The mutant collagen peptide, present in normal or near normal amounts, can still be incorporated into a nascent procollagen triple-helical molecule. As shown in Figure 7.21, the effect of a mutant α_1(I) gene is that *half* of the α_1(I) polypeptide chains but *three-quarters* of the collagen triple helices will be abnormal. These abnormal trimers tend to assemble poorly, may be difficult to export out of the cell, may have altered fibrillar structure, or may be degraded prematurely. The net result is a profound deficiency of normal collagen. Thus, a qualitative abnormality in the protein product of the *COL1A1* gene leads to a more severe phenotype than a quantitative abnormality. This mechanism, aptly denoted "protein suicide," provides a general explanation for the severe phenotype of a mutation affecting a subunit of a multimeric protein, provided that the inclusion of one abnormal subunit leads to loss or decreased function of the entire multimer.

Type II OI is a lethal disorder incompatible with reproduction. Because most cases appeared to be sporadic, it was formerly thought to represent an autosomal recessive disorder. However, molecular analysis has indicated that affected individuals are usually heterozygous for a new mutation in the *COL1A1*, or less commonly, *COL1A2* collagen genes. Because these new mutations may occur in early embryonic development as well as in the development of the gametes, gonadal mosaicism (see chapter 3) has been described in the parents of infants with Type II OI. Such couples have a 5 to 10% risk of having a second child with Type II OI. When the molecular defect has been defined in an affected child, prenatal diagnosis by DNA analysis is available;

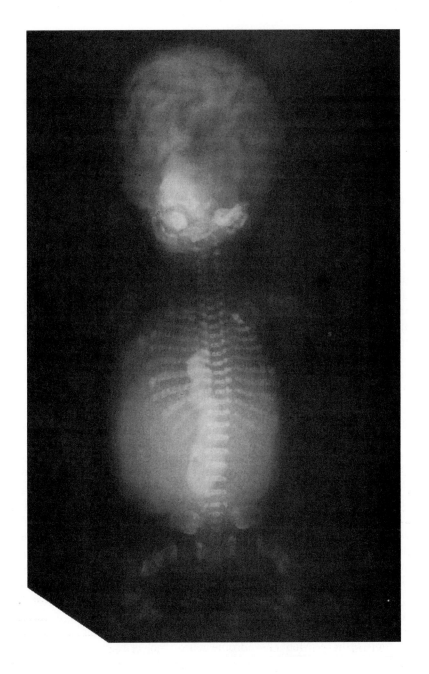

Figure 7.22.   X-ray of an infant with the perinatal lethal form of osteogenesis imperfecta (OI type II).   Note the compressed femurs that include multiple fractures.

the bony abnormalities can also be recognized in the fetus by ultrasound examination.

Ehlers-Danlos Syndrome

Like OI, Ehlers-Danlos syndrome (EDS) has been classified into a large number of clinical subtypes. The hallmark of this set of disorders is increased tissue elasticity and fragility, characterized by joint laxity and thinness of the skin with abnormal scarring, but additional features vary widely from one type to another (Table 7.3). Figure 7.23 shows an individual with type I EDS, which is an autosomal dominant disorder characterized by dramatic hyperextensibility of skin and joints. The skin is thin and heals poorly, resulting in atrophic "cigarette paper" scars after relatively minor trauma.

The strength of major blood vessels, however, is in general preserved. The molecular defect in type I EDS may be a mutation in *COL5A*, the gene encoding the $\alpha1(V)$ chain of the fibrillar Type V collagen.

The best understood and most dangerous form of EDS, type IV, displays less skin elasticity and joint hypermobility, and is characterized by thin, almost translucent, skin and easy bruising. The major serious consequences, however, arise from the dramatic fragility of major arteries, with sudden death from rupture of the aorta, the splenic artery, or a renal artery. Spontaneous perforation of the sigmoid colon is also common. Surgical attempts to repair these catastrophes are often extremely difficult, as the supporting tissues are found to be fragile and hold sutures poorly.

Virtually all families with type IV EDS, which is inherited in an autosomal dominant fashion, have been shown to have quantitative or qualitative abnormalities of type III collagen, which is a homotrimer of $\alpha1(III)$ chains. (One must be careful to avoid confusing the roman numerals associated with the various types of EDS with the roman numerals used to designate the various collagen subtypes.) In most instances, qualitative abnormalities occur in the *COL3A1* gene product, usually resulting from missense mutations involving glycine codons or exon-skipping mutations. Such mutations result in abnormal structure of 7/8 of the resulting triple helices (by the protein suicide mechanism diagrammed in Fig. 7.22). Thus, as in the case of OI discussed above, qualitative mutations may result in a more severe abnormality in collagen production than do null mutations. Since the collagen biosynthetic defect is expressed in cultured fibroblasts, and the specific mutation can be defined in some patients, it is now possible to establish the diagnosis in affected family members prior to the onset of symptoms, or even prenatally.

Of the other types of EDS, the molecular mechanism of two others, which are not due to mutations in collagen genes, deserves mention. In type VI, a deficiency of the enzyme lysyl hydroxylase has been identified. This enzyme is required for the posttranslational hydroxylation of the lysines located in the Y position of the Gly-X-Y repeat mentioned above. Without that hydroxylation, stabilization and cross-linking of the triple helix are reduced and the collagen fibers lack appropriate strength. In type IX EDS, a deficiency of a different enzyme, lysyl oxidase, has been documented. This enzyme, which requires copper as a cofactor, oxidizes lysine and hydroxylysine and is responsible for further cross-linking of collagen. EDS IX is inherited as an X-linked recessive disorder, and the molecular defect is now known to be in the Menkes syndrome gene, which is involved in copper me-

Table 7.3. Ehlers-Danlos Syndromes[a]

Type	Clinical Features	Inheritance[b]	Defect	Mutant Gene
I, Gravis	Hyperextensible skin, hypermobile joints, cigarette paper scars	AD	Abnormal type V collagen	COL5A
II, Mitis	Similar to type I but milder	AD	Unknown	
III, Familial hypermobility	Marked hypermobility of joints	AD	Unknown	
IV, Arterial	Thin translucent skin, marked bruising, arterial and intestinal rupture	AD	Abnormal type III collagen	COL3A1
VI, Ocular	Soft, velvety skin, ocular fragility	AR	Lysyl hydroxylase deficiency	PLOD
IX, Occipital horn syndrome	Lax skin, occipital horns, bladder diverticulae	XLR	Copper utilization	MNK

[a] Only a partial list is shown; at least 10 types of Ehlers-Danlos syndrome have been described.

[b] AD, autosomal dominant; AR, autosomal recessive; XLR, X-linked recessive.

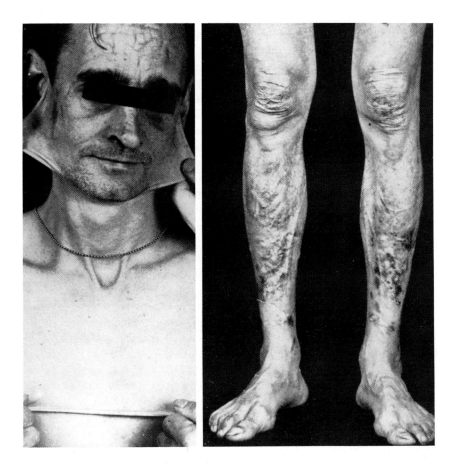

Figure 7.23. Typical appearance of an individual with Ehlers-Danlos syndrome type I. Note the hyperextensible skin and the cigarette paper scars over the lower legs. (Reprinted with permission from McKusick VA. Heritable disorders of connective tissue. 4th ed. St. Louis: Mosby, 1972.)

tabolism. Thus, the Ehlers-Danlos syndromes show evidence of both allelic heterogeneity (different mutations in the *COL3A1* gene in EDS IV) and locus heterogeneity (mutations at different loci causing EDS I, EDS IV, EDS VI, and EDS IX).

Other Collagen Disorders

Mutations in Type II collagen, responsible for the strength of cartilage, have been found to cause a heterogenous group of heritable disorders called chondrodysplasias, characterized by dwarfism, joint deformities, and other skeletal abnormalities. As is the case for OI, various different mutations, including deletions, insertions, or glycine substitutions in the Type II collagen gene (*COL2A1*), can cause these disorders.

LESSONS FROM THE COLLAGEN DISORDERS

Our purpose in discussing this category of disorders is partly to introduce an important group of human genetic diseases, but also to draw some general conclusions about the molecular basis of disease. First, the protein suicide mechanism for dominant disorders, whereby one mutant subunit leads to loss of an entire multimeric protein, first emerged clearly from this analysis of collagen disorders and has subsequently appeared in other contexts. Second, categorization of disease based on clinical criteria, even if elaborate, often underestimates the degree of genetic heterogeneity that is recognized after the molecular basis of the disease has been defined. This is particularly true of the collagen disorders because a number of genetic loci are involved, the genes are large, and the number of potential mutations almost infinite. A natural consequence of this high degree of genetic heterogeneity is that some mutations are likely to cause intermediate phenotypes that do not fit conveniently into any of the clinical classifications. Third, even with a reasonable amount of information about the collagen proteins, it is still not entirely possible to predict the clinical phenotype based on the mutation. Thus, at least at present, accurate prediction of severity is often possible only by reference to other affected family members. Finally, the great variation in phenotype demonstrated by these disorders (OI is a good example) suggests that the less specific phenotypes of such very common adult diseases as osteoporosis ("thinning of bones") and osteoarthritis (degenerative joint disease) may turn out to have their basis in subtle alterations of the collagen genes. There is, in fact, now some evidence that mutations in *COL1A2* may contribute to osteoporosis, and mutations in *COL2A1* have been described in a large family with osteoarthritis. Finally, there are families with aortic aneurysms with mutations in *COL3A1*.

SUGGESTED READINGS

Inborn Errors of Metabolism

Garrod AE. The Croonian lectures on inborn errors of metabolism. Lancet 1908;2:1–7, 73–79, 142–148, 214–200. *The classic publication defining the concept of the inborn errors of metabolism.*
Harris H. The principles of human biochemical genetics. 3rd ed. New York: Elsevier Scientific, 1980. *A beautifully written exposition of the subject in the "premolecular" era.*
Scriver CR, Beaudet AL, Sly WS, Valle D. The metabolic and molecular bases of inherited disease. 7th ed. New York: McGraw-Hill, 1995. *Encyclopedic and authoritative; the standard reference on inborn errors of metabolism and inherited metabolic diseases.*

Alkaptonuria

LaDu BN. Alkaptonuria. In: Scriver CR, Beaudet AL, Sly WS, Valle D, eds. The metabolic and molecular bases of inherited disease. 7th ed. New York: McGraw-Hill, 1995:1371–1386.

Glucose-6-Phosphate Dehydrogenase Deficiency

Luzzatto L, Mehta A. Glucose-6-phosphate dehydrogenase deficiency. In: Scriver CR, Beaudet AL, Sly WS, Valle D, eds. The metabolic and molecular bases of inherited disease. 7th ed. New York: McGraw-Hill, 1995:3367–3398.

α_1-Antitrypsin Deficiency

Cox DW. α_1-Antitrypsin deficiency. In: Scriver CR, Beaudet AL, Sly WS, Valle D, eds. The metabolic and molecular bases of inherited disease. 7th ed. New York: McGraw-Hill, 1995:4125–4158.

Familial Hypercholesterolemia

Goldstein JL, Hobbs HH, Brown MS. Familial hypercholesterolemia. In: Scriver CR, Beaudet AL, Sly WS, Valle D, eds. The metabolic and molecular bases of inherited disease. 7th Ed. New York: McGraw-Hill, 1995:1981–2030.
Motulsky AG. The 1985 Nobel Prize in physiology or medicine. Science 1986;231:126–129. *An excellent perspective on the importance of the familial hypercholesterolemia story to both genetics and medicine.*
Brown MS, Goldstein JL. A receptor-mediated pathway for cholesterol homeostasis. Science 1986;232:34–37. *The Nobel Prize acceptance lecture; an elegant, detailed account of the molecular pathology and genetics of familial hypercholesterolemia.*

Hemophilia

Hoyer LW. Hemophilia A. N Engl J Med 1994;330:38–47.

Collagen Disorders

Byers PH. Disorders of collagen biosynthesis and structure. In: Scriver CR, Beaudet AL, Sly WS, Valle D, eds. The metabolic and molecular bases of inherited disease. 7th ed. New York: McGraw-Hill, 1995;4029–4077.

Beighton P, ed. McKusick's heritable disorders of connective tissue. 5th ed. St. Louis: Mosby, 1993.

Prockop DJ. Mutations in collagen genes as a cause of connective tissue diseases. N Engl J Med 1992;326:540–545.

Cytogenetics

"It is inconceivable that particles of chromatin or any other substance, however complex, can possess the powers which must be assigned to our factors (genes). The supposition that particles of chromatin, indistinguishable from each other and almost homogeneous under any known test, can by their material nature confer all the properties of life surpasses the range of even the most convinced materialism."

—WILLIAM BATESON, 1916 (FROM BOREK E. THE CODE OF LIFE. NEW YORK: COLUMBIA UNIVERSITY PRESS, 1964.)

Chromosome abnormalities are responsible for at least half of spontaneous abortions or miscarriages and are an important cause of congenital malformations. More than 0.5% of newborns are born with significant abnormalities of autosomes or sex chromosomes. Among these, the most common and best known serious chromosomal disorders are trisomy 21, or Down syndrome, and the fragile X syndrome. In addition to constitutional, or germ line, chromosome abnormalities, abnormalities arising in somatic cells play an important role in cancer causation. The structure of chromosomes and their behavior has been described in chapter 2. In this chapter we will examine these topics in more detail and discuss some of the more common abnormalities affecting chromosomes.

Until the 1950s, two salient facts about human chromosomes were recognized, both of them wrong. First, it was believed that human cells contained 48 chromosomes, and second, it was believed that sex was determined, in mammals as it is in the fruit fly *Drosophila*, by the ratio of the number of X chromosomes to autosomes present. Chromosomes could be examined only in actively dividing cells such as tumor cells, cells from the male gonad, cells growing in tissue culture, and bone marrow preparations. The quality of chromosome preparations was nowhere near that which we have today (perhaps accounting for Bateson's skepticism). In 1956, Tjio and Levan clearly demonstrated that human embryonic fibroblasts in culture contained 46 rather than 48 chromosomes.

Within 3 years, three major disorders caused by altered numbers of chromosomes were defined: Down syndrome, Turner syndrome, and Klinefelter syndrome, all of which are discussed later in this chapter.

Cytogenic Methodology

The major advance that facilitated rapid growth of the field of cytogenetics was the development of techniques for examining chromosomes in peripheral blood lymphocytes. In this technique, now standardly used for examining human chromosomes, a small amount of anticoagulated blood is added to tissue culture medium. Phytohemagglutinin, extracted from the red bean, is added to agglutinate red blood cells and stimulate lymphocytes to divide. These dividing cells can be blocked in mitosis using microtubule inhibitors such as colchicine, and the cells lysed in hypotonic buffers. Preparations of metaphase chromosomes can then be stained and examined microscopically for alterations in number and structure (Fig. 8.1). Techniques for radioactively labeling DNA with tritiated thymidine during the S or synthetic phase

Figure 8.1.   A metaphase spread prepared from a human peripheral blood lymphocyte culture and stained by the Giemsa banding method. An intact, nonmitotic lymphocyte nucleus is shown on the *right.*(Courtesy of the University of Michigan Clinical Cytogenetics Service.)

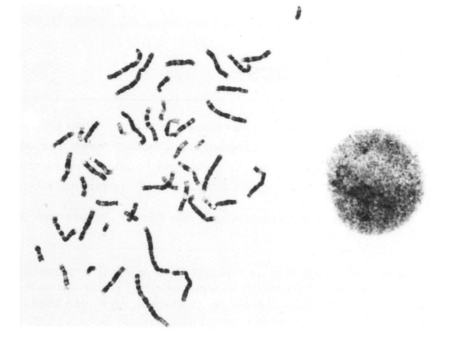

of the cell cycle allowed investigators to examine the timing of chromosome replication. In the 1970s, newer staining and banding techniques were introduced that significantly improved the resolution of chromosome morphology.

CHROMOSOME BANDING AND MORPHOLOGY

The currently most widely used technique, Giemsa banding, or G-banding, involves gentle trypsin treatment of chromosome preparations followed by staining with Giemsa. This results in a pattern of light and dark bands that is unique for each human chromosome and allows the unequivocal definition of each chromosome (Fig. 8.2). By this technique approximately 350–550 bands per haploid set are observed; each band represents approximately $5–10 \times 10^6$ bp of DNA. Because one gene may range from 10^3 bp (α-globin) to more than 2×10^6 bp (e.g., dystrophin), and because it is estimated that there is approximately one gene every 30,000 bp, each band may represent several to hundreds of individual genes. Newer techniques allow examination of chromosomes in prometaphase, at which time the chromosomes are more extended than in metaphase, allowing even higher degrees of resolution (Fig. 8.3). More than 850 bands per haploid set can be distinguished by this technique.

The dark-staining G-bands contain DNA that is AT-rich and are thought to contain fewer active genes. The DNA is in a condensed state in interphase nuclei and is rich in long interspersed DNA sequences (LINES), which are repetitive regions of DNA that do not encode expressed genes. The weakly staining bands, or R-bands (reverse bands), contain DNA that is GC-rich and contains many transcribed genes. The DNA is in a more extended state in interphase nuclei and contains, in addition to transcribed genes, increased numbers of short interspersed DNA sequences (SINES), including *Alu* sequences. Most breakpoints and rearrangements in chromosomes are thought to occur in R-bands.

Chromosome morphology is defined by the position of the centromere, or central constriction, that divides the chromosome into a short arm desig-

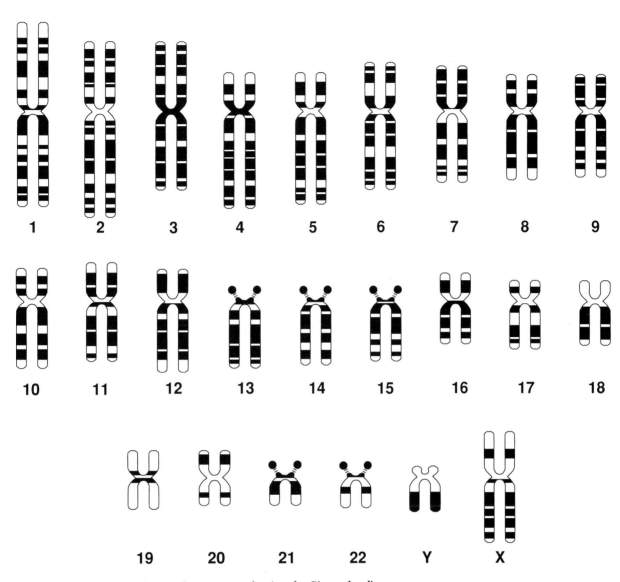

Figure 8.2.   Ideogram of human chromosomes showing the Giemsa banding patterns, arranged and numbered according to the Paris classification of 1971.   (Reprinted with permission from deGrouchy J, Turleau C. Clinical Atlas of Human Chromosomes. 2nd ed. New York: John Wiley & Sons, 1984.)

nated **p** for petite and a long arm designated **q** (Fig. 8.4). Chromosomes are metacentric if the centromere lies in the middle of the chromosome, submetacentric when the centromere is somewhat distant from the center, and acrocentric when the centromere lies near the end of the chromosome. The human acrocentric autosomal chromosomes (chromosomes 13–15, 21, and 22) have short arms that consist mainly of a satellite and a thin stalk, regions that form the nucleolus of the resting cell and contain multiple tandemly repeated copies of the genes for ribosomal RNA.

Two structural features deserve special attention. The **centromere** holds **sister chromatids** together for proper segregation at mitosis and meiosis, and is the site of formation of the kinetochore, the structure that binds spindle microtubules and regulates chromosome movements during cell division. Centromeres also contain "satellite" DNA, short, tandemly re-

Color Plates

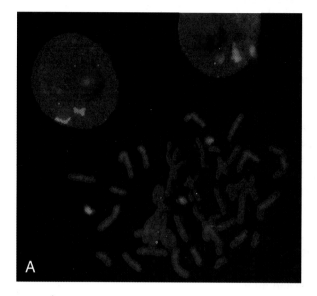

A

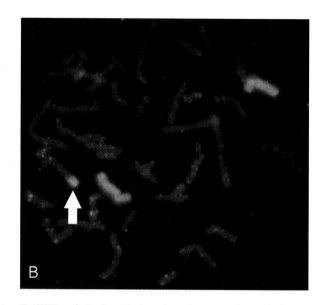

B

Figure 8.8. Examples of FISH.
A. FISH analysis, using a chromosome 21 painting probe, applied to a metaphase and two interphase cells from a patient with trisomy 21 Down syndrome. In the metaphase cell, the chromosome 21 long arms are painted along their entire lengths. The painting probe does not include sequences from the chromosome 21 short arm because probes to this region cross-hybridize to other acrocentric chromosomes. In the interphase cells, three clear "domains" are evident, even though the individual chromosomes cannot be identified. (Courtesy of DL Van Dyke and A Wiktor, Henry Ford Health Sciences Center.)

B. FISH analysis of a metaphase from a patient with an unbalanced autosomal translocation involving chromosome 10. By standard Giemsa staining, the origin of the extra material on chromosome 10 could not be defined. Using a chromosome 9 painting probe, the two normal chromosomes 9 are painted along their entire length, and the abnormal chromosome 10 (*arrow*) can be shown to contain a duplicated segment of chromosome 9 material translocated to the long arm of chromosome 10. (Courtesy of DL Van Dyke and A Wiktor, Henry Ford Health Sciences Center.)

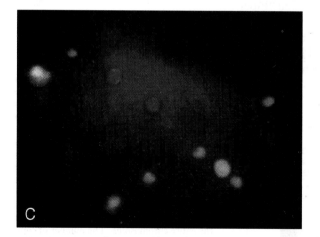

C

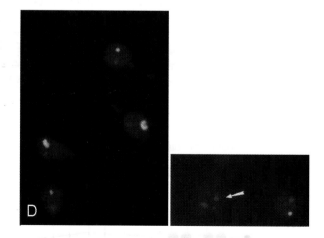

D

C. Multicolor FISH of an interphase cell (an uncultured amniotic fluid cell) using 5 centromeric probes. There are two signals each for chromosomes 13 (*red*) and 21 (*green*), but three signals for chromosome 18 (*pink*), and 2 X-chromosome (*yellow*) plus 1 Y-chromosome (*white*) signals. Thus, this cell shows trisomy for both chromosome 18 and the sex chromosomes. The karyotype is 48,XXY,+18. (Reprinted with permission from Ried T, Landes G, Dackowski W, Klinger K, Ward DC: Multicolor fluorescence *in situ* hybridization for the simultaneous detection of probe sets for chromosomes 13, 18, 21, X and Y in uncultured amniotic fluid cells. Hum Mol Genet 1992;1:307–313.)

D. FISH analysis of nondisjunction in human sperm. Three-color hybridization, using centromeric probes for chromosome 8 (*red*), the Y chromosome (*yellow*), and the X chromosome (*green*), shows four normal haploid sperm on the left, and a sperm (*arrow*) disomic for chromosome 8 on the right. (Reprinted with permission from Williams BJ, Ballenger CA, Malter HE, Bishop F, Tucker M, Zwingman TA, Hassold TJ: Non-disjunction in human sperm: results of fluorescence *in situ* hybridization studies using two and three probes. Hum Mol Genet 1993;2:1929–1936.)

E. Spectral imaging of a normal human metaphase spread after hybridization with 24 different chromosome painting probes labeled with combinations of 5 different fluorochromes. (Courtesy of T Ried, National Center for Human Genome Research.)

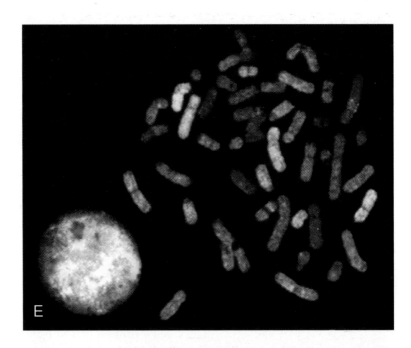

F. Karyotype, using 24-color multiplex FISH (M-FISH), from a patient with a reciprocal translocation involving the short arm of chromosome 2 and the long arm of chromosome 14. (Reprinted with permission from Speicher MR, Ballard SW, Ward DC: Karyotyping human chromosomes by combinatorial multi-fluor FISH. Nat Genet 1996;12:368–75.)

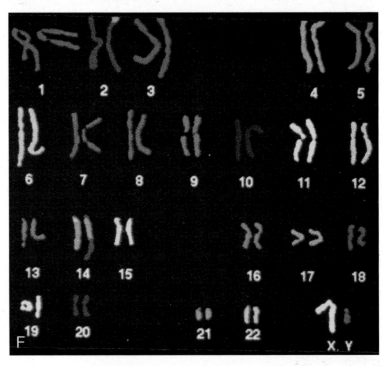

G. FISH diagnosis of the interstitial deletion in Prader-Willi syndrome using a locus-specific cosmid probe (*red, solid arrow*) within the critical deletion region. The two chromosome 15 homologs are identified by a chromosome 15-specific centromeric probe (*green*), and the deleted homolog (*open arrow*) shows no hybridization to the PWS region cosmid probe. (Courtesy of D Ledbetter, National Center for Human Genome Research.)

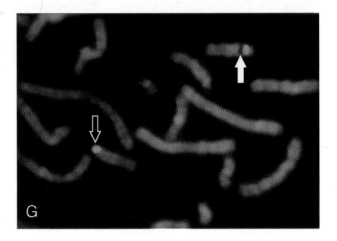

The diagnostic applications of FISH technology include the detection and definition of both numerical and structural chromosomal abnormalities in metaphase spreads. Numerical chromosome abnormalities can also be readily detected in interphase cells from virtually any tissue. Therefore, these techniques have important applications in the clinical evaluation of constitutional chromosome disorders and of certain leukemias, lymphomas, and solid tumors, as well as in prenatal diagnosis. Specific examples will be discussed later in this chapter. FISH can also be applied to haploid cells such as sperm to obtain information on the frequency of chromosome abnormalities in gametes (Fig. 8.8F).

Chromosome Abnormalities

Chromosome abnormalities may be numerical or structural. In discussing numerical chromosome abnormalities it is important to define ploidy. **Euploid** refers to any exact multiple of N, the number of chromosomes in a normal haploid gamete. The number of chromosomes in a normal somatic cell is **diploid** or 2N. Euploid chromosome constitutions need not be normal; for example, triploidy (69 chromosomes) is a euploid chromosome abnormality commonly found in spontaneous abortions (Fig. 8.9). **Aneuploid** refers to any number of chromosomes that is noneuploid and, for constitutional chromosome disorders, usually refers to an extra copy of a single chromosome, i.e., **trisomy** (as in trisomy 21 Down syndrome), or the absence of a single chromosome, i.e., **monosomy** (as in 45,X Turner syndrome).

NUMERICAL ABNORMALITIES

Aneuploidy is the result of **nondisjunction,** or failure of chromosomes to separate normally during cell division, and can occur during meiosis or mitosis. Although the causes of nondisjunction are not known, it is appreciated that the risk of meiotic nondisjunction increases with increasing maternal age. When nondisjunction occurs after fertilization, that is, mitotic nondisjunction, one expects to see mosaicism, or two or more populations of chromosomally different cells.

Figure 8.9. Peripheral blood lymphocyte karyotype from a newborn with triploidy. This abnormality is usually the result of fertilization of the egg by two sperm. (Courtesy of the University of Michigan Clinical Cytogenetics Service.)

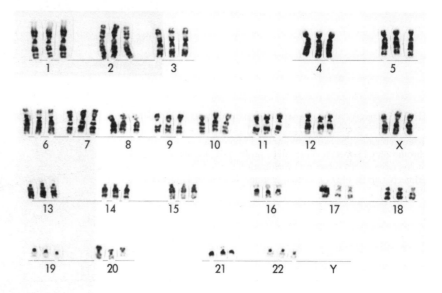

Meiotic nondisjunction can occur in either the first or second meiotic divisions with quite different consequences, as indicated in Figure 8.10. If nondisjunction occurs during the first meiotic division, the gametes formed will contain *both* the parental chromosomes (maternal *and* paternal) that failed to separate, or neither. When nondisjunction occurs in the second meiotic division, the gametes will contain two copies of *one* parental chromosome (maternal *or* paternal), or neither. Thus, the resulting offspring from a mating in which one of the gametes has undergone meiotic nondisjunction in the first meiotic division will have a copy of homologous chromosomes derived from *both* the grandfather and grandmother. In contrast, when meiotic nondisjunction has occurred in the second meiotic division there will be two copies of *either* the grandpaternally or grandmaternally derived chromosome. Note that these two copies will *not* be genetically *identical* because of recombination occurring at the 4-chromatid stage of meiosis I (chapter 2). Also note that monosomic zygotes can also arise from nondisjunction occurring in either the first or second meiotic division.

STRUCTURAL ABNORMALITIES

Structural abnormalities of chromosomes may involve either one or two (or more) chromosomes (Fig. 8.11). When only one chromosome is involved, it may have a deletion or duplication of a portion of the chromosome, a pericentric (involving the centromere) or paracentric (not involving the centromere) inversion, or the formation of a ring chromosome or isochromosome. Structural abnormalities involving two or more chromosomes may result in insertions of material from one chromosome into another, or, more commonly, translocation or exchange of chromosomal material between two or more chromosomes. Two major forms of chromosome translocation are recognized: reciprocal translocation (Fig. 8.12A) and Robertsonian transloca-

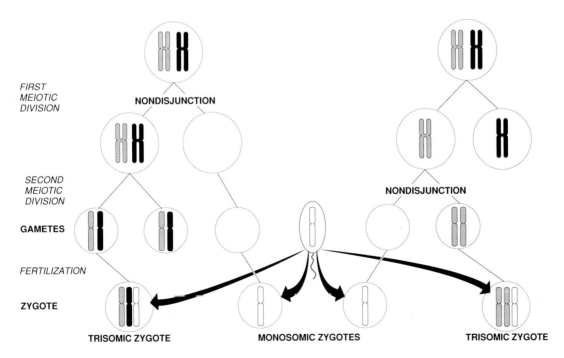

Figure 8.10.   Chromosomal consequences of nondisjunction occurring in the first or second meiotic division.   See text for details.

Figure 8.11. Structural abnormalities of chromosomes. *Inversions* involve two breaks in a single chromosome. If the breaks bracket the centromere, this is a pericentric inversion; if they do not, it is paracentric. *Insertions* result from at least three breaks in at least two chromosomes. Karyotypically unbalanced offspring have pure duplications or pure deletions of the inserted region. *Isochromosomes* arise from abnormal centromere division and result in either duplication of the short arm and deletion of the long arm (*ISO p*), or duplication of the long arm and deletion of the short arm (*ISO q*). The latter does occur for the X chromosome.

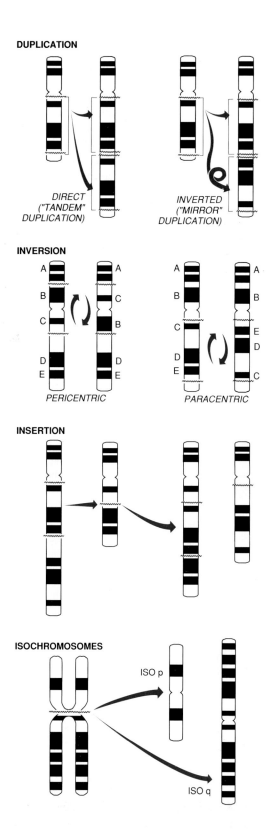

tion or centric fusion (Fig. 8.13A). In both of these cases, if no essential chromosome material is lost and no genes are damaged by the breakage and reunion, the individual carrying such a translocation will be clinically normal. However, such individuals are at increased risk of having chromosomally unbalanced offspring. This is illustrated in Figures 8.14 and 8.15.

A.

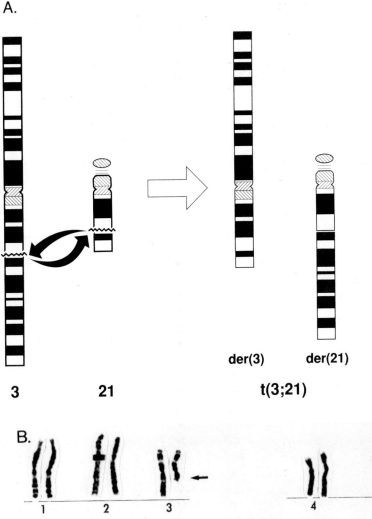

der(3)   der(21)

3   21   t(3;21)

Figure 8.12.   Reciprocal translocation be-tween chromosomes 3 and 21.   The break-points on the long arm of each chromosome are indicated by the *red wavy line* in the dia-gram (**A**). Chromosome 21 material is shown in *red*. The translocation chromosomes (der (3) and der (21)) are indicated by *arrows* on the karyotype (**B**).

B.

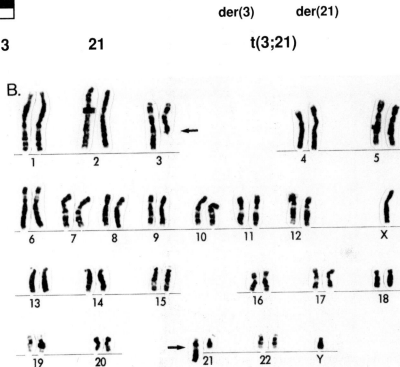

In the example shown in Figures 8.12 and 8.14, there has been a recip-rocal translocation between chromosomes 3 and 21 involving a portion of the long arm of each chromosome. At meiosis, a cross-shaped or quadrira-dial structure is formed (Fig. 8.14) and the homologous chromosomes can separate in several different ways. In alternate segregation, the two normal chromosomes go to one daughter cell and the translocation chromosomes to the other. In this case, two kinds of gametes are formed: normal gametes

Figure 8.13. Robertsonian translocation or centric fusion involving the long arms of chromosomes 14 and 21.   Chromosome 21 material is shown in *red* in the diagram (**A**). The translocation chromosome is indicated by the *arrow* on the karyotype (**B**).

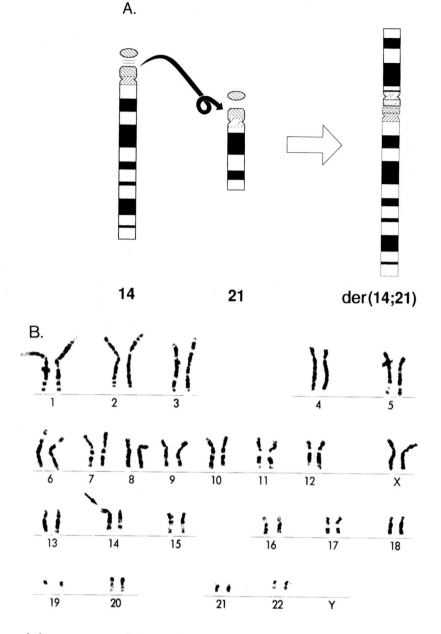

and those carrying a balanced reciprocal translocation. Fertilization of the normal gamete results in a normal offspring, whereas fertilization of the gamete with the balanced translocation results in an offspring with a balanced reciprocal translocation who should be clinically normal just as is the parent. However, if separation of the chromosomes at meiosis results in the production of gametes containing one normal chromosome and one translocation chromosome as in the so-called adjacent 1 or adjacent 2 segregation, then an unbalanced chromosome constitution is transmitted by that gamete.

In adjacent 1 segregation, homologous centromeres segregate from one another. Fertilization of an unbalanced gamete results in an offspring who has an extra copy of the end of the long arm of chromosome 3 and is missing a portion of the long arm of chromosome 21, or an individual with the reciprocal arrangement, that is, the absence of a portion of the long arm of chromosome 3 and the addition of material from the long arm of chromo-

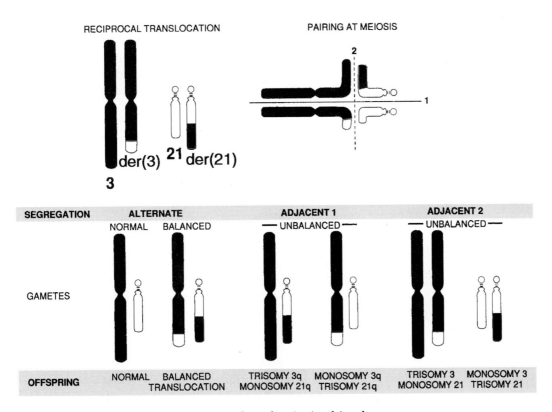

Figure 8.14. Meiotic segregation in a reciprocal translocation involving chromosomes 3 and 21. See text for details.

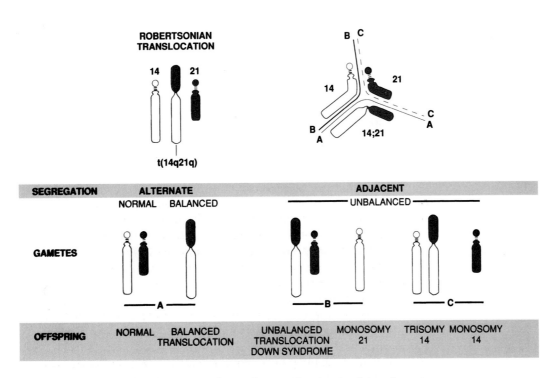

Figure 8.15. Meiotic segregation in Robertsonian translocation involving chromosomes 14 and 21. See text for details.

some 21. Fertilization of gametes produced by adjacent 2 segregation, in which homologous centromeres do not segregate, results in this example in virtually total monosomy for one of the two chromosomes and a partial trisomy of the other. This degree of chromosome abnormality is generally incompatible with viability even in early embryonic life and results in spontaneous abortion, so that this outcome is rarely seen.

It is clear that certain segregation patterns (e.g., adjacent 2) usually produce a greater degree of chromosomal imbalance than others and are thus observed less frequently in liveborn offspring or even fetuses because they are less likely to survive. However, it appears that the different segregations also do not occur with equal frequency in meiosis. Using the technique of in vitro fertilization of hamster oocytes with human sperm, it is possible to examine karyotypes of sperm from men heterozygous for balanced translocations. Approximately 50% of sperm karyotypes were found to be balanced, resulting from alternate segregation, with the expected equal frequency of normal and balanced translocation complements. Adjacent 1 segregation was responsible for the majority of chromosomally unbalanced gametes. Unbalanced karyotypes were more frequent in sperm than in fetuses and liveborns, again indicating intrauterine selection against chromosomally abnormal zygotes.

Figure 8.13 shows a typical Robertsonian translocation or centric fusion between chromosome 14 and chromosome 21. Such translocations involve chromosomes in the D and G groups, that is, chromosomes 13, 14, 15, 21, and 22. These are acrocentric chromosomes with short arms consisting of a satellite and stalk containing the nucleolar organizing region and tandemly repeated ribosomal RNA genes. These chromosomes tend to cluster during meiosis and will more often than other chromosomes undergo breakage and recombination with loss of the short arms and fusion of the long arms of the involved chromosomes. At the *molecular* level, such fusion chromosomes are unbalanced because they lack the short arms of both chromosomes, but at the *phenotypic* level, they are "balanced" because the redundancy of ribosomal RNA genes makes the loss of these short arms irrelevant. The loss of the short arms is also not clinically significant because individuals with so-called balanced Robertsonian translocations are clinically normal. However, they are at significant risk for having offspring with a clinically significant "unbalanced" translocation. In the example, shown in Figure 8.15, of an individual with 45 chromosomes and a fusion of the long arm of 14 with the long arm of 21, the involved chromosomes line up in a triradial configuration at meiosis. There are three possible ways the chromosomes can segregate during meiosis and these are shown in Figure 8.15.

During alternate segregation at meiosis (indicated by the *line* marked *A*), one gamete will receive one copy each of the normal chromosome 21 and normal chromosome 14, whereas the other gamete will receive the derivative, or translocation, chromosome carrying the long arms of 14 and 21. Fertilization of these gametes by a normal gamete will result, respectively, in a normal karyotype with 46 chromosomes, and a balanced translocation karyotype with a total of 45 chromosomes like that of the translocation carrier parent. These offspring are clinically normal.

If, on the other hand, adjacent segregation occurs as indicated by *line B*, one gamete will receive a normal chromosome 14 but no chromosome 21. Fertilization by a normal gamete will result in a karyotype with 45 chromosomes but only a single copy of chromosome 21 and hence, monosomy 21, which is generally not viable. The other gamete formed will contain the normal copy of chromosome 21 plus the translocation chromosome. Upon fertilization with a normal gamete, this zygote will contain 46 chromosomes including two copies of the normal chromosome 21, one copy of the normal 14, and the translocation chromosome containing the long arms of chromosomes 14 and 21. Functionally, this individual has three copies of the long arm of chromosome 21, and hence will have the clinical phenotype of Down syndrome. His karyotype (assuming, for example, a male) would be written as 46,XY,+21,der(14;21)(q10;q10).

Finally, in the adjacent segregation indicated by *line C*, one gamete will receive the normal copy of chromosome 14 plus the translocation chromosome. Fertilization of such a gamete by a normal gamete results in a zygote containing 46 chromosomes and functionally trisomic for chromosome 14, which is not viable. The other gamete will receive the normal chromosome 21 but no chromosome 14. Upon fertilization by a normal gamete, this zygote will contain only 45 chromosomes and be lacking one copy of chromosome 14. Monosomy 14 is also not viable.

Because monosomy 21 and monosomy 14 as well as trisomy 14 are not viable, one might expect three possible outcomes in the offspring of a 14q;21q translocation parent: normal, balanced translocation, and unbalanced translocation causing Down syndrome. These three types of progeny do not occur with the expected equal frequency, however. Instead, when the mother is the carrier of the 14q;21q translocation, approximately 10–15% of offspring are affected with Down syndrome because they carry two copies of the normal chromosome 21 plus the translocation chromosome, approximately half are balanced translocation carriers like the mother, and 40% are chromosomally normal. For reasons that are not known, when the father is the carrier of the translocation, the risk that a child will be affected is considerably lower, less than 5%. The lower-than-expected frequency of trisomy 21 among liveborn offspring is thought to reflect the high frequency of spontaneous abortion of trisomic fetuses.

SPONTANEOUS ABORTIONS

Numerically speaking, the major clinical consequence of chromosomal abnormalities occurs before birth; approximately 50% or more of spontaneously aborted fetuses have major chromosomal abnormalities. Because approximately 15% of recognized pregnancies end in spontaneous abortion or miscarriage, generally in the first trimester of pregnancy, this indicates that, at a minimum, 7.5% of conceptions have major chromosome abnormalities. Furthermore, it is now estimated that as many as 50% of conceptions end in spontaneous abortion (many of which are so early as to be recognized only by hormone assays), suggesting that at least 25% of all conceptions are afflicted with major chromosome abnormalities.

The major types of chromosome abnormalities found in abortuses are indicated in Table 8.2. Trisomies, as a group, are the most common abnormality; individually, the most common aberrations are monosomy X (45,X), triploidy, and trisomy 16. It is interesting that whereas trisomy 16 is never seen in liveborn infants and triploidy is only rarely seen in liveborns who tend to die very early in infancy, 45,X is seen in liveborn females, but only with a frequency of approximately 1 in 5000 and is the cause of Turner syndrome. Thus, there is significant loss of conceptions with major chromosomal abnormalities.

Trisomy 13, 18, and 21 are found in about 9% of chromosomally abnormal abortuses, in approximately 2.5% of all stillborn fetuses, but in only

Clinical Consequences of Chromosome Abnormalities

Table 8.2. Relative Frequencies of Different Abnormalities in Chromosomally Abnormal Abortuses[a]

Type		Frequency (%)
Trisomy		52
	16	15
	13, 18, 21	9
	XXX, XXY, XYY	1
	All others	27
45, X		18
Triploidy		17
Tetraploidy		6
Other		7
Total		100

[a] Modified from Hassold TJ: Chromosome abnormalities in human reproductive wastage. Trends Genet 2:105–110, 1986.

0.1% of liveborns, again indicating a high rate of loss of chromosomally abnormal zygotes. Most of this loss occurs early in gestation, as indicated by the much higher frequency of chromosome abnormalities among spontaneous abortuses (50%) than among stillborns, defined as losses after 28 weeks gestation (5%).

BIRTH DEFECTS

The second major clinical consequence of constitutional chromosome abnormalities is birth defects. The frequency of various chromosome aberrations found in newborn surveys is indicated in Table 8.3. Balanced rearrangements, which usually cause no clinical abnormality but which may predispose a carrier adult to bearing a chromosomally unbalanced offspring, are the most common, affecting 1 in 500 individuals. However, various unbalanced chromosome constitutions are not uncommon and the burden of chromosome abnormalities is clearly a significant one, with more than 0.5% of all newborns affected with serious chromosome abnormalities. Although the clinical findings in chromosome abnormalities can vary considerably, the general features are a triad of **growth retardation, mental retardation,** and **specific somatic abnormalities.**

Down Syndrome

One of the best recognized and most common serious chromosomal disorders is Down syndrome, which is usually caused by an extra copy of chromosome 21 or trisomy 21. The clinical features of this condition include growth retardation, varying degrees of mental retardation, and a spectrum of somatic abnormalities including head and facial features, which resulted in this condition being given the unfortunate designation of mongolism in the past. These features include a flattened face and occiput, upward slanting of the eyes, an extra skin fold at the medial aspect of the eyes (epicanthal folds), a large tongue, and small ears (Fig. 8.16).

In addition, Down syndrome babies are often very floppy or hypotonic, 40% have significant congenital heart disease (often atrioventricular canal defects), and 5% have serious gastrointestinal anomalies, including duodenal stenosis. There is a 15- to 20-fold increased risk of leukemia, an increased susceptibility to infections, and an increased frequency of cataracts, thyroid dysfunction, and signs of premature aging. Virtually all individuals

Table 8.3.   Incidence of Chromosomal Abnormalities in Newborn Infants[a]

	Number	Approximate Incidence
Sex chromosome abnormalities in 28,580 males		
XXY	30	1/1000
XYY	26	1/1100
Other	17	1/1700
Total	73	1/400
Sex chromosome abnormalities in 14,976 females		
45,X	2	1/7500
XXX	13	1/1200
Other	5	1/3000
Total	20	1/750
Autosomal abnormalities in 43,556 babies		
+D (trisomy 13)	3	1/15,000
+E (trisomy 18)	4	1/11,000
+G (trisomy 21)	45	1/900
Other trisomies	2	1/22,000
Total	54	1/800
Structural rearrangements		
Balanced	81	1/500
Unbalanced	21	1/2100
Total	102	1/400
Total chromosomal abnormalities	249	1/170

[a] Data from six surveys in Scotland, Denmark, Canada, and the United States. Reprinted with permission from Jacobs PA, Melville M, Ratcliffe S, Keay AJ, Syme J: A cytogenetic survey of 11,680 newborn infants. Ann Hum Genet 37:359–376, 1974 © Cambridge University Press.

with Down syndrome who live beyond 35 years show pathologic features of Alzheimer's disease. The most serious health problem faced by children with Down syndrome is congenital heart disease. With improved medical and surgical care for these problems, and with changed attitudes toward the care of children with Down syndrome, the average life expectancy has increased from approximately 9 years in 1930 to almost 60 years today.

The chromosomal basis for Down syndrome in approximately 95% of affected individuals is trisomy 21 secondary to nondisjunction during meiosis. By using DNA polymorphisms, it is possible in most families to determine in which parent and at which meiotic step nondisjunction has occurred (Fig. 8.17). In 95% of cases, the extra chromosome 21 is maternal in origin, and in almost 80% of these cases, nondisjunction occurred in meiosis I. It has long been recognized that there is a strong association between maternal age and the risk of bearing a child with trisomy 21 (or other trisomies such as 13 and 18) (Fig. 8.18), but not Down syndrome secondary to translocation; the basis for this association, however, remains unknown.

Approximately 4% of cases of Down syndrome are the result of an unbalanced translocation; 9% of Down syndrome babies born to mothers younger than 30 years of age have an unbalanced translocation, whereas fewer than 2% of those born to mothers older than 35 years do. Approximately 60% of such translocations involve the long arm of a D group chromosome (chromosome 13, 14, or 15) fused to the long arm of 21; most of these involve chromosome 14. Although about half of such unbalanced translocations represent *de novo* events occurring during gametogenesis in a parent (usually the mother) of the affected child, the remainder are the result of inherited translocations. This latter fact is important because it indicates that other family members may also be translocation carriers and at significant risk of bearing a child with Down syndrome. Approximately 40% of translocations involve only the G group chromosomes, 21 and 22. Ninety percent of these are apparent 21q;21q translocations (actually 21q isochromosomes) and nearly all of these represent

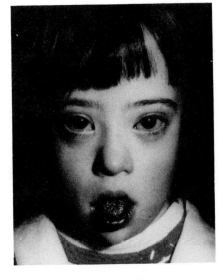

Figure 8.16.   A girl with Down syndrome. Note the straight hair, flattened face, open mouth with large tongue, and upward slanting eyes with epicanthal folds.

Figure 8.17. Determination of the site of nondisjunction in Down syndrome using DNA polymorphisms. D21S1, D21S111, and D21S17 are anonymous polymorphic marker loci on chromosome 21. The polymorphism recognized by D21S1 is compatible *only* with maternal nondisjunction, but does not allow differentiation between meiosis I or II. The polymorphisms recognized by D21S111 and D21S17 are compatible with nondisjunction in paternal meiosis I or II, or maternal meiosis I, but not maternal meiosis II. Taken together, these results are most consistent with nondisjunction in maternal meiosis I.

	MOTHER	FATHER	CHILD	
D21S1	2,2	1,1	1,2,2	MATERNAL
D21S111	1,2	1,1	1,1,2	IF MATERNAL, THEN I
D21S17	1,2	2,2	1,2,2	IF MATERNAL, THEN I

de novo events. In those rare circumstances in which the parent is a carrier of a 21q;21q translocation, the only viable offspring such an individual could have would necessarily have Down syndrome. Finally, less than 3% of individuals with Down syndrome are mosaics in that they have a 47,+21 line of cells in addition to a normal euploid line. These individuals often have milder manifestations of Down syndrome.

The empirical recurrence risks to parents who have had a child with trisomy 21 are approximately 1%; the reasons for this increased risk are unknown. For carriers of a balanced translocation, the risks that a child will be affected are approximately 10–15% if the mother is a carrier but less than 5% if the father is carrier. Again, it is important to recognize that there is a similar risk to other relatives if the translocation is inherited. Each first-degree relative of a balanced translocation carrier has approximately a 50% chance of also being a carrier of that same translocation.

Chromosome 21 is one of the smallest of the chromosomes, containing approximately 1.7% of the total cellular DNA or approximately 1500 genes. From studies of individuals with trisomy for only a part of chromosome 21, it is thought that only the distal one-third of the long arm of chromosome 21, specifically bands q21.2 to q22.3, must be present in an extra copy to cause Down syndrome. A large number of genes have now been mapped to this region of chromosome 21, and a gene dosage effect has been demonstrated for several of these in trisomy 21. The genes for amyloid precursor protein, superoxide dismutase-1, certain purine synthetic enzymes, a human oncogene *ETS-2*, and alpha-A crystallin, a protein found in the lens (Fig. 8.19), are of particular interest in that patients with Down syndrome develop

Figure 8.18. The relationship between maternal age and incidence of Down syndrome due to trisomy 21. (Redrawn from Hamerton JL. Human Cytogenetics. Vol. II, New York: Academic Press, 1971.)

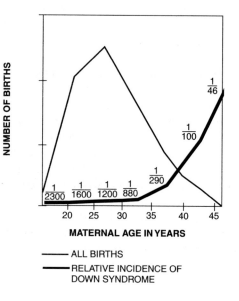

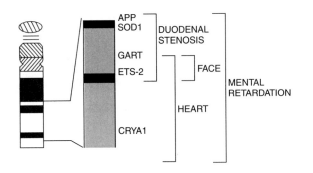

Figure 8.19. Phenotypic map of human trisomy 21 based on molecular and cytogenetic analyses of patients with triplication of part of chromosome 21. Only a few of the genes mapped to 21q21.2 to q22.3 are shown. (Redrawn from Epstein CJ. Down syndrome (trisomy 21). In: Scriver CR, Beaudet AL, Sly WS, Valle D, eds. The Metabolic and Molecular Bases of Inherited Disease. 7th ed. New York: McGraw-Hill, 1995:749–794.)

Alzheimer's disease early in life, and they frequently have increased levels of purines, an increased risk of acute leukemia, and a higher frequency of cataracts. However, whether any of these phenotypic features can be correlated directly with trisomy of specific genes on the long arm of chromosome 21 remains to be determined.

Other Autosomal Abnormalities

Other serious chromosome abnormalities include a number of trisomies and partial trisomies. One example is trisomy 13 with a frequency of approximately 1 in 15,000 live births. Approximately one-half of these babies die within the first month of life. Characteristically they have a failure of normal brain development called holoprosencephaly, in which there is an absence of normal formation of the frontal cortex. There are associated abnormalities of the skull and face including severe cleft lip and palate and midfacial abnormalities (Fig. 8.20). Peculiar punched-out scalp defects are characteristic of this syndrome, as is polydactyly (extra fingers and toes). As is the case with other major chromosome abnormalities, these babies are growth retarded and severely developmentally retarded.

Other chromosome abnormalities involve structural defects such as partial trisomies or partial monosomies; that is, extra pieces or missing pieces of a chromosome resulting in alterations in dosage of multiple genes. **Microdeletion syndromes, or contiguous gene syndromes,** are usually sporadic, but occasionally familial, syndromes with a consistent but complex phenotype associated with a small (usually < 5 Mb) chromosomal deletion. For example, hemizygosity for an interstitial deletion of chromosome 22q11.2 is associated with a variable clinical syndrome called CATCH 22 (*C*ardiac defect, *A*bnormal facies, *T*hymic hypoplasia, *C*left palate, *H*ypocalcemia, and *22q11* deletions), and encompasses a spectrum of disorders including DiGeorge syndrome (thymic hypoplasia, parathyroid hypoplasia, facial abnormalities, and conotruncal [ventricular outflow tract] cardiac defects) and velocardiofacial syndrome (cleft palate, abnormal nose, developmental delay, and conotruncal defects). As a group, these 22q11 deletions are thought to have an incidence of 1/5000 and to play a role in 5% of all congenital heart defects. Genes in this region must be important in the development of third and fourth pharyngeal pouch derivatives, which include the thymus, parathyroids, and conotruncus. Although microdeletions are sometimes detectable by high-resolution prometaphase chromosome analysis, and were originally defined by association with a chromosome abnormality, FISH analysis is both more sensitive and more practical. Probes targeted to the critical chromosomal region in an affected individual will show hybridization to only one of the two homologous chromosomes in a metaphase spread, and only one rather than two signals in an interphase nucleus (Fig. 8.21).

Figure 8.20. An infant with trisomy 13. Note the facial malformation and severe cleft lip and palate (**A**) and polydactyly (**B**).

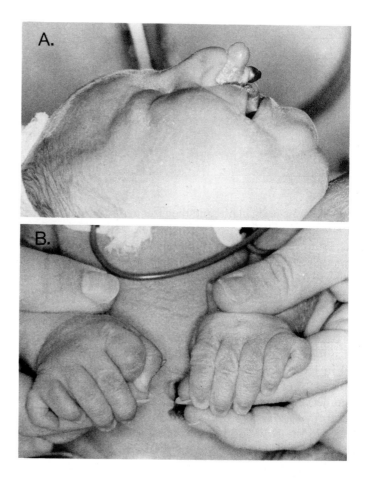

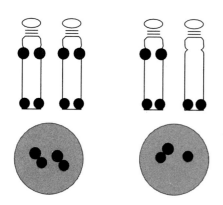

Figure 8.21. Detection of the microdeletion in the CATCH 22 syndrome by FISH analysis. Diagramatic representation of the analysis, using locus-specific probes, in both metaphase chromosomes and interphase nuclei, in normal (*left*) and affected (*right*) individuals. A control probe (*black*) that recognizes the distal end of the long arm of chromosome 22 is used to mark that chromosome. Note that in normal individuals, both chromosomes 22 have hybridization signals with the 11q22 probe (*red*), whereas in affected individuals only one chromosome 22 is labeled. (Redrawn from Emanuel BS. The use of fluorescence *in situ* hybridization to identify human chromosomal anomalies. Growth Genet Horm 1993;9:6–12.)

Genomic Imprinting

Two other microdeletion syndromes, Prader-Willi syndrome and Angelman syndrome, are of particular importance because they illustrate the newly recognized phenomenon of **genomic imprinting,** the differential expression of alleles depending on the parent of origin. Prader-Willi syndrome (PWS), affecting 1/10,000 liveborns, is characterized by mild to moderate mental retardation, hypotonia and poor feeding in infancy, short stature, small hands and feet, and small external genitalia, and by marked hyperphagia (compulsive overeating) and massive obesity beginning after the age of about two years (Fig. 8.22). By prometaphase analysis, approximately half of PWS patients were found to have a microdeletion of chromosome 15q11-q13. Analysis of DNA polymorphisms showed, remarkably, that *all* of these deletions affected the chromosome 15 inherited from the father. Angelman syndrome (AS) is characterized by more severe mental retardation with absence of speech, but also by seizures, jerky gait, inappropriate laughter, protruding tongue, and enlarged jaw. Surprisingly, many AS patients were found to have the *same* microdeletion on chromosome 15 as PWS patients, but in this case the deletion was always in the chromosome inherited from the mother. These observations suggested that certain autosomal genes might be differentially expressed depending on whether they were inherited from the father or from the mother.

It is now known, from FISH analyses, that approximately 70–75% of patients with PWS have a microdeletion of the paternal 15q11-q13. An additional 20–25% of patients were found by DNA polymorphism analysis to

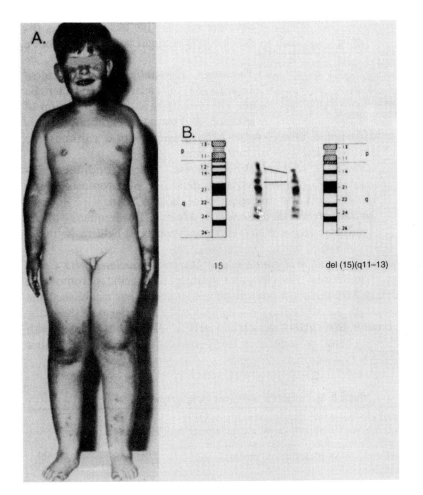

15   del (15)(q11–13)

Figure 8.22.   Prader-Willi syndrome.   A. A 9½ year-old boy with obesity, small penis, and small hands and feet. (Reprinted with permission from Jones KL. Smith's Recognizable Patterns of Human Malformations. 4th ed. Philadelphia: WB Saunders, 1988.) **B.** Schematic diagram and a partial karotype from a patient with the Prader-Willi syndrome showing the interstitial deletion of bands 11 to 13 in the long arm of chromosome 15 (15q11–13). (Courtesy of the University of Michigan Clinical Cytogenetics Service.) FISH diagnosis of the interstitial deletion in PWS is shown in Figure 8.8G.

have two copies of the maternal chromosome 15 and no copy of the paternal chromosome, a condition called **uniparental disomy** (Fig. 8.23). This situation presumably arises from a zygote with trisomy 15, with two maternal chromosomes and one paternal chromosome. Trisomy 15 would be expected to be lethal, but the loss of one chromosome 15 might allow survival and the birth of a viable infant. If the single paternal chromosome were lost in such a trisomy, the infant would be born with maternal uniparental disomy for chromosome 15 and would have Prader-Willi syndrome. Rare patients with AS (< 5%) were found to have paternal uniparental disomy for chromosome 15. These accidents of nature indicate that maternal and paternal genetic contributions of autosomal genes are not necessarily equivalent, and that genetic contributions from both parents are necessary for normal development.

More striking evidence for genetic imprinting comes from studies on early mouse embryos. After fertilization of the mouse egg, the sperm and egg pronuclei remain separate for some time and can be distinguished microscopically. Experimentally, one pronucleus (for example, the paternal) can be removed and another pronucleus, of maternal origin, inserted into the egg. Embryos with two maternally derived nuclei (gynogenetic) develop more or less normally for a time, but have very poorly developed extra-embryonic membranes. Embryos with two paternally derived nuclei (androgenetic) have relatively normal extra-embryonic membranes, but highly abnormal embryonic structures. Neither of these conditions is compatible

PRADER-WILLI SYNDROME

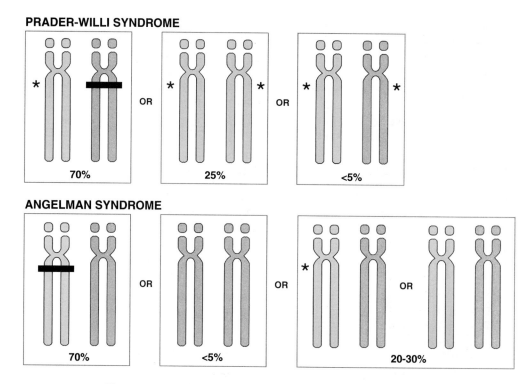

ANGELMAN SYNDROME

Figure 8.23.   Molecular basis for Prader-Willi syndrome (PWS) and Angelman syndrome (AS). Approximately 70 to 75% of patients with PWS have a detectable microdeletion (*black bar*) of a portion of the paternal chromosome 15 (*gray*). The maternal chromosome 15 (*light red*) is methylated (*red asterisk*) at several loci on 15q11–13. About 20 to 25% of PWS patients have maternal uniparental disomy with both maternal homologs methylated and transcriptionally silent. A small number of patients have biparental inheritance of chromosome 15 without a detectable deletion, but show maternal methylation at several loci in the critical region on both chromosomes 15. In AS, 70% of patients have a detectable microdeletion of the maternal chromosome 15; but only less than 5% of patients have paternal uniparental disomy. Biparental inheritance of chromosome 15 with no deletion and with a normal methylation pattern is the most common situation in familial AS. It is assumed that these patients may have point mutations or other subtle abnormalities in the as yet unidentified AS gene on the maternal chromosome 15. Finally, some patients with AS have biparental inheritance with abnormal methylation (absence of normally methylated maternal allele. (Redrawn from a figure provided by D Ledbetter, National Center for Human Genome Research.)

with normal embryonic and fetal development to term. Both maternal and paternal genetic contributions are necessary for normal development and are complementary, consistent with the view that some genes may be differentially activated or inactivated (that is, imprinted) during gametogenesis in the male and female parents. Thus at different loci, only the maternal or paternal gene may be expressed. Further evidence comes from two human conditions. Hydatidiform moles are human placental tumors that have two paternally derived haploid sets of chromosomes, and no maternal chromosomes. Ovarian teratomas, benign tumors that contain multiple differentiated tissues, arise from cells bearing only maternally derived chromosomes in the absence of paternal chromosomes. These conditions again illustrate that the absence of genes from one of the parents results in abnormal development.

The mechanism of imprinting is thought to involve differential methylation of genes during male and female gametogenesis, resulting in transcriptional inactivation. Thus, the deletion of the active allele of a gene (e.g., the paternal allele in PWS) results in structural monosomy for that region, but functional nullisomy, because the maternal allele is not expressed. Uniparental disomy for the chromosome homologue carrying the inactive allele (e.g., maternal disomy in PWS) would result in functional nullisomy despite structural disomy. Genomic imprinting may help to explain differences in the phenotype of chromosome deletion syndromes depending on the parental origin of the deletion, and, for some autosomal dominant disorders, may help to explain incomplete penetrance and differences in severity of the phenotype depending on the parental origin of the mutant allele.

CHROMOSOMAL CHANGES IN NEOPLASIA

In addition to germ line, or constitutional, chromosome abnormalities, there is a growing recognition of the role of somatic cell chromosome abnormalities in a variety of solid cancers and leukemias. One particularly well-understood example is the Burkitt's lymphoma in which there is frequently a reciprocal translocation of a piece of the long arm of chromosome 8 with the long arm of chromosome 14, or less frequently, with the long arm of chromosome 22 or 2. In chronic myelogenous leukemia, a form of leukemia in adults, there is almost always a reciprocal translocation between the long arms of chromosome 9 and 22 (Ph[1] or Philadelphia chromosome). The mechanisms by which these translocations cause malignancy is discussed in chapter 11. Because specific and consistent chromosomal changes are seen in many types of leukemias and lymphomas, chromosome studies, including FISH, are important diagnostic and prognostic tools in their clinical management.

In addition to the somatic cell chromosome abnormalities in cancer, discussed above, there is a group of rare recessively inherited disorders characterized by an abnormally high rate of spontaneous, or induced, chromosomal breakage and an increased risk of leukemia and solid cancers. The mapping and cloning of the genes for these disorders, including Bloom syndrome, Fanconi anemia, and ataxia-telangiectasia, discussed in chapter 11, should improve our understanding of the genetic bases of malignancy.

SEX CHROMOSOMES

"It is as if in the evolution of sex a fragment at one time broke away from an X chromosome . . . and thereafter in relation to the other chromosomes was helpless to prevent them from expressing themselves in the form of an incomplete female, the creature we call the male! It is largely to this original X-chromosome deficiency of the male that almost all the troubles to which the male falls heir may be traced. . ."

—ASHLEY MONTAGU (REPRINTED WITH PERMISSION FROM MONTAGU, ASHLEY. THE NATURAL SUPERIORITY OF WOMEN. MACMILLAN PUBLISHING COMPANY. © 1952, 1953, 1968, 1974 ASHLEY MONTAGU.)

Sex Chromosomes and Sexual Differentiation

The X chromosome is large, containing 6% of the total DNA; the Y chromosome is usually much smaller, though it can vary in size reflecting different amounts of heterochromatin. Almost 250 diseases have been shown to be X-linked, but less than 20 to be Y-linked. More than 300 functional genes and over 10,000 DNA markers have been mapped to the X chromosome, with most of the genes encoding somatic functions. In contrast, although there are now more than 700 DNA markers mapped to the Y chromosome, only 26 genes thus far have been assigned to this chromosome. However, one of these, named *SRY*, plays the critical role of determining gonadal sex.

In early embryonic life, the human fetal gonad is undifferentiated. Germ cells migrate from the yolk sac into the gonad during the 4th week of development, and at approximately 6–7 weeks of development, the gonad undergoes sexual differentiation (Fig. 8.24). In the presence of a Y chromosome the central portion, or medulla, of the gonad develops to become the testis. The testis elaborates two inducers. One is the androgen testosterone, which causes wolffian duct proliferation. These ducts become the male internal genitalia. The other inducer is a nonsteroid glycoprotein called müllerian inhibitory substance, which causes regression of müllerian duct structures. In the absence of a Y chromosome, as in the human XX female, the outer portion or cortex of the gonad develops into the ovary. There is no production of testosterone or of müllerian inhibitory substance. Therefore, there is regression of the wolffian duct structures and proliferation of müllerian duct structures, which form the female internal genitalia including the upper portion of the vagina, the uterus, and the oviducts or fallopian tubes. It is usually the presence or absence of the testis that determines sexual differentiation rather than whether or not an ovary is present. Removal of the gonad in early mammalian fetuses results in development of female internal genitalia.

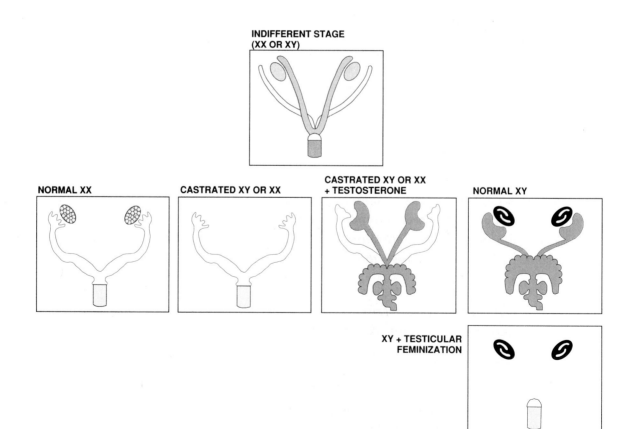

Figure 8.24. Human sexual differentiation. See text for details.

The mechanism of sex determination has been the subject of scientific speculation and investigation since antiquity. It was assumed that sex was determined in humans, as in *Drosophila*, by the ratio of the number of X chromosomes to autosomes. Only in 1959 was it realized that it is the presence or absence of a Y chromosome that determines sex. This was based on the discovery of 47,XXY Klinefelter syndrome individuals who were phenotypically male, and the finding that mice with only a single X chromosome were female.

The specific gene on the Y chromosome responsible for development of the testis has been sought by a study of rare exceptions to the rule that it is the Y chromosome that determines gonadal sex. Males with a 46,XX chromosome constitution, who are phenotypically normal except that they have small testes without spermatogenesis, as in the Klinefelter syndrome discussed below, were studied using a series of DNA probes mapped to various portions of the Y chromosome. It had been hypothesized that these individuals had cryptic Y chromosome sequences on the paternal X chromosome because of a translocation between the X and Y chromosomes. Unlike autosomes, the X and Y chromosomes do not line up side-by-side along their lengths during male meiosis, but rather align in an almost head-to-head orientation (Fig. 8.25). The terminal ends of the short arms of the X and Y chromosomes contain the 2.6-Mb long, so-called pseudoautosomal regions, which are highly homologous, and between which there is extensive recombination during meiosis. It was suggested that a recombination event on the short arm of the Y chromosome, near the pseudoautosomal region boundary, might result in translocation of the testis-determining factor from the Y onto the X. In fact, about 85% of XX males were found to have Y-derived sequences. A 35-kb region of the Y chromosome, immediately adjacent to the pseudoautosomal region, was shown to be the minimal amount of Y chromosome DNA necessary to cause sex reversal in 46,XX individuals (Fig. 8.26). Sequencing of this region identified a single gene, which was named *SRY* for *S*ex-determining *R*egion *Y*. This

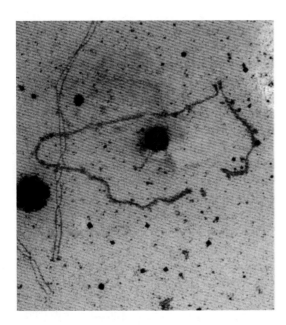

Figure 8.25.   Electron micrograph of the X chromosome (*left*) and Y chromosome (*right*) during the pachytene stage of meiosis I. Note that pairing is limited to the pseudoautosomal region at the end of the short arms of the two chromosomes. (Reprinted with permission from Connor JM, Ferguson-Smith MA. Essential Medical Genetics. 4th ed. Oxford: Blackwell Scientific Publications, 1993.)

Figure 8.26.   Map of the sex-determining region on the Y chromosome. The pseudoautosomal region is shown in *black* and the *SRY* gene in *red*. The *red line* indicates the minimal amount of Y chromosome DNA found in 46,XX males, and the *black line* delineates the region deleted in a 46,XY female. (Redrawn from Affara NA. Sex and the single Y. BioEssays 1991;13:475–478.)

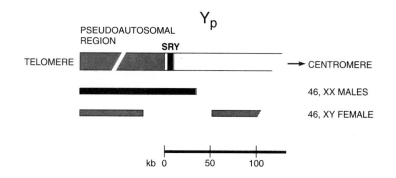

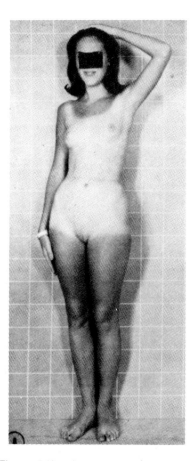

Figure 8.27.   A patient with testicular feminization.   Note the normal female phenotype except for decreased axillary and pubic hair. (Reprinted with permission from Grumbach MM, Van Wyk JJ. Disorders of sex differentiation. In: Wilson JD, Foster DW, eds. Textbook of Endocrinology. 7th ed. Philadelphia: WB Saunders, 1985.)

gene contains a highly conserved DNA-binding domain, homologous to the so-called high mobility group (HMG) protein box, which is known to cause DNA bending and activate gene transcription. Analysis of the pattern of expression of the mouse homologue of this gene, *Sry*, indicated that it was expressed only in somatic cells of the gonadal ridge immediately before the differentiation of the testis, as would be expected for a testis-determining factor. Note that, by convention, human gene symbols are in all capitals (e.g., *SRY*), whereas rodent gene symbols are in lower case except for the first letter (e.g., *Sry*). Proof that *SRY/Sry* is, in fact, the testis-determining factor came from studies in which a 14-kb fragment that included the mouse *Sry* gene was used to produce transgenic mice that contained the normal female XX chromosomes plus 14 kb of the Y chromosome bearing the *Sry* gene. Some of these chromosomal females developed into phenotypic males with testes and normal male mating behavior. Interestingly, these mice were infertile, as is the case with human XX males.

Studies on 46,XY females demonstrated that some had deletions of the *SRY* gene, but others had point mutations or small deletions in the *SRY* gene, virtually all occurring in the HMG box DNA-binding region. More than 20 mutations in the *SRY* gene have now been described, but such mutations account for only 15–20% of XY females. This suggests that mutations in other genes in the testis-determining pathway might account for this phenotype. This is also consistent with *SRY* being a transcription factor, which must activate other genes in the testicular differentiation pathway for normal development of the internal genitalia to occur. Investigation of other rare sex-reversal disorders should help elucidate the steps in this pathway.

External sexual differentiation is the result of the influence of an androgen derivative, 5α-dihydrotestosterone, which causes differentiation of male external genitalia. In individuals with the X-linked mutation testicular feminization, there is androgen insensitivity secondary to an abnormal or deficient androgen receptor and these individuals fail to develop normal male external genitalia. They have testes and a normal female external phenotype (Fig. 8.27) but lack female or male internal genital structures. These women are often detected clinically when they fail to menstruate and investigation reveals a 46,XY karyotype and the presence of testes, usually found in the inguinal region.

X-CHROMOSOME INACTIVATION

Although males are hemizygous for the X chromosome (have only a single copy), the mean amounts of gene products of X-encoded genes such as red blood cell G6PD activity (Fig. 8.28) are the same as in females who have two

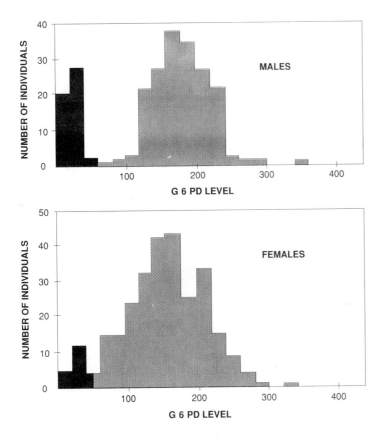

Figure 8.28. Distribution of red cell G6PD activity in a population of black male and female subjects from Nigeria. *Black bars* indicate G6PD-deficient individuals. Note that the distribution of G6PD activity in nondeficient individuals (*red-shaded area*) is essentially the same in males and females. (Redrawn from Harris H. The Principles of Human Biochemical Genetics. 2nd ed. Amsterdam: North-Holland Publishers, 1975.)

X chromosomes. Therefore, there must be some mechanism of dosage compensation. The independent investigations of four geneticists, Mary Lyon, Lianne Russell, Ernest Beutler, and Susumo Ohno, resulted in an understanding of this mechanism that now is called the "Lyon hypothesis" after Mary Lyon, a British geneticist. The Lyon hypothesis (Fig. 8.29) states that in *somatic* cells (*a*) X inactivation occurs **early** in embryonic life (late blastocyst stage in humans); (*b*) the inactivation is **random;** that is, either the paternal or maternal X chromosome may be inactivated; (*c*) X inactivation is **complete,** in that virtually all of the X chromosome is inactivated; and (*d*) X-chromosome inactivation is **permanent and clonally propagated;** that is, if the paternally derived X chromosome is inactivated in a given cell, all of the progeny of that cell will express an active maternally derived X whereas the paternally derived X remains inactive. The result of lyonization is that the female is a **mosaic** (Fig. 8.30) of cells, each functionally hemizygous for one or the other X chromosome.

It should be noted that there are exceptions to the above statements about X inactivation. Although X inactivation is usually random, a structurally abnormal X, e.g., an X chromosome bearing a deletion, is preferentially inactivated. On the other hand, in individuals with balanced X-autosome translocations, it is usually the normal X chromosome that is preferentially inactivated (see chapter 9). Although X inactivation is extensive, it is not complete; more than 16 human genes are known to escape inactivation (Fig. 8.31). These include genes in or near the pseudoautosomal region, as well as genes distant from it. Some, but not all, of these genes have functional Y homologues that might preserve equal dosage between the sexes. It is estimated that up to one-third of genes on the human X chromosome may escape complete inactivation. Finally, it should be noted that

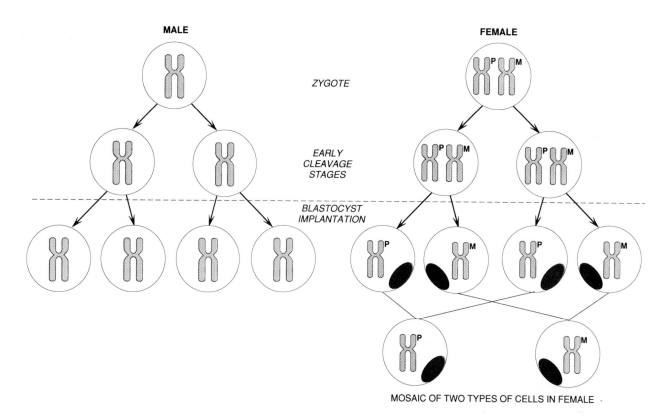

Figure 8.29.   Schematic diagram of the Lyon hypothesis.   *P* represents the paternally derived X chromosome, and *M*, the maternally derived X in the female; the single X in the male must be inherited from the mother. The inactive X is shown as the *dark mass.*

while X inactivation is permanent in most somatic cells, it must be reversible in the development of germ cells.

Several lines of evidence support the Lyon hypothesis. The first came from genetic studies in mice. Female mice heterozygous for an X-linked coat color mutation, e.g., tortoiseshell, were always found to have a mottled coat; that is, they showed patches of tortoiseshell fur and of wild-type fur (Fig. 8.32). In contrast, males hemizygous for this mutant showed uniform tortoiseshell coat color. Calico cats are another familiar example of this phenomenon. Female mice heterozygous for two nonallelic, mutant coat color genes expressed patches of fur containing only one or the other mutant color when the genes were in repulsion (on opposite chromosomes), but patches

Figure 8.30.   Mosaic from the floor of a Roman villa at Pompeii.   Note patches of only black stones and patches of only white.

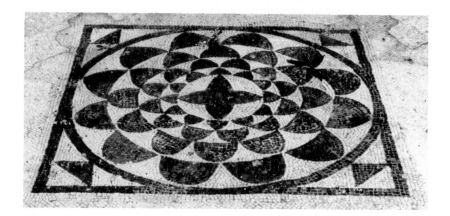

containing a blend of both mutant colors or patches of wild-type fur when the genes were in coupling (on the same X chromosome).

The cytologic evidence for lyonization came first from the serendipitous discovery of sex chromatin, or the Barr body. The Canadian cytologist Murray Barr, studying the morphologic effects of repetitive electrical stimulation on neurons in the cat, noted that the nuclei of neurons from some cats contained an extra dark-staining chromatin body and that these chromatin bodies were found only in female cats. Subsequent studies in humans, using epithelial cells scraped from the buccal mucosa, indicated that the number of sex chromatin bodies is equal to the number of X chromosomes minus one. Normal males who have only one X chromosome have no sex chromatin, whereas normal females with two X chromosomes have one (Fig. 8.33). Individuals with three X chromosomes have two Barr bodies. Later studies showed that during prophase one of the two X chromosomes appeared to be heteropyknotic, i.e., dense and dark-staining, suggestive of inactive chromatin. Finally, studies using thymidine labeling of chromosomes in cultured cells indicated that one of the two X chromosomes replicated late during the S phase of the cell cycle.

The biochemical evidence supporting lyonization came initially from studies on the expression of G6PD in cultured skin fibroblasts from women heterozygous for G6PD A, the common electrophoretic variant of G6PD, and the wild-type G6PD B allele. Mass cultures of fibroblasts expressed both the A and B forms of this enzyme, whereas clones of skin fibroblasts, that is, cell lines derived from a single cell precursor, expressed *either* A or B but never both (Fig. 8.34). Similar clonal expression of biochemical markers has been defined for other X-linked genes, including ornithine transcarbamylase (Fig. 8.35). The correlation of this biochemical evidence with cytologic evidence came from studies in mules, the female hybrid offspring of a cross between a horse and a donkey. Because horse and donkey X chromosomes can be distinguished cytologically and the G6PD activity differentiated electrophoretically, one could correlate, in individual lines of skin fibroblasts cultured from mules, the presence of the horse G6PD when the donkey X chromosome was inactive and vice versa. Taken together, the genetic, cytologic, and biochemical evidence strongly supports the hypothesis that in every somatic cell in a female mammal, only one X chromosome is active.

The significance of the Lyon hypothesis is severalfold. First, it helps to understand the manifestations of X-linked genes and diseases in humans and it accounts for the much greater variability of clinical manifestations in heterozygous females than in hemizygous males. By the same token, it helps explain the considerable difficulties that arise in biochemical carrier detection techniques aimed at identifying female carriers of X-linked diseases. It should be noted that whereas X inactivation is generally random, in any given cell lineage in an individual, significantly skewed patterns of X inactivation may be found. X-chromosome inactivation has also been used as a marker for studies of differentiation and malignant transformation. For example, in a study of uterine fibroids (common, benign smooth muscle tumors arising in the uterus), it was shown that in women heterozygous for G6PD A and B that each fibroid tumor expressed only A or B type G6PD but never both. This was interpreted to indicate that each tumor most likely arose from a single cell. The power of this technique has been markedly increased by the use of X-linked DNA markers. Perhaps most importantly, X inactivation provides an interesting model for the study of gene regulation because it provides an example in which many genes on a chromosome are permanently inactivated.

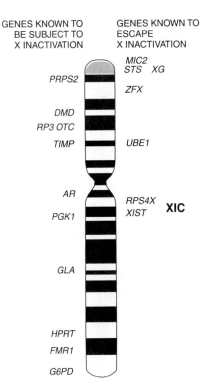

Figure 8.31. Partial map of the human X chromosome depicting genes subject to X inactivation and others that escape X inactivation. *DMD*, dystrophin, the gene that is abnormal in Duchenne muscular dystrophy; *OTC*, ornithine transcarbamylase; *AR*, androgen receptor; *HPRT*, hypoxanthine phosphoribosyltransferase; *G6PD*, glucose-6-phosphate dehydrogenase; *MIC2* and *XG*, genes that encode cell surface proteins; *STS*, steroid sulfatase; *ZFX*, zinc finger X; *RPS4X*, ribosomal subunit protein 4; *XIST*, X-inactive specific transcript. The X-inactivation center (XIC) is the *dark red* band on Xq; the pseudoautosomal region is the *light red* region at Xpter. (Redrawn from Davies K: The essence of inactivity. Nature 1991;349:15–16.)

The mechanism of X inactivation is not fully understood, but certainly involves altered chromatin structure, including differential methylation of DNA and acetylation of histones. The CpG islands (clusters of CpG dinucleotides in the 5′-upstream region of genes) associated with silenced genes on the inactive X chromosome are heavily methylated, whereas their homologous sequences on the active X chromosome are unmethylated; the CpG islands associated with those genes that escape inactivation on the inactive X also remain unmethylated. Genetic analyses of X-chromosome translocations and deletions that alter the pattern of X inactivation have identified an X-inactivation center (XIC) at Xq13.2 (Fig. 8.31), which appears to be required in *cis* for X inactivation to occur. Within the XIC is a candidate gene, *XIST* (*X Inactive-Specific Transcript*, pronounced "exist"), which is uniquely expressed from the *inactive*, but not the active, X chromosome. Thus, its expression is female-specific in karyotypically normal individuals; but in individuals with X-chromosome aneuploidy, the amount of *XIST* transcript is directly proportional to the number of X chromosomes minus one. Inactivation of the *Xist* gene (the mouse homologue of *XIST*) by homologous recombination completely prevents inactivation of the targeted chromosome, demonstrating the requirement for *Xist/XIST* for X inactivation. The *XIST* gene is transcribed into a 17-kb mRNA, which contains no conserved open reading frames (i.e., it contains many stop codons); thus, the product of the *XIST* locus appears to be an untranslated RNA, which may serve a structural role rather than encoding a protein. Interestingly, the *XIST* transcript has been found to be specifically associated with the Barr body in interphase nuclei. The mechanism by which *XIST* initiates and/or maintains X inactivation is as yet unknown.

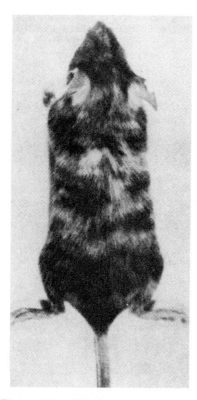

Figure 8.32. Female mouse heterozygous for the X-linked coat color mutation tortoiseshell. (Reprinted with permission from Thompson MW. Genetic consequences of heteropyknosis of an X chromosome. Can J Genet Cytol 1965;7: 202–213.)

Figure 8.33. Sex chromatin body in human buccal mucosa cells. Note that a Barr body (*arrow*) is present in the nucleus of a cell from a female subject (*left*) but not from a male (*right*). (Reprinted with permission from Grumbach MM, Van Wyk JJ. Disorders of sex differentiation. In: Wilson JD, Foster DW, eds. Textbook of Endocrinology. 7th ed. Philadelphia: WB Saunders, 1985.)

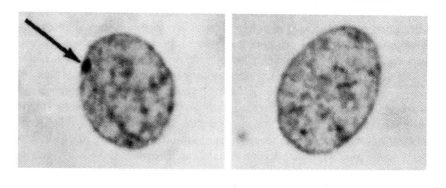

Figure 8.34. Electrophoretic analysis of G6PD in fibroblast cultures from a woman heterozygous for an electrophoretic variant *A* of G6PD. Note that in the mass culture of fibroblasts (*lane 1*) both G6PD A and B are expressed. Clonal isolates of fibroblasts from this mass culture (*lanes 2–10*) express only G6PD A or only B but never both electrophoretic types. (Redrawn from Davidson RG, Nitowsky HN, Childs B. Demonstration of two populations of cells in the human female heterozygous for glucose-6-phosphate dehydrogenase variants. Proc Natl Acad Sci USA 1963;50:481–485.)

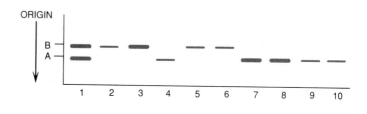

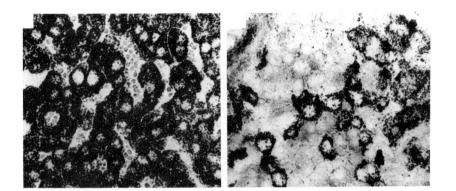

Figure 8.35.   Histochemical staining of or-nithine transcarbamylase (OTC) activity in a liver biopsy from a normal woman (*left*) and a woman heterozygous for OTC defi-ciency (*right*).   The latter had 21% of normal OTC activity as assayed biochemically in this liver biopsy; however, individual cells have ei-ther normal activity (dark staining) or are de-void of activity. (Reprinted with permission from Ricciuti FC, Gelehrter TD, Rosenberg LE: X-Chromosome inactivation in human liver: confirmation of X-linkage or ornithine transcarbamylase. Am J Hum Genet 1976;28: 332–338.)

DISORDERS OF SEX CHROMOSOMES

Klinefelter Syndrome

The Klinefelter syndrome, which occurs in approximately 1 per 1000 male live births, is characterized by postpubertal testicular failure. The patient is a phenotypic male with small testes, hyalinized testicular tubules, and azoospermia (failure to produce normal amounts of sperm), resulting in in-fertility and variable signs of hypogonadism. These individuals are normal in appearance before puberty, but after puberty are recognized by their small testes and occasionally by enlargement of the breasts (gynecomastia) and ab-normal body proportions (Fig. 8.36). Interestingly, individuals with this syn-drome have a greater-than-expected frequency of social pathology, which can range from lack of normal social adjustment to actual difficulties with the law. Significant mental retardation is not usually part of this syndrome, although average IQ may be somewhat reduced. Individuals with the Kline-felter syndrome typically have a 47,XXY chromosome constitution. Their cells are chromatin-positive (that is, they contain a Barr body) and there are at least two Xs and one Y in at least some of their cells. This form of X-chro-mosome aneuploidy is thought to arise from meiotic nondisjunction, occur-ring equally often in the father or mother. Paternal nondisjunction events (which must occur in meiosis I) and maternal meiosis I nondisjunctions show a parental age effect. Some men with the Klinefelter syndrome have been found to have more than two copies of the X chromosome plus a Y, imply-ing more than one nondisjunction event. The more X chromosomes the pa-tient has, the greater the likelihood that there is mental retardation associ-ated with this syndrome.

XYY Syndrome

Because of the social pathology associated with the Klinefelter syndrome, studies were undertaken in mental-penal institutions in the United King-dom to assess the frequency of the 47,XXY karyotypes among inmates in such institutions. This led to the discovery of individuals with aneuploidy of the Y chromosome, for example 47,XYY and 48,XXYY. 47,XYY occurs in approximately 1 in 1000 male live births but was found in 4–20 per 1000 in-mates of mental-penal institutions. The frequency of 48,XXYY, which is as-sociated with the Klinefelter phenotype, was 50 times as high among in-mates as in the newborn population. This has raised the question of whether the extra Y chromosome is causally associated with behavior abnormalities. XYY males have normal sexual development and are fertile. The only phe-notype uniformly associated with the XYY karyotype is tall stature; the mag-

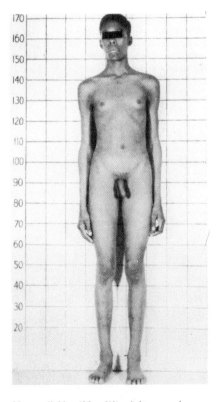

Figure 8.36.   The Klinefelter syndrome. Note that the patient has a normal phallus but has gynecomastia (female-like breast develop-ment). (This photo appeared in J Chronic Dis (July 1960) Feinstein AR, ed., and in Medical Genetics 1958–1960. St. Louis: Mosby, 1961. Reprinted with permission of the editors of the Journal of Chronic Diseases.)

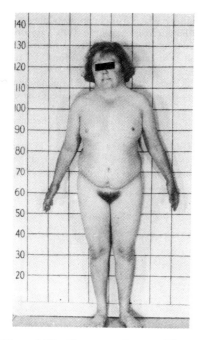

Figure 8.37.   Turner syndrome.   The patient has short stature, webbed neck, shield-shaped chest with wide-spaced nipples and underdeveloped breasts, and an increased carrying angle of the arms. (This photo appeared in J Chronic Dis (July 1960) Feinstein AR, ed., and in Medical Genetics 1958–1960. St. Louis: Mosby, 1961. Reprinted with permission of the editors of the Journal of Chronic Diseases.)

nitude of the increased risk, if any, of social pathology associated with this syndrome is as yet unclear. Aneuploidy of the Y chromosome must arise from meiotic nondisjunction in paternal meiosis.

Turner Syndrome

The Turner syndrome is characterized by a phenotypic female with gonadal dysgenesis and sexual immaturity. Characteristically, these women have primary amenorrhea (failure to menstruate) and infertility. The typical syndrome is also associated with short stature (usually less than 5 feet) and a host of somatic abnormalities including webbing of the neck, swelling of the hands and feet in infancy, increased carrying angle at the elbow, and cardiovascular and renal abnormalities (Fig. 8.37). The frequency of Turner syndrome in liveborn girls is about 1/5000, but the frequency of monosomy X (see below) in conceptuses may be as high as 4%. It is estimated that more than 99% of 45,X conceptuses are spontaneously aborted.

Karyotypically, there is something wrong with the second sex chromosome in at least some of the cells of individuals with Turner syndrome (Table 8.4). Slightly more than half of patients with Turner syndrome are monosomic for the X, i.e., 45,X, and are chromatin-negative. Approximately 15% have structural abnormalities of the X chromosome, including isochromosome X, deletions of portions of the X or ring chromosomes. These individuals have 46 chromosomes and are chromatin-positive; i.e., a Barr body would be present. Another 15% are mosaic for 45,X/46,XX, and an additional 15% are mosaic for a 45,X cell line plus a 46,X, abnormal X cell line or a 47,XXX cell line. The presence of mosaicism indicates that nondisjunction must have occurred during mitosis after fertilization rather than during meiosis. Thus, Turner syndrome can arise from either meiotic nondisjunction (in approximately 80%, the nondisjunction is in paternal meiosis) or from mitotic nondisjunction, the latter resulting in mosaicism.

From studies of patients with Turner syndrome with an abnormal X chromosome it has been suggested that monosomy of the short arm of the X chromosome is responsible for the short stature and somatic abnormalities accompanying this syndrome. However, genes on the long arm of the X may be critical for ovarian development and maintenance. Because only one X chromosome is normally active in the somatic cells of the female, the question arises as to why Turner syndrome occurs at all. It would appear that a gene or genes on the inactive X chromosome (and on the Y chromosome, because XY individuals do not have Turner syndrome) can prevent the clinical manifestations of Turner syndrome. Many years ago, Ferguson-Smith

Table 8.4. Abnormal Karyotypes in Turner Syndrome		
45,X		
46,X, abnormal X		
Deletion	X,Xp−	
Isochromosome	X,i(Xq)	
		Monosomy short arm
		Trisomy long arm
Ring		
Mosaicism		
X/XX		
X/XY		Virilization, gonadoblastoma
X/X, abnormal X		
X/XXX		
X/XX/XXX, etc.		

hypothesized that the genes responsible for Turner syndrome would be X-linked genes that escape X-chromosome inactivation, and that have Y-linked homologues. The *RPS4* gene, which encodes a ribosomal protein subunit, escapes inactivation on the X and has a homologue on the Y, and has been suggested as a possible candidate gene to explain some of the clinical abnormalities in Turner syndrome. It is also possible that two active X chromosomes are required for normal ovarian development in early fetal life; it is known that the inactive X chromosome is reactivated in oogonia when meiosis begins during fetal life.

The ovary is an unusual organ in that there is programed destruction of its major product, eggs. The fetal ovary is thought to contain some 7 million oocytes, which have decreased in number to 3 million at the time of birth. By the time of menarche, or onset of menses, the number has fallen to approximately 400,000 and by menopause it is around 10,000. Individuals with Turner syndrome have oocytes during fetal life but they are virtually gone by the age of 2 years; menopause has occurred before menarche.

From the study of patients with Turner syndrome with mosaicism, it is known that the presence of a normal 46,XX cell line mollifies the disorder and there have been rare patients with 46,XX/45,X mosaicism who have had normal menses and even fertility. The presence of an XY cell line (found in approximately 5% of patients with Turner syndrome) may be associated with virilization at birth and again at puberty, and more significantly, a 20% risk of malignancy of the dysgenic gonad. It is interesting to consider that women with 46,XY/45,X Turner syndrome mosaicism must have arisen as male zygotes who then underwent a mitotic nondisjunctional event resulting in Turner syndrome.

X-Linked Mental Retardation and Fragile X

When peripheral blood lymphocyte cultures are deprived of folate, or thymidine metabolism is perturbed, apparent breaks or gaps in chromosomes, so-called fragile sites, can be observed. Using these techniques, a folate-sensitive fragile site was described at Xq27.3 in males affected with a form of X-linked mental retardation that came to be known as the fragile X syndrome. The fragile X syndrome is characterized by facial abnormalities, including a narrow face with prominent forehead, jaw, and ears (Fig. 8.38), macroorchidism (large testes) in 90% of postpubertal affected males, mild connective tissue abnormalities, and most importantly, moderate to severe mental retardation. Affected females usually have milder manifestations. Cytogenetically, the fragile site, designated FRAXA (*FRA*gile site, *X* chromosome, *A* site) at Xq27.3 is demonstrable in about 50% of metaphase spreads in virtually all clinically affected males and most affected females (Fig. 8.39). The fragile X syndrome affects approximately 1 per 1250 males and approximately 1 in 2000 females, and affects all ethnic groups. Thus, the fragile X syndrome is the most common inherited form of mental retardation in humans.

Although the pattern of inheritance of the fragile X syndrome is clearly X linked, there are a number of features at variance with simple X-linked inheritance. Most males who carry the mutation are mentally retarded and show the cytogenetic abnormality, but fully 20% of obligatory carrier males are phenotypically and cytogenetically normal, so-called normal transmitting males. On the other hand, as many as one-third of heterozygous females are clinically affected, but mental retardation occurs in such a carrier female only if the mutation is inherited from her mother, not when it is inherited

Figure 8.38. Forty-five-year-old man with fragile X syndrome. Note the long face with prominent ears, jaw, and forehead. (Reprinted with permission from Jacobs PA, Glover TW, Mayer M, Fox P, Gerrard JW, Dunn HG, Herbst DS. X-Linked mental retardation: a study of 7 families. Am J Med Genet 1980;7:471–489.)

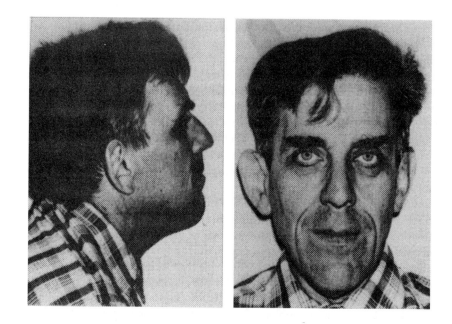

from a normal transmitting father. Most strikingly, the risk of mental retardation is much higher in the grandchildren of a normal transmitting male than in his siblings. Thus, the penetrance of the disorder, or risk of clinical manifestations, appears to be a function of position in the pedigree, and appears to increase in successive generations showing the phenomenon of anticipation. This unusual behavior of the fragile X syndrome in pedigrees has been called the **Sherman paradox** (Fig. 8.40).

The explanation for this paradox came from the cloning and characterization of the gene involved, designated *Fragile X Mental Retardation-1* (*FMR1*). The *FMR1* gene occupies 38 kb at Xq27.3, contains 17 exons, and appears to encode an RNA-binding protein. In the untranslated first exon,

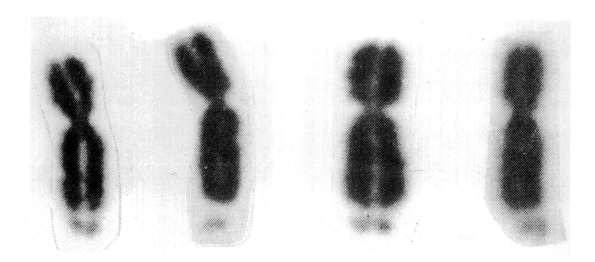

Figure 8.39. Partial karyotype (showing only the X chromosome) from peripheral blood leukocyte cultures from four males with mental retardation and the fragile X syndrome. (Reprinted with permission from Jacobs PA, Glover TW, Mayer M, Fox P, Gerrard JW, Dunn HG, Herbst DS. X-Linked mental retardation: a study of 7 families. Am J Med Genet 1980;7:471–489.)

a polymorphic CGG triplet repeat was found, which normally varies in size from 6 to 52 repeats, with a mode of 30 (Fig. 8.41). In affected patients with the fragile X syndrome, this repeat has undergone a massive expansion to hundreds or even thousands of CGG repeats. When the number of repeats exceeds about 230, the 5′ end of the *FMR1* gene becomes hypermethylated and transcription is shut off. The absence of *FMR1* mRNA and protein is thought to be responsible for the clinical manifestations of this syndrome. The expanded repeat is also highly unstable during mitosis, and affected individuals show extensive somatic mosaicism with respect to the number of repeats in different tissues. All males who have the full mutation are clinically affected, as are approximately 50% of females who are heterozygous for the full mutation; presumably, the probability of females being clinically affected reflects the pattern of X inactivation.

Most female carriers of the fragile X syndrome have intermediate numbers of CGG repeats, ranging from approximately 50 to 230. In this range, the 5′ region of the FMR1 gene is unmethylated and the gene is transcriptionally active. This situation, called a *premutation*, is also found in normal transmitting males. The premutation is unstable when transmitted, and for unknown reasons, the number of repeats appears to increase more strikingly when the premutation is transmitted by the mother than when it is transmitted by the father. The risk that there will be expansion from the premutation to full mutation in maternal meiosis is proportional to the number of repeats; this risk is less than 20% when the number of repeats is less than 70, but is greater than 99% for repeat lengths more than 90. Thus, no full mutations arise from normal length repeats, but only from premutations. Affected females are the daughters of premutation mothers and not premutation fathers; and, because the size of the triplet repeat tends to increase as it is transmitted through a pedigree, the penetrance of the clinical syndrome appears to increase in subsequent generations. Thus, the triplet repeat expansion explains the Sherman paradox.

The diagnosis of fragile X syndrome should be considered in any child with undiagnosed developmental retardation or mental retardation. Now that the molecular basis of this condition is understood, molecular diagnostic

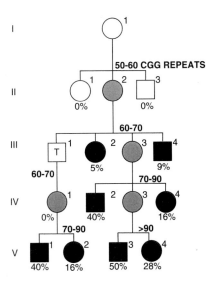
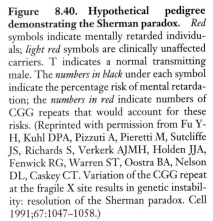

Figure 8.40. Hypothetical pedigree demonstrating the Sherman paradox. *Red* symbols indicate mentally retarded individuals; *light red* symbols are clinically unaffected carriers. T indicates a normal transmitting male. The *numbers in black* under each symbol indicate the percentage risk of mental retardation; the *numbers in red* indicate numbers of CGG repeats that would account for these risks. (Reprinted with permission from Fu Y-H, Kuhl DPA, Pizzuti A, Pieretti M, Sutcliffe JS, Richards S, Verkerk AJMH, Holden JJA, Fenwick RG, Warren ST, Oostra BA, Nelson DL, Caskey CT. Variation of the CGG repeat at the fragile X site results in genetic instability: resolution of the Sherman paradox. Cell 1991;67:1047–1058.)

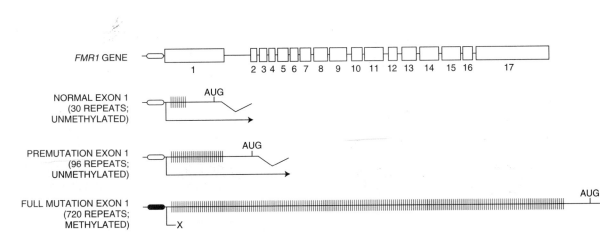

Figure 8.41. Diagram of the *FMR1* gene and the first exon in normal, premutation, and full mutation alleles. The *oval* immediately to the left of the start site of transcription represents the promoter region of the *FMR1* gene. The *open* symbol represents active transcription, and the *black* symbol, silenced transcription. The *vertical lines* indicate CGG trinucleotides upstream of the methionine codon (AUG) at the translational start site. (Reprinted with permission from Warren ST, Nelson DL. Advances in molecular analysis of fragile X syndrome. JAMA 1994;271:536–542.)

techniques are available that are considerably more efficient and reliable than cytogenetic analyses. The preferred method for detecting the full mutation is Southern blot analysis of DNA from blood or other tissue obtained postnatally or prenatally. The DNA is typically digested with two restriction enzymes, one of which is sensitive to the methylation state of the DNA so that analysis of methylation can be carried out, as well as assessment of the size of the triplet repeat (Fig. 8.42). Accurate determination of the repeat size of normal and of premutation alleles, however, is best carried out by PCR techniques (Fig. 8.43). Unlike many of the genetic diseases discussed in this book, fragile X syndrome is atypical in that the vast majority of patients have a defined type of mutation, namely expanded triplet repeats, in a specific location within the *FMR1* gene, the 5′ untranslated first exon. This greatly simplifies molecular diagnostic testing. Standard cytogenetic analysis, however, should still be carried out to rule out any other chromosome abnormalities that might explain a patient's clinical state. Because of the high frequency of the fragile X syndrome, genetic screening programs are under consideration. Preliminary studies using antibodies to FMR1 protein suggest that it may be possible to screen for the presence or absence of the gene product.

The discovery of the molecular basis of the fragile X syndrome, and the role of triplet repeats and dynamic mutations in this condition, not only explained the peculiar patterns of inheritance encompassed by the Sherman paradox, but was quickly followed by the discovery of triplet repeat expansion in a number of other genetic diseases (Fig. 8.44). The role of CTG repeats in the 3′ untranslated region of the myotonin gene in myotonic dystrophy has been discussed in chapter 3, as was the expansion of CAG repeats

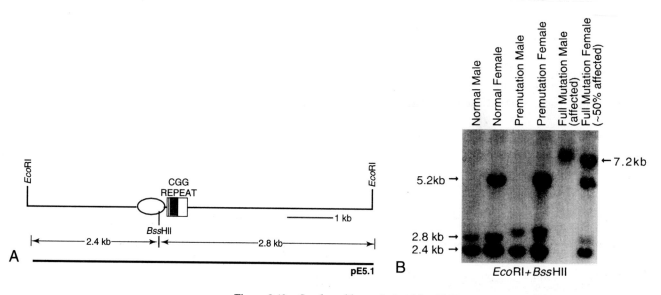

Figure 8.42. Southern blot analysis of the *FMR1* gene. The *left panel* shows a diagram of the *FMR1* gene. The *oval* represents the promoter region; the *box*, the first exon, with the region of triplet repeats in *red*. The *Eco*RI fragment is normally 5.2 kb in length. *Bss*HII activity is sensitive to the methylation status of the DNA, and cuts only unmethylated DNA. The *right panel* shows an example of a Southern blot of DNA cleaved with both *Eco*RI and *Bss*HII, and hybridized with the probe pE5.1. A 5.2-kb band is observed from the inactive X (on which *FMR1* is normally methylated), whereas two smaller (2.8- and 2.4-kb) bands are observed from the active X of the female and the single X of the normal male. As seen in the diagram, the CGG repeat lies within the 2.8-kb fragment, and, thus, premutation males and females show a slightly larger band than the normal 2.8-kb band. Full mutation males demonstrate a markedly enlarged and methylated band, while full mutation females display the three bands of the normal female pattern plus an additional larger band reflecting the methylated and expanded *FMR1* mutation. (From Warren ST, Nelson DL. Advances in molecular analysis of fragile X syndrome. JAMA 1994;271:536–542.)

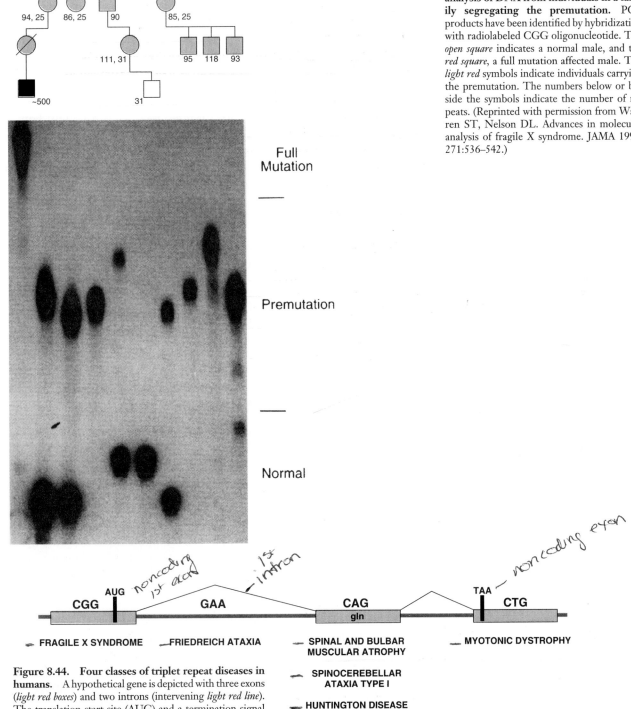

Figure 8.43. Polymerase chain reaction analysis of DNA from individuals in a family segregating the premutation. PCR products have been identified by hybridization with radiolabeled CGG oligonucleotide. The *open square* indicates a normal male, and the *red square*, a full mutation affected male. The *light red* symbols indicate individuals carrying the premutation. The numbers below or beside the symbols indicate the number of repeats. (Reprinted with permission from Warren ST, Nelson DL. Advances in molecular analysis of fragile X syndrome. JAMA 1994; 271:536–542.)

Figure 8.44. Four classes of triplet repeat diseases in humans. A hypothetical gene is depicted with three exons (*light red boxes*) and two introns (intervening *light red line*). The translation start site (AUG) and a termination signal (TAA) are indicated by the *red vertical bars*. In fragile X syndrome, CGG repeats are found in 5'-untranslated region of the first exon of *FMR1*. In Friedreich's ataxia, GAA repeats are found in the first intron of *X25*, the gene encoding frataxin. In Huntington's disease and the other neurodegenerative diseases listed, CAG repeats are found in exons, and encode an elongated polyglutamine tract. In myotonic dystrophy, CTG repeats are found in the 3'-untranslated region of the last exon of the DM protein kinase (myotonin) gene. (Redrawn from Warren ST: The expanding world of trinucleotide repeats. Science 1996;271:1374–1375.)

encoding polyglutamine tracts in the coding region of genes involved in Huntington disease and other neurodegenerative diseases. It is noteworthy that the mechanism by which the triplet repeat causes disease is apparently different among these conditions. In fragile X syndrome, there is hypermethylation and silencing of transcription resulting in a loss of function; in the case of the dominantly inherited neurodegenerative disorders, an abnormal protein is produced, and in the case of myotonic dystrophy, the pathogenesis, while not yet understood, may involve altered mRNA stability. Very recently, a unique fourth class of triplet repeat diseases has been discovered. Friedreich ataxia, an autosomal *recessive* neurodegenerative disease characterized by ataxia (incoordination), dysarthria (slurred speech), and cardiac problems, is caused by expansion of a GAA repeat in the first *intron* of the X25 gene encoding frataxin. This expansion, from 10–20 copies in normal individuals to 200–900 copies in patients, may interfere with processing of frataxin heterogeneous nuclear RNA by creating multiple AG splice acceptor sites, resulting in absence of mature mRNA in the cytoplasm.

X-Autosome Translocations

Occasionally, reciprocal translocation can occur between the X chromosome and one of the autosomes. These accidents of nature have turned out to be very useful for gene mapping (as discussed in chapter 9 with respect to Duchenne muscular dystrophy) and in understanding karyotype-phenotype correlations. Presumably, during the breakage and rejoining of chromosomal segments there is either loss of some chromosomal material or breakage within a gene on the X chromosome. Because the normal X chromosome is preferentially inactivated in cases of X-autosome translocation, females heterozygous for such a translocation may express X-linked recessive diseases otherwise observed only in hemizygous males.

Indications for Chromosome Analysis (Table 8.5)

1. Known or Suspected Chromosome Abnormality. It is imperative that any patient with a known or suspected chromosome abnormality have the diagnosis made or confirmed by a karyotypic analysis. Even experienced physicians may miss the diagnosis of Down syndrome in a newborn, for example. These serious disorders deserve the most accurate diagnostic procedures available and there is no reason not to perform such a study. As discussed above, it is also important in the case of Down syndrome to determine whether the individual has trisomy 21 or an unbalanced translocation that might be inherited from a balanced carrier parent.

2. Multiple Congenital Anomalies, Especially When Associated with Growth and/or Mental Retardation. Because the characteristic phenotype of major chromosome abnormalities is the combination of growth retardation, mental retardation, and somatic abnormalities, this combination

Table 8.5. Indications for Karyotype
Known or suspected chromosome abnormality
Multiple congenital anomalies and/or growth and mental retardation
Disorder of sexual differentiation
Undiagnosed mental retardation
Selected hematologic malignancies
Multiple miscarriages

should always suggest the possibility of a chromosome abnormality and a karotype should be done. Subtle abnormalities may require prometaphase analysis or FISH, when available, for microdeletion syndromes.

3. Disorders of Sexual Differentiation. These conditions, discussed earlier in this chapter, require a definition of chromosomal sex for accurate diagnosis and management of the condition. Rapid and accurate diagnosis of aneuploidy of sex chromosomes and autosomes can be accomplished by FISH analysis of mitotic or interphase cells.

4. Undiagnosed Mental Retardation. The frequency of the fragile X syndrome requires that this condition be sought in both X-linked mental retardation as well as in any patient with undiagnosed mental retardation. Chromosome analysis is an essential part of the evaluation, in addition to molecular diagnostics.

5. Hematologic Malignancies and Diseases Associated with Chromosome Instability. The frequent finding of specific chromosome abnormalities in certain hematologic malignancies has established the value of chromosome studies in diagnosis and in prognosis of these disorders. In addition there are certain genetic diseases associated with chromosome instability and a high risk of leukemia and other malignancies.

6. Multiple Miscarriages. In approximately 5% of couples who have had two or more spontaneous abortions, one or the other parent carries a balanced translocation. The assumption is that the unbalanced state might account for the spontaneous abortions, although this has rarely been proven. Nevertheless, the detection of such couples would be an indication to monitor future pregnancies by prenatal diagnosis.

Finally, chromosome studies are not usually indicated in cases of clearcut Mendelian diseases, which generally do not have detectable chromosome abnormalities. In rare instances, however (see chapter 9), a chromosomal translocation breaking within a single gene may produce a dominantly inherited disorder, and it should be remembered that a small chromosomal deletion may segregate within a family in exactly the same fashion as a single gene, dominant Mendelian trait. With the development of newer techniques for improved resolution of structural abnormalities of chromosomes, diseases not previously thought to be associated with chromosomal changes may indeed be found to have such changes.

SUGGESTED READINGS

Belmont JW. Genetic control of X-inactivation and processes leading to X-inactivation skewing. Am J Hum Genet 1996;58:1101–1108. *A concise, current review of the mechanism of X chromosome inactivation and its variations.*

Emanuel BS. The use of fluorescence *in situ* hybridization to identify human chromosomal anomalies. Growth Genet Horm 1993;9:6–12. *A clear discussion, with useful diagrams, of the rationale and uses of FISH analysis.*

Epstein CJ. Down syndrome (trisomy 21). In: Scriver CR, Beaudet AL, Sly WS, Valle D, eds. The Metabolic and Molecular Bases of Inherited Disease. 7th ed. New York: McGraw-Hill, 1995:749–794. *A thoughtful and comprehensive review of the clinical, cytogenetic, and molecular aspects of Down syndrome.*

Ferguson-Smith MA, Goodfellow PN. SRY and primary sex-reversal syndromes. In: Scriver CR, Beaudet AL, Sly WS, Valle D, eds. The Metabolic and Molecular Bases of Inherited Disease. 7th ed. New York: McGraw-Hill, 1995:739–748. *A brief summary of sex reversal syndromes, and a clear explanation of the experiments leading to the discovery of SRY.*

Gardner RJM, Sutherland GR. Chromosome Abnormalities and Genetic Counseling. New York: Oxford University Press, 1989. *A useful book for dealing with counseling issues related to chromosome abnormalities; unfortunately written before the discovery of triplet repeat disorders, or of the use of FISH.*

Hassold TJ. Chromosome abnormalities in human reproductive wastage. Trends Genet

Figure 9.1. Linkage of the Duffy blood group to chromosome 1. A pair of number 1 chromosomes from two different individuals is shown in **A.** These studies, done before the advent of chromosome banding, detect a remarkable increase in length below the centromere, referred to as a heteromorphism, in one of the pair of chromosomes on the *left.* The chromosomes on the *right* show the more usual morphology. The pedigree in **B** shows the pattern of inheritance for the Duffy blood group and the chromosome 1 heteromorphism. The half-solid *symbols* indicate the presence of the heteromorphism on chromosome 1, and the *a* and *b* designations indicate the Duffy blood group genotypes. Although the individuals in generation I are of unknown status, in the rest of the pedigree it can be seen that the chromosome with the heteromorphism universally travels with the a allele at the Duffy locus. (Adapted from Donahue RP, Bias WB, Renwick JH, McKusick VA. Probable assignment of the Duffy blood group locus to chromosome 1 in man. Proc Natl Acad Sci USA 1968;61:949–955.)

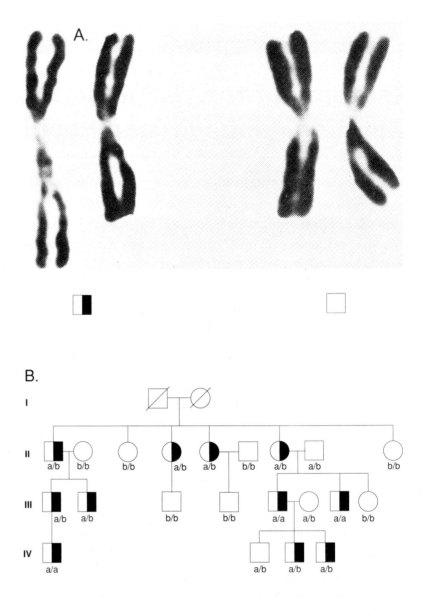

Since Donahue's observation in 1968, dramatic advances in molecular genetic technology have led to the successful mapping of more than 16,000 human genes. Most of these genes have been placed on the human genetic map very recently through the large-scale, cooperative efforts of the Human Genome Project (see chapter 10).

Linkage Analysis

Donahue's localization of the Duffy blood group locus to chromosome 1 is an early example of genetic linkage analysis. This approach maps a gene by analysis of its proximity to another locus on the same chromosome. Such loci are then said to be "linked."

Donahue's method could hardly be generalized to the mapping of large numbers of genes, depending as it did on the occurrence of a visible chromosome heteromorphism that does not occur on most chromosomes. Mapping of human disease genes is currently performed primarily by genetic linkage studies using a well-characterized set of polymorphic DNA markers much more abundant and informative than the single chromosome 1 heteromorphism used by Donahue, but nonetheless relying on the same fundamental genetic principles.

In order to understand the concept of linkage analysis, it is essential to have a firm grasp on the events that occur during meiosis I, especially as regards crossing over. In Figure 9.2, a pair of homologous chromosomes is shown undergoing meiosis. In the *left-hand* part of the figure, the two loci being followed, designated A (or a) and B (or b), are far apart on the chromosome, which makes it likely that a crossover will occur between them. Such a crossover, shown at the *bottom*, produces chromosomes that have swapped or recombined their alleles. In this example, what began as a chromosome with A and B alleles and a chromosome with a and b alleles results in all 4 possible combinations after meiosis.

The same crossover is shown on the *right-hand side* of the figure, now with the two loci closer together. As a result, A stays with B and a with b. As this figure illustrates, recombination between two loci is less common, the closer they are to each other. Thus, recombination between two loci can be used as a rough measure of their distance apart.

The use of this approach to follow the inheritance of a Mendelian disease is illustrated in Figure 9.3. The principle of the approach is simple: if the disease locus is quite close to a polymorphic locus (often called the "**marker locus**") whose inheritance can be followed in an affected family, it is possible to predict who is going to be affected by following the inheritance of the marker locus. The chance of being mistaken in this analysis is a function of how far apart the marker locus and the disease locus are. In the figure, the father is affected with a dominant disorder; hence, his genotype is DN at the disease locus, whereas his normal wife is NN. At the marker locus, he happens to be Aa, whereas his wife is AA. Looking at his offspring, all but II-4 show perfect linkage of the disease locus and the marker locus, because all of those who have inherited the father's A allele have also inherited the disease gene, and all who inherited the a allele inherited the normal allele at the disease locus. In fact, one would need this sort of information to determine that the disease gene in the father is on the same chromosome as the A allele at the marker locus; this is called "determining the **phase**" of these two loci.

Individual II-4, however, is an exception. This offspring is affected with the disease, but inherited an a allele from his father. This is an example of **recombination** between these two loci.

It is important to appreciate in this sort of analysis that the allele at the marker locus is not in itself the cause of the disease. Thus, for example, finding an individual with genotype AA at the marker locus in some other family with no history of this disease would not indicate that that individual has the disease (I-2 is an example of this). An important corollary is that linkage analysis to follow the inheritance of a disease gene can in general only be performed when several family members are available, including some who are affected with the disease. Furthermore, the analysis shown in Figure 9.3 would have been impossible if the father were homozygous AA or aa because, in that instance, one could not distinguish his two chromosomes at the marker locus. Hence, in linkage analysis, the most useful marker loci are those that are highly polymorphic.

The distance between two loci is defined in genetic terms in units of **centiMorgans** (cM). If two loci are 1 cM apart, there is a 1% chance of recombination between these loci as the chromosome is passed from parent to child. Thus, one can think of centiMorgans as a rough unit of distance along the chromosome, although the relation to physical distance is not truly lin-

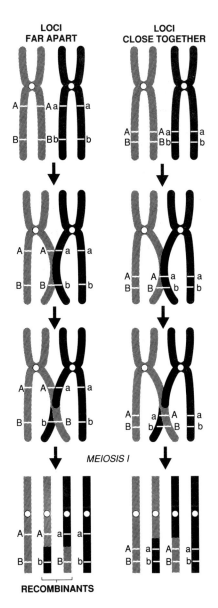

Figure 9.2. Crossing over between homologous chromosomes in meiosis. On the *left* is shown an example in which two loci are relatively far apart, such that recombination is likely to occur between them. On the *right* is shown a situation in which two loci are close together, such that recombination between them will be a rarer event.

Figure 9.9.   Use of human-rodent somatic cell hybrids for gene mapping.   The human chromosome content of human-mouse hybrid clones prepared as illustrated in Figure 9.7 are determined by karyotype analysis. A gene of interest can now be mapped by analyzing DNA prepared from the individual hybrid clones by Southern blotting or PCR to identify those clones that contain the sequence of interest. The Southern blot hybridization or PCR reaction must identify specific bands unique to the human sequence, distinguishing it from the endogenous mouse sequence. Similarly, protein prepared from the cells can be analyzed to identify hybrid clones containing the human gene of interest, as long as it is expressed in these cells and a specific assay exists to distinguish the human and mouse proteins. In the example shown here, a starch gel electrophoresis assay distinguishes the human marker from the endogenous mouse protein. Those hybrids giving a positive signal for the human DNA sequence or protein must contain the chromosome from which this is derived. (Adapted from Shows TB, Sakaguchi AY, Naylor SL. Mapping the human genome, cloned genes, DNA polymorphisms, and inherited disease. Adv Hum Genet 1982;12:341–452.)

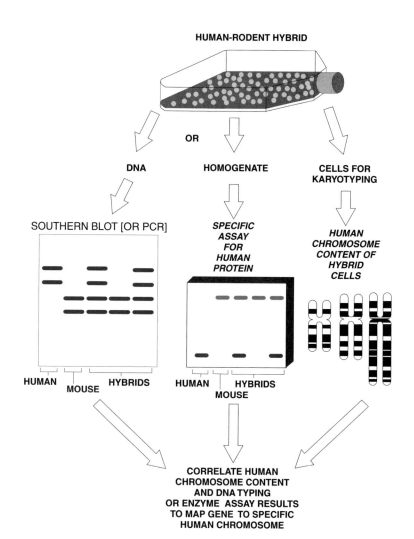

grate into the rodent chromosomes and subsequently be stably carried in the corresponding cell line. The hybrid cells are referred to as radiation hybrids. When a large panel of radiation hybrid cell lines is screened by Southern blotting or PCR for the presence of two genes of interest, as illustrated in Figure 9.10, the frequency with which the two genes are identified in the same cell line will depend on how close to each other they were on the original human chromosome. The farther apart the two genes, the greater the likelihood that they will be separated by the radiation fragmentation procedure. In contrast, genes that are very close to each other will almost always be located on the same fragment. This analysis could be viewed as a specialized form of linkage. Since each hybrid cell line contains many different human chromosome fragments from multiple chromosomes, interpretation of these data is very complex and requires sophisticated computer programs. However, this approach can provide powerful information about the relative positions of large numbers of genes and has become an important tool in the Human Genome Project.

DOSAGE

It is also possible to map a gene to a specific chromosome if cell lines are available that have varying numbers of that particular chromosome. This has

Table 9.1.   Mapping a DNA Probe Using Somatic Cell Hybrids

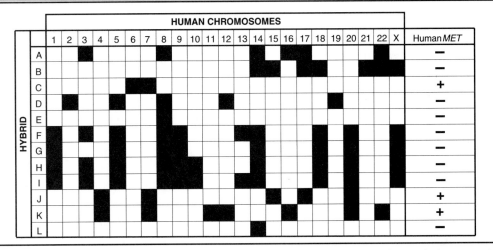

		1	2	3	4	5	6	7	8	9	10	11	12	13	14	15	16	17	18	19	20	21	22	X	Human *MET*
HYBRID	A																								−
	B																								−
	C																								+
	D																								−
	E																								−
	F																								−
	G																								−
	H																								−
	I																								−
	J																								+
	K																								+
	L																								−

A panel of somatic cell hybrids (A-L), each of which contains 1–11 human chromosomes in a rodent background, has been used to score for the presence of the cloned human *MET* oncogene. The *MET* probe is positive in hybrids C, J, and K, which could occur only if the *MET* gene is on chromosome 7. (Used with permission from Cooper CS, Park M, Blair DG, et al. Molecular cloning of a new transforming gene from a chemically transformed human cell line. Nature 1984;311:29–33. © 1984, Macmillan Magazines Ltd.)

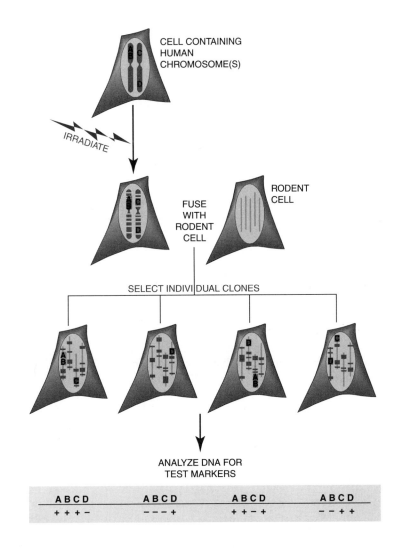

Figure 9.10.   Generation of a radiation hybrid mapping panel.   The preparation of radiation hybrids is similar to the process described for whole chromosome somatic cell hybrids in Figure 9.7. A full set of human chromosomes can be used as the source, or alternatively, the procedure can start with a somatic cell hybrid carrying only one or a few human chromosomes. The human chromosomes are fragmented by irradiation, with higher doses creating smaller fragments. After fusion to a rodent cell, multiple human chromosomal fragments are stably incorporated into the rodent chromosomes. Each resulting somatic cell hybrid line carries many human fragments from multiple chromosomes. Two genes located near each other in the human chromosome are more likely to end up together on the same fragment. Loci that are very close together, indicated by the "A" and "B" in the red segment, will almost always be contained in the same fragment, whereas loci that are farther apart, such as "C" and "D", will more often be separated by the random fragmentation of the irradiation process. Thus, very much like linkage analysis, the frequency with which two genetic loci are identified in the same somatic cell hybrid clone is inversely related to their physical separation in the genome. In practice, a radiation hybrid mapping panel generally contains hundreds of individual clones.

Figure 9.11. Use of dosage to map a DNA probe to the X chromosome. DNA in *lane 1* was obtained from an individual with a 49,XXXXY karyotype, whereas that depicted in *lane 2* is from a normal female, and that in *lane 3* is from a normal male. *Lane 4* contains DNA from a male (B.B.) with a small deletion within the short arm of the X chromosome (see Figure 9.19). Probe p4B12 is on an autosome and therefore detects similar intensity signals in all *four lanes*. Probe pERT87 is located on the short arm of the X chromosome within the region deleted in B.B. It can be seen that the intensity of the signal in the other *three lanes* is a function of the number of X chromosomes, confirming that this probe is located on the X. (Used with permission from Kunkel LM, Monaco AP, Middlesworth W, et al. Specific cloning of DNA fragments absent from the DNA of a male patient with an X chromosome deletion. Proc Natl Acad Sci USA 1985;82:4778–4782.)

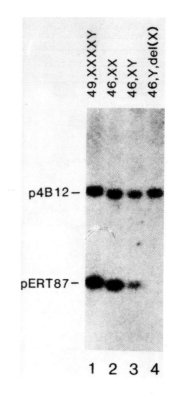

been most useful for the X chromosome, by taking advantage of cell lines from individuals who have anywhere from one to four X chromosomes, as shown in Figure 9.11. If the amount of DNA in each lane of the Southern blot has been carefully kept constant, a probe located on the X chromosome (pERT87) will be four times more intense in the 49,XXXXY cell line than in the 46,XY line. An autosomal probe (p4B12), on the other hand, will look the same in all of these lanes.

The Human Major Histocompatibility Complex

We have considered the general features of polymorphic loci in humans, as well as their usefulness in genetic mapping. The human major histocompatibility complex (MHC, also frequently called HLA for human leukocyte antigen), first introduced in chapter 4, is worthy of special attention because of its high degree of polymorphism and relation to disease, particularly immunologic disorders. The structure of the HLA locus is shown schematically in Figure 9.12. The human MHC is located on the short arm of chromosome 6, occupying about 4 megabases of DNA.

The MHC class I and class II genes encode closely related proteins that reside on the cell surface and are members of the immunoglobulin supergene family. They are involved in the processing and presentation of self and foreign protein, respectively, as antigens to the immune system. These functions are essential for the control of the T-cell immune response as well as antibody production by B cells. The HLA class III region is a segment of approximately 1 megabase between class I and class II that contains at least 12 genes, many of which also play roles in host defense, including three complement genes and the genes for the cytokines tumor necrosis factor α and β. There are at least 23 class II genes and 15 class I genes, although the functions of many of these genes remain to be determined.

The class I and class II genes are the most polymorphic loci in the mammalian genome. There are at least 57 variants of HLA-A, 111 for HLA-B,

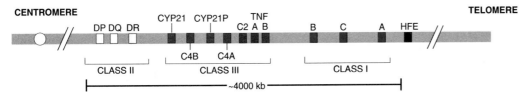

Figure 9.12.   Diagram of the human major histocompatibility complex on the short arm of chromosome 6.   Though not drawn to scale, the relative locations of some of the important genes in this complex are illustrated here, including the HLA A, B, and C class I genes and the DP, DQ, and DR class II genes. Congenital adrenal hyperplasia as a result of 21-hydroxylase deficiency has long been known to be linked to HLA. The molecular basis for this disease is often a rearrangement between the 21-hydroxylase gene, CYP21, which lies in the class III region, and its nearby, highly homologous pseudogene, CYP21P. C2, C4A, and C4B are components of the complement system and the TNFA and B genes encode the cytokines tumor necrosis factor α and β. (The latter is now referred to as lymphotoxin A.) HFE is the gene for genetic hemochromatosis.

and 34 for HLA-C. The high degree of polymorphism in the HLA genes may be maintained by natural selection as the result of differences among the various alleles in the level of protection against infectious disease pathogens. Differences between the HLA genes of mother and child may also be an important factor in the maintenance of fetal and placental tissues during pregnancy.

The inheritance of HLA alleles precisely follows the expectation for a codominant Mendelian system. Figure 9.13 shows a nuclear family with a typical inheritance pattern. HLA typing is used in a number of clinical settings, most importantly for identifying potential donors for organ transplantation. For this analysis, the specific alleles are routinely identified at the HLA-A, HLA-B, HLA-C (all class I) and at the HLA-DR (class II) loci. HLA analysis was originally performed by serotyping using antibodies that specifically identified each allele. These antibodies were generally derived from the sera of women after multiple pregnancies in which antibodies had developed against the foreign HLA antigens of the fetus. Serotyping techniques are gradually being replaced with DNA-based analysis. Crossovers

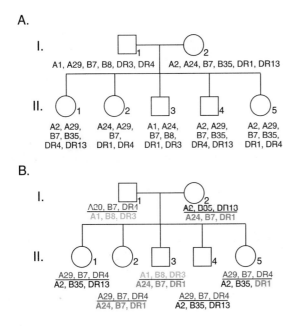

Figure 9.13.   Analysis of HLA typing data. **A** shows the results of HLA typing of two parents and five offspring. The typing itself does not completely establish the genotype, as one must determine which A, B, and DR alleles are on the same chromosomes. This is referred to as "haplotyping," and has been done in **B.** Haplotyping is accomplished by inspection of the alleles present in the offspring and parents. For example, individual II-1 must have inherited the A29, B7, and DR4 alleles from her father and the A2, B35, and DR13 alleles from her mother. This establishes A29, B7, DR4 as one of the haplotypes for I-1 and, as a result, A1, B8, DR3 as the other haplotype. Similar reasoning unambiguously establishes the haplotypes for all of the individuals in this pedigree. Individual II-5 demonstrates a recombination on the maternal haplotype, between B35 and DR13. This figure only shows HLA typing for the A, B, and DR loci. However, in clinical practice, typing information is often also available for C and DQ.

occurring between the most telomeric of these genes (HLA-A) and the most centromeric (DR) do occur, because the genetic distance between them is approximately 3 cM (corresponding well to the known physical distance of approximately 3 megabases). Such recombination events can be expected in approximately 3% of meioses.

As illustrated in Figure 9.13, by inspection of the HLA typing results in a family it is usually possible to deduce the paternal or maternal origin of the alleles for each of the HLA genes and in this way to determine how they are associated together on the parental chromosomes. For example, because individual II-1 inherited A29, B7, and DR4 from her father, and individual II-3 inherited A1, B8, and DR3 from the father, we can deduce that one of the father's chromosomes carries A29, B7, and DR4 whereas the other carries A1, B8, and DR3. This set of polymorphic, linked alleles that are inherited together are referred to as a **haplotype.** The four distinct parental haplotypes can easily be deduced for this pedigree. Note that each of the haplotypes has been passed on intact through meiosis to generation II, with one exception. Individual II-5 has inherited an A2, B35, DR1 allele from her mother that would appear to represent a recombination. This event exchanged material from the two maternal chromosomes and must have occurred somewhere between the B and DR genes.

Individual II-1 is suffering from acute leukemia and is in need of a bone marrow transplant. A close match between the patient and the bone marrow donor at the HLA locus is an important factor in determining the success of the transplantation procedure. Analysis of the HLA haplotype data in Figure 9.13B reveals that the patient's brother II-4 is a perfect match, having inherited the identical paternal and maternal HLA haplotypes as the patient. II-4 is referred to as an HLA-identical sibling match. Individual II-5 has also inherited the same two haplotypes but is a less optimal match because of the recombination event in the maternal allele. Sibling II-2 shares the paternal haplotype but not the maternal and is thus referred to as **haploidentical.** Sibling II-3 is a complete mismatch, having inherited the opposite allele from both parents. The probability of any two siblings being HLA identical is 25%. Though a haploidentical sibling can be used as a bone marrow donor in some situations, a full match is preferable. HLA matching is also important, though less critical, for kidney and other organ transplants.

Because the HLA complex is so polymorphic, it makes an ideal marker for linkage studies. Furthermore, as noted above, the various alleles could be detected by a panel of serologic antibodies beginning approximately 30 years before the genes involved were cloned. A large number of genetic analyses have been carried out in the past several decades using HLA as the marker, testing this against a variety of diseases. As expected, most of those disorders did not show linkage. However, in several important examples, including hemochromatosis described below, linkage to HLA was in important step in the identification of the corresponding disease gene.

Hemochromatosis is an autosomal recessive disease in which excessive iron accumulation occurs in affected adults. Homozygous individuals absorb iron from the gastrointestinal tract at high rates throughout their life. The normal control of iron in the body operates at the level of intestinal absorption, but the mechanism that would normally act to slow absorption in the setting of adequate iron stores is defective. The excess iron deposits in the heart, liver, pancreas, skin, and endocrine system, leading to a variety of symptoms, including heart failure, cirrhosis, pituitary hormone deficiency, and "bronze diabetes" (skin pigmentation and pancreatic endocrine insufficiency). Females often do not show symptoms until after menopause, as menstrual blood loss protects against iron accumulation. Males, however, often show evidence of disease by middle adulthood. The most effective treatment is periodic removal of blood, since this is a simple way to remove iron. As this is usually successful, it is always a tragedy to miss this diagnosis. Because the disease is recessive, it is essential to examine other members in a family at risk, especially siblings, when one individual is diagnosed.

As shown in Figure 9.12, the gene for idiopathic hemochromatosis (HFE) is located near the MHC, distal to the A gene of the class I cluster. Even before the hemochromatosis gene itself was cloned, assessment of risk was often possible through linkage to HLA. In a given family with multiple affected individuals, inheritance of a particular HLA haplotype can be used to track the segregation of the hemochromatosis gene, using the same principle illustrated for the polymorphic marker and NF1 in Figure 9.5. Because of the extremely high polymorphism of the HLA locus, informative analysis can generally be performed in any family with one or more clearly affected individual. In addition, as early as 1975 a strong association between a specific HLA type and hemochromatosis was noted. Specifically, the majority of hemochromatosis mutant alleles were noted to travel on a chromosome also carrying the A3 HLA allele. This preferential occurrence of a disease gene in association with specific alleles of linked markers is called **linkage disequilibrium.** This linkage disequilibrium probably indicates that most chromosomes carrying the hemochromatosis mutation are descended from a common ancestor. The mechanism for the generation of linkage disequilibrium is diagramed in Figure 9.14. This sort of disequilibrium generally implies that (*a*) most of the disease chromosomes carry the same mutation, and (*b*) the markers being tested are quite close to the disease gene. There is considerable linkage disequilibrium across the entire HLA locus. The A3 allele is in linkage disequilibrium with the B7 and B14 alleles, and as a result B7 and B14 are also highly associated with hemochromatosis. Thus, HLA typing alone can significantly alter the estimate of risk for hemochromatosis, even if other family members are not available for formal linkage analysis.

The hemochromatosis gene (denoted HFE) has recently been cloned. As predicted by the linkage disequilibrium observation, a single mutation accounts for 85% of hemochromatosis chromosomes (a cysteine to tyrosine substitution at codon 282, denoted C282Y). DNA analysis for this mutation provides a direct test to detect this very common disease (approximately 1:500). Although reliable tests to indicate the presence of iron overload are available, DNA testing is capable of detecting the presence of the disease even *before* iron overload occurs, which allows ideal management of this preventable and potentially curable disease. For this reason, widespread population screening is under consideration.

As predicted by the 1:500 frequency of hemochromatosis homozygotes (q^2), approximately 8.5% of the population are heterozygotes (2 pq). Heterozygosity for this mutation does not appear to be associated with significant clinical problems, except when the individual also has another coexistent form of liver disease such as hepatitis. It has been suggested that hemochromatosis heterozygotes may have had a selective advantage in the past because of their slightly increased iron stores, which could perhaps explain the high frequency of this allele in the population. Positive selection pressure may have also contributed to the rapid expansion of a single founder mutation allele, accounting for the linkage disequilibrium described above.

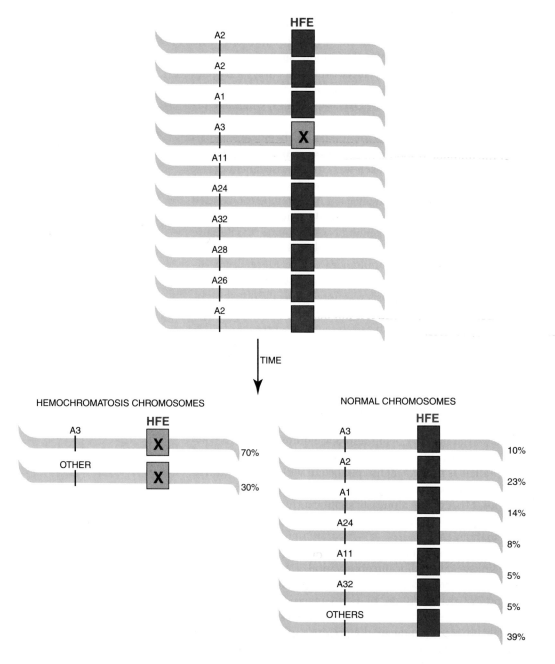

Figure 9.14.   Mechanism for the occurrence of linkage disequilibrium.   In this example, the hemochromatosis gene (HFE) mutation (indicated by an X) is shown as having arisen only once on an ancestral chromosome, which carried the HLA A3 allele. In the next few generations after the mutation arose, all chromosomes carrying the mutation also have the A3 allele. With time, little recombination has occurred between these two loci, so that the HFE gene mutation is still associated with the HLA A3 allele on 70% of hemochromatosis chromosomes, even though the HLA A3 allele only makes up 10% of normal chromosomes. The strength of the linkage disequilibrium is related to the genetic distance separating the two loci as well as the amount of time that has passed since the occurrence of the initial mutation event. As would be predicted, other polymorphic markers at a greater distance from the HFE gene, such as the HLA B, C, and DR loci, show considerably weaker evidence for linkage disequilibrium with hemochromatosis.

As discussed in chapter 4, a number of other diseases, particularly several "autoimmune" disorders, show associations with specific HLA alleles, ankylosing spondylitis and the HLA-B27 allele being a striking example. The meaning of these associations is still not entirely clear, but several hypotheses have been proposed. One is that the HLA protein itself is responsible for the predisposition to disease. This could occur if a particular HLA product in combination with a particular foreign agent such as a virus were incapable of inducing an effective immune response, so that a chronic infection resulted. If the immune response to the foreign agent in the context of a particular HLA allele in some way crossreacted with the host and led to destruction of normal cells, an autoimmune situation would be created. An alternative mechanism is that the HLA loci themselves are not responsible for the predisposition to disease, but this phenomenon derives from other as yet unidentified loci within this cluster, which are in linkage disequilibrium with HLA. The latter hypothesis suggests that autoimmune diseases are similar to idiopathic hemochromatosis, except that they do not follow strict Mendelian inheritance patterns. At the very least, one would have to propose the presence of reduced penetrance, other modifier genes, or an interaction with the environment. At present, it is not possible to distinguish between these various hypotheses.

Identifying Human Disease Genes

Until the mid-1980s, scientists studying a human genetic disease could only hope to identify the responsible gene through careful analysis of the pathophysiology of the disease in patients. The hemoglobinopathies, arising as a consequence of mutations in the hemoglobin genes (discussed in detail in chapter 6), were the first human diseases to be characterized at the molecular genetic level. The hemoglobinopathies were particularly amenable to study because the pathology of the disease could be localized to the red blood cell and the corresponding hemoglobin protein was available in virtually unlimited quantities through the collection of peripheral blood. Until recently, the standard paradigm for the study of human genetic diseases followed this pattern and began by identifying the functional defect in the patient. Characterization of the deficient protein or enzyme could subsequently lead to cloning of the responsible gene using the cDNA and genomic cloning methods outlined in chapter 5. This general approach, moving from the basic biochemical defect to the responsible gene, has been referred to as "functional cloning" (Fig. 9.15). Unfortunately, this model was only applicable to a limited number of human disease genes for which the biochemical defect could be directly determined. As of 1986, the specific causative genes had only been identified for approximately 200 human diseases and many of the most important ones remained unapproachable. By

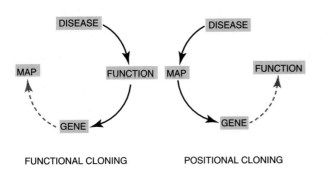

FUNCTIONAL CLONING   POSITIONAL CLONING

Figure 9.15. Comparison of the steps in functional and positional gene cloning. In traditional functional cloning, the study of gene function precedes gene identification. In positional cloning, gene mapping comes first, eventually leading to gene identification. After the gene has been identified, this then permits an optional study of gene function. The solid arrows indicate required steps in the approach and dotted arrows indicate optional steps. (Adapted from Collins FS. Positional cloning: let's not call it reverse anymore. Nat Genet 1992;1:3–6.)

the late 1980s, the powerful techniques of modern molecular genetics made it possible to locate the gene responsible for a human disease based solely on its map position, without the benefit of any functional information. This approach is referred to as "positional cloning" (Fig. 9.15).

Positional Cloning

The magnitude of the positional cloning problem is illustrated in Figure 9.16. The total size of the human genome is approximately 3×10^9 base pairs and is estimated to contain approximately 100,000 genes. A chromosome contains from $50-260 \times 10^6$ bp, corresponding to approximately 1500–8000 genes. Positional cloning begins at the level of the whole genome (3×10^9 base pairs) and ends at single base pair resolution, permitting identification of subtle point mutations causing human disease. There are two major bottlenecks in this process. The first is mapping the gene to a specific chromosomal region by cytogenetic approaches or linkage analysis. This generally places the gene within a region of several million base pairs, often containing on the order of 100 genes. The second major obstacle is identifying the correct gene among all the possible candidates within that interval.

The first genes to be identified by positional cloning took advantage of chromosomal aberrations that pointed to a specific gene location. An important example is provided by the cloning of the Duchenne muscular dystrophy (DMD) gene.

DUCHENNE MUSCULAR DYSTROPHY

Duchenne muscular dystrophy is an X-linked condition with onset of weakness in affected boys in early childhood. These boys are usually wheelchairbound before the age of 10 years and death usually occurs from complications of muscle degeneration by about age 20 years.

Because DMD is an X-linked recessive disease, finding a female affected with this disease is very unusual. Possible explanations would include homozygosity for the disease gene or extremely skewed X chromosome inactivation (see chapter 8). A third possibility was identified by cytogenetic studies on several such affected girls that revealed X-autosome translocations; the autosome involved in each case was different, but the breakpoint on the X chromosome was always in band p21 (Fig. 9.17). The simplest explanation for this phenomenon is that the translocation has actually broken within the DMD gene in each of these cases. One might wonder, therefore, why these girls would be affected, since they also carry a normal X chromosome. The answer lies in the phenomenon of X inactivation; in all cases, the normal X chromosome is inactivated and the translocation X remains active, leaving no functioning copy of the normal gene at the DMD locus (Fig. 9.18). Thus, the discovery of these rare individuals led to the conclusion that the DMD gene most likely maps to Xp21. This conclusion was also supported by standard linkage analysis in a number of other families.

Not only translocations, but also deletions, can assist in the mapping of a gene for human disease. Again, DMD provides an instructive example. Even small chromosomal deletions are likely to involve a number of genes (a contiguous gene syndrome, see chapter 8), so a clue to the possible presence of a chromosomal deletion is the occurrence of more than one genetic defect in a single individual. A boy (B.B.) with no family history of any genetic disorder was discovered to have DMD, chronic granulomatous disease (CGD, a disorder of white cells that seriously impairs the ability to fight off infection), and two other X-linked traits. The simultaneous occurrence of

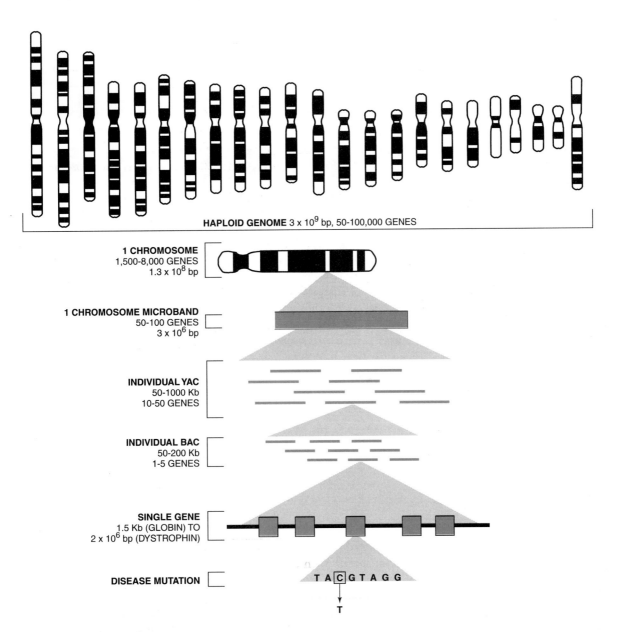

Figure 9.16.   The scale of the positional cloning problem.   Positional cloning begins with all 23 chromosomes of the haploid human genome as depicted at the top and aims to move to the single nucleotide resolution at the bottom, which is required for the identification of disease-causing mutations. **Yeast artificial chromosomes** (YACs) are specialized cloning vectors grown in yeast that can carry from 50 to 1000 kb of foreign DNA. YACs have proved very valuable for the mapping of large regions of DNA. **Bacterial artificial chromosomes** (BACs) are specialized cloning vectors maintained in bacteria that can hold 50–200 kb of DNA. Though smaller than YACs, BACs offer a number of technical advantages over YACs and are another important tool for the positional cloner.

these four X-linked conditions led to a careful cytogenetic analysis, which revealed an extremely small deletion of band Xp21.2 (see Fig. 9.19). Because neither parent carried such a deletion, this appeared to be a de novo occurrence, allowing the mapping of these four X-linked conditions to that part of the X chromosome. This unique individual also provided a critical clue in the puzzle that led to the cloning of the CGD and DMD genes and the beginnings of a molecular understanding of both of these diseases.

Figure 9.17. Karyotype of a female with Duchenne muscular dystrophy. As indicated by the *arrows*, there is an apparently balanced translocation between chromosome 21 and one of the X chromosomes in this female. In the *bottom row* are shown high-resolution pictures. On the *left* is the normal X chromosome. Next to that is a derivative X that has exchanged the top half of the short arm with a small piece of chromosome 21. Next to that is the other counterpart of the translocation, a chromosome 21 that has distal Xp attached to its short arm. On the *right* is the normal chromosome 21. The breakpoint on the X chromosome is at p21, which turns out to be the location of the muscular dystrophy gene. (Used with permission from Verellen-Dumoulin C, Freund M, DeMeyer R, et al. Expression of an X-linked muscular dystrophy in a female due to translocation involving Xp21 and non-random inactivation of the normal X chromosome. Hum Genet 1984;67:115–119.)

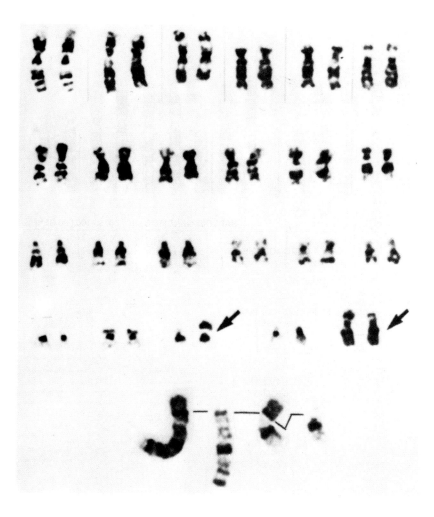

Cloning of the DMD gene was accomplished by two groups of researchers using two different approaches. One group was able to clone a portion of the gene by working with the X-autosome translocation shown in Figure 9.17, in which the translocation connects X-chromosome sequences to DNA from the short arm of chromosome 21. This region, like the short arms of chromosomes 13, 14, 15, and 22, contains ribosomal genes, which are repeated sequences coding for the ribosomal RNAs. Because those sequences were known, it was possible with some ingenuity to clone the breakpoint in this affected female, which connected ribosomal sequences to DNA from the X chromosome. As expected, this X-chromosome sequence turned out to lie within the DMD gene.

Another approach was taken by another group of researchers using DNA from the boy with the small Xp21.2 deletion (Fig. 9.19). Using a clever subtraction technique, they were able to obtain cloned fragments of DNA that are present on a normal X chromosome but absent in this boy's DNA. One such clone, pERT87, was used for the Southern blot shown in Figure 9.11; the 46,Y,del(X) *lane* is DNA from the boy with the Xp21.2 deletion. When they tested these clones on boys who had DMD with *no* visible cytogenetic deletion, pERT87 was also missing in the DNA from some of these boys (Fig. 9.20). This suggested that this fragment of DNA might include part of the DMD gene itself. The cloned segment of DNA was extended to include about 140,000 bp and probes from this region detected deletions at

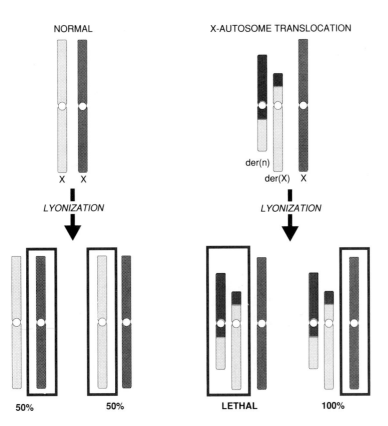

Figure 9.18.   The consequences of X-inactivation in the presence of an X-autosome translocation.   In the normal situation, about 50% of the cells will have inactivated each X chromosome. (Inactivation is indicated by the *closed box* around a chromosome.) In the presence of an X-autosome translocation, however, cells that inactivate the X chromosome involved in the translocation also inactivate the attached autosomal material, which is presumably lethal to the cell. As a result, virtually 100% of the somatic cells of such an individual are found to have inactivated the normal X. This explains the occurrence of Duchenne muscular dystrophy in a female with an X-autosome translocation interrupting the DMD gene on Xp21, even though such a person carries a normal DMD gene on the normal X. For simplicity, only the X chromosomes and the translocated autosomes are shown in this diagram.

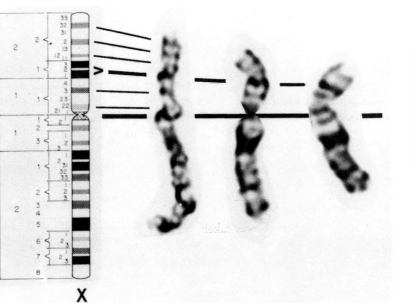

Figure 9.19.   Occurrence of a small interstitial deletion in Xp21.2 in a boy (B.B.) with Duchenne muscular dystrophy, chronic granulomatous disease, and two other X-linked conditions.   On the *left* is shown a diagram of the normal banding pattern, and on the *right* are three representations of the X chromosome from this boy. A very subtle decrease in the size of the Xp21 band is present, and the light band Xp21.2 is never visible. (Courtesy of Dr. U. Francke Howard Hughes Medical Institute at Stanford University.)

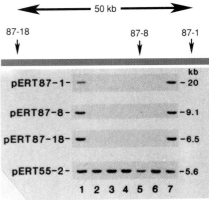

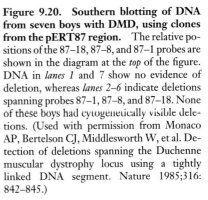

Figure 9.20.   Southern blotting of DNA from seven boys with DMD, using clones from the pERT87 region.   The relative positions of the 87–18, 87–8, and 87–1 probes are shown in the diagram at the *top* of the figure. DNA in *lanes 1* and *7* show no evidence of deletion, whereas *lanes 2–6* indicate deletions spanning probes 87–1, 87–8, and 87–18. None of these boys had cytogenetically visible deletions. (Used with permission from Monaco AP, Bertelson CJ, Middlesworth W, et al. Detection of deletions spanning the Duchenne muscular dystrophy locus using a tightly linked DNA segment. Nature 1985;316:842–845.)

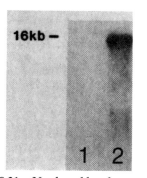

Figure 9.21.   Northern blot, demonstrating a 16-kb transcript in RNA obtained from fetal skeletal muscle (*lane 2*) but not in a non-muscle cell RNA sample (*lane 1*). The probe is a cDNA clone that was derived by screening a cDNA library with a clone from the pERT87 region. This is a very large mRNA, and represents the normal transcript of the DMD gene. (Used with permission from Monaco AP, Neve RL, Colletti-Feener C, et al. Isolation of candidate cDNAs for portions of the Duchenne muscular dystrophy gene. Nature 1986;323:646–650.)

both sides of this interval in boys with DMD, suggesting that the DMD gene is very large. Several fragments within this region were then tested to see whether any of them might include exons of the DMD gene, and eventually a 16-kb muscle-specific transcript was detected on Northern blots (Fig. 9.21). The cDNA for this gene was subsequently cloned, and it was determined that the genomic DNA sequence encoding the DMD gene is truly mammoth. The largest human gene identified to date, the DMD gene contains 79 exons and occupies 2.3 million bp, or more than 1% of the X chromosome!

The protein encoded by the DMD gene has been termed dystrophin, a very large protein (427 kDa) that is involved in the contractile apparatus of muscle cells. Biochemical studies of dystrophin have identified a number of other cytoskeletal proteins that interact with dystrophin, referred to as the dystrophin-associated protein complex (Fig. 9.22). Mutations in several of these genes have recently been shown to result in autosomal forms of muscular dystrophy. Cloning of the DMD gene also revealed the molecular basis for a milder form of X-linked muscular dystrophy termed Becker muscular dystrophy (BMD). Becker muscular dystrophy turned out also to be caused by mutations within the DMD gene. However, BMD generally results from mutations or deletions that maintain the translation reading frame, resulting in the production of some dystrophin protein (Fig. 9.23), though of reduced quantity or altered size. Mutations in the severe form of DMD generally result in no dystrophin expression, or production of a truncated or nonfunctional protein (Fig. 9.23).

Approximately two-thirds of DMD and BMD patients have a deletion of one or more exons of the DMD gene. Though it is not generally practical to sequence the entire dystrophin gene, a number of techniques, such as multiplex PCR (Fig. 9.24) have been developed to screen for deletions

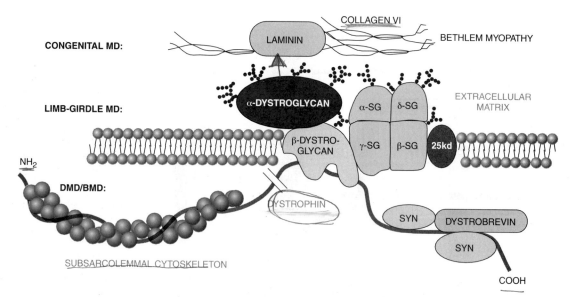

Figure 9.22.   Model for assembly of dystrophin and the dystrophin-associated protein complex.   Dystrophin, shown as a thick black line, interacts at its N-terminus with the subsarcolemmal cytoskeleton. The C-terminal domain interacts with β-dystroglycan, which links dystrophin to the extracellular matrix protein, laminin. Other associated proteins include the sarcoglycans (SG), syntrophins (SYN), and dystrobrevin. Mutations in the sarcoglycans, laminin, and collagen type VI lead to autosomal forms of limb-girdle muscular dystrophy, a congenital form of muscular dystrophy, and Bethlem myopathy, respectively. (Courtesy of Dr. J.S. Chamberlain, University of Michigan.)

Normal   BMD

DMD   DMD

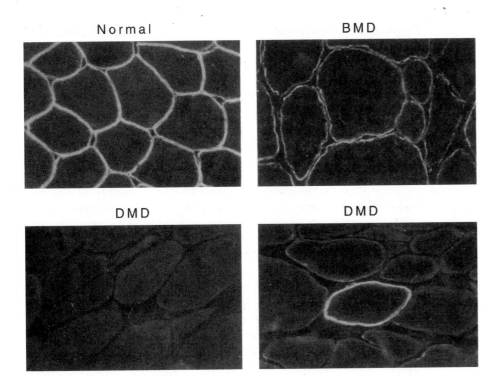

Figure 9.23.   Detection of dystrophin by immunofluorescence.   Frozen sections of muscle from a normal control and BMD and DMD patients were labeled with an anti-dystrophin monoclonal antibody by immunofluorescence. The intense staining seen around the periphery of the normal muscle fibers in the *upper left* is completely absent from the DMD fibers at the *lower left*, whereas the BMD muscle at the *upper right* shows markedly reduced dystrophin. Note the single dystrophin-positive fiber in the *lower right* DMD muscle section. Such infrequent positive fibers are occasionally seen in DMD muscle and are thought to represent rare "revertents," in which a second somatic mutation event has partially or completely restored the protein coding sequence. (Used with permission from Nicholson, LV, Davison K, Johnson MA, et al. Dystrophin in skeletal muscle. II. Immunoreactivity in patients with Xp21 muscular dystrophy. J Neurol Sci 1989;94:137–146.)

within the gene. Analysis of dystrophin protein in muscle biopsy samples by immunolabeling techniques is also a useful diagnostic tool, as illustrated in Figure 9.23.

HUNTINGTON DISEASE

Huntington disease is an autosomal dominant disorder affecting about 1 in 20,000 individuals. The average age of onset is not until 37 years, though penetrance is high (essentially 100% by age 80). Symptoms consist of personality changes, memory loss, and a peculiar series of motor problems including chorea (involuntary movements of the arms and legs). Pathologically, those who have died of the disease are found to have dramatic neuronal

Figure 9.24.   Multiplex PCR to screen for dystrophin gene deletions.   For this diagnostic test, a patient's DNA sample is simultaneously amplified in one PCR reaction using primers spanning nine different segments of the dystrophin gene. The products from each of nine DMD patients are separated in *lanes A-I* of the gel. The nine amplified fragments, from *top* to *bottom*, correspond to exons 45, 48, 19, 17, 51, 8, 12, 44, and 4, respectively. No deletions are detected in patients A, C, F, and I, with all nine bands present. *Lane B* detects a deletion involving exon 44 and *lane D* a deletion spanning exons 8, 12, 17, and 19. The deletion in *lane G* is similar to *lane D*, except that exon 8 is still present. The deletions in *lanes E* and *H* both span exons 45 and 48, with the *lane E* deletion also including exon 51. This multiplex PCR analysis will detect deletions in approximately half of all DMD and BMD patients (Used with permission from Chamberlain JS, Chamberlain JR, Fenwick RG, et al. Diagnosis of Duchenne and Becker muscular dystrophies by polymerase chain reaction: a multicenter study. JAMA, 1992; 267:2609–2615.)

A   B   C   D   E   F   G   H   I

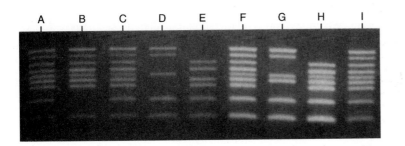

loss in parts of the basal ganglia of the brain, especially the caudate nucleus. Despite years of research, no evidence for any specific protein abnormality was ever obtained in comparing tissues from Huntington patients with normal tissues. Thus, there were no clues as to the underlying genetic defect in Huntington disease to allow a functional cloning approach. There were also no chromosomal abnormalities in any patients to point to a specific region.

Huntington disease was the first genetic disorder to be mapped through a systematic screening of polymorphic genetic markers for linkage. This approach, often referred to as a genome scan, has become the standard first step toward positional cloning of human disease genes. With the realization in the early 1980s of the utility of DNA RFLPs for this type of analysis, Huntington disease became a leading target because of its autosomal dominant inheritance, high penetrance, and the availability of large families. Researchers thus began the arduous process of collecting family material and developing a series of probes, expecting that 100–300 such probes would have to be tried out before a linkage was found. By good fortune, the 12th probe that was tried, called G8, turned out to be tightly linked to the Huntington disease (HD) locus. This fortunate finding provided immediate impetus for other investigators to enter the field of linkage analysis using DNA polymorphisms. The G8 marker detects two polymorphic *Hin*dIII sites, as diagramed in Figure 9.25. Because there are two polymorphic sites, there are four possible chromosome patterns (haplotypes), denoted A, B, C, and D, depending on which sites are present or absent. All possible genotypes have been observed, as shown by Southern blot in Figure 9.25.

Figure 9.26 shows a portion of a very large Venezuelan pedigree in which Huntington disease is occurring. Because of the large number of affected individuals in this pedigree, it was of enormous use in carrying out the linkage analysis. Indicated on the pedigree are the genotypes at the G8 locus as determined by RFLP analysis. Inspection reveals that all individuals with Huntington disease have inherited the C allele from their affected parent, except for the shaded individual in generation IV, who must represent a recombinant. Again, note that the RFLP analysis simply helps one track the Huntington chromosome in this family, and having the C allele does not equate with having Huntington disease, as should be obvious from the fact that several unrelated spouses also have a C allele. LOD score calculations from this pedigree and others indicate that the genetic distance between G8 and the Huntington disease locus is about 3 cM. Combining all families being studied throughout the world, the linkage between G8 and HD was absolutely unquestionable, with odds in favor of linkage reaching more than 1080 to 1 (a LOD score of 80)! Such a high LOD score could only have been obtained by studying a very large number of affected individuals within families. The G8 marker was mapped to the tip of the short arm of chromosome 4, indicating that HD must also be close to this location.

Though linkage of G8 to HD was first reported in 1983, it would take another 10 years to complete the positional cloning process leading to the identification of the Huntington disease gene itself and the characterization of the HD genetic defect. However, as soon as G8 and other polymorphic markers closely linked to HD had been identified, it became possible to perform predictive DNA testing in individuals at risk for HD well before they had developed symptoms and long before diagnosis would have been possible with standard medical approaches. This presymptomatic DNA diagnosis opened up a new series of complex clinical and ethical questions, some of which are addressed in chapters 12 and 14.

Cloning of the HD gene in 1993 permitted characterization of the re-

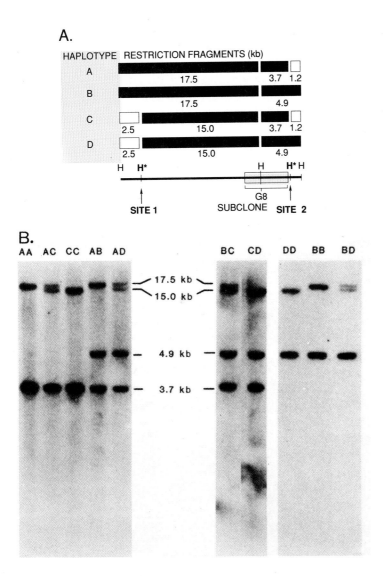

A.

HAPLOTYPE   RESTRICTION FRAGMENTS (kb)

Figure 9.25.   Analysis of the G8 RFLP.
A. Diagram of the G8 locus. This RFLP is more complex than others we have described, because it detects two polymorphic *Hind*III sites. The polymorphic sites are marked with *asterisks* and invariant sites are also shown. Depending on whether sites 1 or 2 are present or absent, a total of four different patterns can appear from each chromosome. These are designated by haplotypes A, B, C, and D. The position of the probe is indicated at the *bottom* of the diagram. Notice that the 2.5-kb band from haplotype C and D and the 1.2-kb fragment from haplotypes A and C will not be visualized on the Southern blot using this probe, because the probe does not overlap these fragments. **B.** Southern blot showing each of the 10 possible genotypes at the G8 locus. Note that the pattern observed for the genotype AD is identical to that for BC, so these can only be distinguished by typing close relatives. (Used with permission from Gusella JF, Tanzi RE, Anderson MA, et al. DNA markers for nervous system diseases. Science 1984;225:1320–1326.)

sponsible genetic mutation. This was the end result of years of effort to characterize genes near G8 and identify an alteration that distinguished affected from unaffected individuals. Huntington disease results from a triplet-repeat expansion in the amino terminus of the HD protein, referred to as huntingtin (see chapter 8, Fig. 8.44). Though the function of the huntingtin protein is still unknown, cloning of the HD gene has provided powerful new research tools that should ultimately lead to improved understanding of HD pathophysiology and the development of new therapies.

Expansion of the HD triplet repeat is detected directly by PCR of the HD locus as shown in Figure 9.27. The CAG repeat ranges from 10–30 copies in length in normal chromosomes and from 36–121 on HD chromosomes. Measurement of the length of the CAG repeat in the HD gene provides a direct diagnosis of HD without the need to test other family members, as required for linkage analysis, and without the concern of possible recombination. There is a general correlation between the length of the CAG repeat and the age of onset of symptoms (longer repeats predict earlier onset), but this is not precise enough to be useful clinically.

The development of molecular diagnosis for HD has served as a valu-

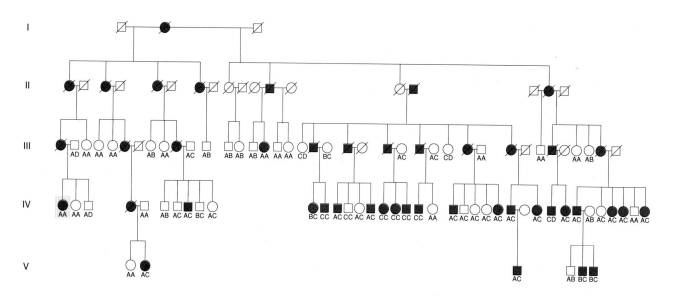

Figure 9.26. A portion of a large Venezuelan pedigree of individuals affected with Huntington disease.   Note that many individuals in the earlier generations are deceased. It is still possible, however, to carry out linkage analysis by allowing the computer program to consider all possible genotypes for deceased individuals that are consistent with Mendelian inheritance. Note that all affected individuals have a C allele for G8, except for the *shaded* individual in generation IV. (Used with permission from Gusella JF, Tanzi RE, Anderson MA, et al. DNA markers for nervous system diseases. Science 1984;225:1320–1326.)

able model for the general approach to presymptomatic testing for other adult-onset diseases. The complex ethical issues raised by DNA testing for HD (chapters 12 and 14) have become of much more general concern with the recent identification of highly prevalent genetic mutations contributing to common diseases such as breast and colon cancer (see chapter 11).

CYSTIC FIBROSIS

Cystic fibrosis (CF) is one of the most common autosomal recessive diseases of white populations, affecting approximately 1 in 2500 newborns. From Hardy-Weinberg considerations, one can calculate that the frequency of heterozygous carriers is about 1 in 25 individuals. The disease is character-

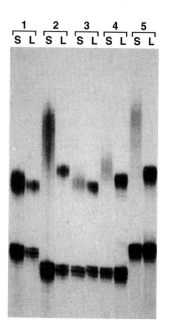

Figure 9.27. PCR analysis of the expanded triplet repeat in HD gene. The PCR primers are designed to amplify a segment at the 5′ end of the *HD* coding sequence containing the CAG repeat. The DNAs were obtained from five members of the Venezuelan HD pedigree shown in Figure 9.26. Lanes marked "S" are the results using DNA prepared from sperm and lanes marked "L" used lymphoblast DNA. The *lower bands* in each lane are derived from the normal chromosome and contain between 19 and 24 copies of the CAG repeat. The *upper bands* in each lane are the products from the chromosome carrying the *HD* gene mutation. When measured in the lymphoblast DNA lanes, these expanded alleles range in length from 45 (lane 1-L) to 52 copies of the triplet repeat (lanes 2-L and 5-L). Thus, all 5 of these individuals (ages 24–30 years at the time of this study) carry the HD mutation and can be expected to develop Huntington disease. Notice that the expanded alleles amplified from the sperm DNA samples show a range of sizes, generally larger than the same allele amplified from lymphoblast DNA. This is because of the particular instability of this triplet repeat during male meiosis, which frequently results in expansion of the HD allele and accounts for the clinical observation that early onset of HD is more likely when the disease is paternally inherited. Each of the normal alleles (*lower band*) actually consists of a cluster of closely spaced bands. This is an artifact of the PCR caused by "slippage" of DNA polymerase during amplification. (Used with permission from Duyao M, Ambrose C, Myers R, et al. Trinucleotide repeat length instability and age of onset in Huntington disease. Nat Genet 1993;387–392.)

ized clinically by sticky viscous secretions of the pancreas and lungs. It may be recognizable at birth by a condition called "meconium ileus," which is an intestinal obstruction. The diagnosis is commonly made by demonstrating an elevation of chloride in sweat. This is both a highly sensitive and specific finding in CF. Children with this disorder usually experience pancreatic insufficiency, which can be managed with enzyme supplementation. Their chronic pulmonary infections are more difficult to manage, however, and in spite of gains in survival based on vigorous treatment of the chest infections with antibiotics and physical therapy, the current average survival is about 30 years. Decades of research failed to identify the specific gene product involved in cystic fibrosis, although considerable evidence was collected indicating an abnormality in ion transport across cell membranes.

Because of its clinical importance and the failure of functional cloning approaches, CF was also a prime target for gene mapping by linkage analysis. Linkage to markers on chromosome 7 was first demonstrated in 1985. With the testing of additional markers on chromosome 7, the CF gene was found to lie close to the markers *MET* and J3.11. Physical mapping techniques indicated that the distance between these markers was about 1.6 million bp, which is a large enough region to contain approximately 50 genes. Additional markers were subsequently obtained within this interval and allowed the position of the CF gene to be narrowed down even further.

As polymorphic markers were identified closer and closer to the CF gene, an increasing degree of linkage disequilibrium was observed, similar to that described earlier for hemochromatosis and HLA. In this and similar situations, the degree of linkage disequilibrium can sometimes provide useful information about the actual location of the gene. Greater than 70% of CF chromosomes were observed to have a specific pattern of polymorphic alleles that was only found in about 25% of normal chromosomes.

The cystic fibrosis gene was eventually cloned by careful study of the approximately 500,000-bp candidate interval defined by genetic analysis. Without the availability of major rearrangements, which were so helpful in the DMD search, a major problem was to identify the *correct* gene. In fact, three possible genes from this region were studied, which turned out *not* to be responsible for CF, before the correct gene was finally cloned.

As shown in Figure 9.28, Northern blotting with the fourth candidate gene as probe detected a transcript in lung, pancreas, sweat glands, intestine, and liver, all of which are affected in CF. This gene is large, containing 26 exons and stretching across 250,000 bp of DNA (Fig. 9.29). The mRNA transcript is 6129-bp long and encodes a 1480-amino acid protein. The sequence of this protein, termed CFTR for cystic fibrosis transmembrane regulator, suggested that it is anchored in the cell membrane and binds ATP, based on similarities to other known proteins. These predictions have been borne out by subsequent experiments, which have also shown that the protein functions as a chloride channel.

To prove the correctness of this candidate gene, it was necessary to identify mutations that correlate with disease. Cloning and sequencing a cDNA prepared from sweat glands of a CF patient revealed an unequivocal difference from the normal sequence in exon 10: a 3-bp deletion was found, which would have the effect of deleting a single amino acid (a phenylalanine) at residue 508 (Fig. 9.30). That this represents a mutation *causative* of CF, and not a neutral polymorphism, was subsequently demonstrated by functional analysis of recombinant proteins carrying either the normal sequence or the codon 508 deletion (denoted ΔF508). It is interesting to note that the

Figure 9.28.   Northern blot showing the pattern of expression of the cystic fibrosis gene.   The probe for the blot is a fragment of a cDNA prepared from normal human sweat glands. *Each lane* of the Northern blot contains RNA from a different normal human tissue. A 6.2-kb mRNA is apparent in lung, pancreas, and sweat gland, but not in all tissues (e.g., brain). This is consistent with expectations of the CF gene transcript, which presumably performs an important normal function in these organs; when both copies of the gene are defective, CF is the result. (Used with permission from Riordan JR, Rommens JM, Kerem B, et al. Identification of the cystic fibrosis gene: cloning and characterization of complementary DNA. Science 1989;245:1066–1073.)

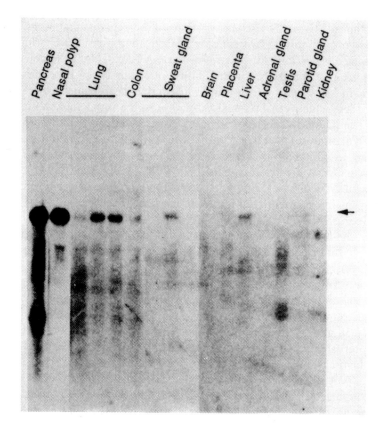

ΔF508 mutation is present on 70% of CF chromosomes, but on nearly all CF chromosomes with the common polymorphism haplotype previously shown to be in linkage disequilibrium with CF (see above). ΔF508 is thus the ancestral or founder mutation whose existence was first suggested by linkage analysis, before the cloning of the CF gene.

The cloning of the CF gene has had major consequences. Most immediately, it has made it possible to readily detect heterozygotes for this autosomal recessive disease (4% of whites), thus allowing many couples at risk for having an affected child to obtain this information before starting their families (see discussion of genetic screening in chapter 12). As noted above, approximately 70% of CF alleles carry ΔF508. More than 600 other mutations have been identified within the gene through the study of numerous patients. As discussed in chapter 12, DNA testing for CF carriers by screening with a panel of 70 of the most common CF mutations can detect 90% of heterozygous carriers among northern European whites, and between 60% and 98% of carriers in other selected populations. A recent expert panel has recommended offering CF carrier testing to all couples contemplating or already engaged in a pregnancy.

Second, the cloning of the CF gene has led to important advances in understanding the biology of the disease. Continued progress in basic research should lead to new approaches to treatment, in both the pharmaceutical and gene therapy arenas (chapter 13). Finally, the success in identifying the CF gene by positional cloning, even in the absence of gross genetic rearrangements to lead the way, demonstrated the feasibility of this approach for identifying the genes for a large number of human disorders for which no information exists about function of the normal gene.

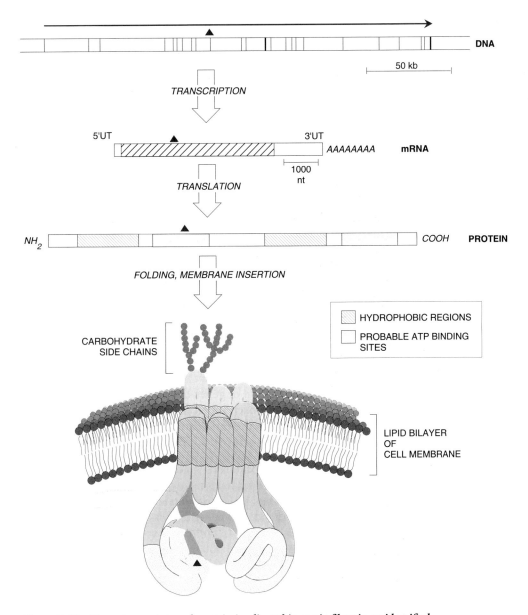

Figure 9.29.   Gene, transcript, and protein implicated in cystic fibrosis, as identified by positional cloning.   The folding of CFTR shown here is hypothetical, based on similarities to other known proteins. The *red triangle* indicates the location of the 3-bp deletion in exon 10, which represents the common mutation in CF. This leads to a loss of a single amino acid in the protein product, also indicated by a *red triangle*.

NORMAL

DNA	.. GAA	AAT	ATC	ATC	TTT	GGT	GTT	TCC ..
PROTEIN	Glu	Asn	Ile	Ile	Phe	Gly	Val	Ser
POSITION	504	505	506	507	508	509	510	511

CYSTIC FIBROSIS

DNA	.. GAA	AAT	ATC	AT-	--T	GGT	GTT	TCC ..
PROTEIN	Glu	Asn	Ile	Ile		Gly	Val	Ser

Figure 9.30.   The common mutation responsible for cystic fibrosis.   A deletion of CTT in exon 10 results in the loss of a phenylalanine at position 508 of the 1480-amino acid protein. The isoleucine at 507 is unaltered because ATC and ATT both code for isoleucine.

Table 9.2. Disease Genes Identified by Positional Cloning[a]

1986
Chronic granulomatous disease
Duchenne muscular dystrophy
Retinoblastoma

1989
Cystic fibrosis

1990
Wilms tumor
Neurofibromatosis type 1
Testis determining factor
Choroideremia

1991
Fragile X syndrome
Familial polyposis coli
Kallmann syndrome
Aniridia

1992
Myotonic dystrophy
Lowe syndrome
Norrie syndrome

1993
Menkes disease
X-linked agammaglobulinemia
Glycerol kinase deficiency
Adrenoleukodystrophy
Neurofibromatosis type 2
Huntington disease
Von Hippel-Lindau disease
Spinocerebellar ataxia 1
Lissencephaly
Wilson disease
Tuberous sclerosis

1994
McLeod syndrome
Polycystic kidney disease, type 1

Dentatorubral pallidoluysian atrophy
Fragile X RES
Achondroplasia
Wiskott Aldrich syndrome
Early onset breast/ovarian cancer (BRCA1)
Diastrophic dysplasia
Aarskog-Scott syndrome
Congenital adrenal hypoplasia
Emery-Dreifuss muscular dystrophy
Machado-Joseph disease

1995
Spinal muscular atrophy
Chondrodysplasia punctata
Limb-girdle muscular dystrophy
Ocular albinism
Ataxia telangiectasia
Alzheimer disease (chromosome 14)
Alzheimer disease (chromosome 1)
Hypophosphatemic rickets
Hereditary multiple exostoses
Bloom syndrome
Early onset breast cancer (BRCA2)

1996
Friedreich's ataxia
Progressive myoclonic epilepsy
Treacher Collins syndrome
Long QT syndrome (chromosome 11)
Barth syndrome
Simpson-Golabi-Behmel syndrome
Werner syndrome
X-linked retinitis pigmentosa (RP3)
Polycystic kidney disease, type 2
Basal cell nevus syndrome
X-linked myotubular myopathy
Anhidrotic ectodermal dysplasia
Hemochromatosis
Chédiak-Higashi syndrome
Rieger syndrome
Maturity-onset diabetes of the young (chromosome 12)

[a]As of December 9, 1996. This list excludes genes identified primarily by a candidate gene approach or on the basis of somatic mutation in cancer cells.

led to the development of powerful computer resources for accessing these data and rich interconnections between the various databases. The Online Mendelian Inheritance in Man (OMIM), **http://www.ncbi.nlm.nih.gov/Omim/,** the outgrowth of the pioneering efforts of Dr. Victor McKusick to catalog human genetic diseases, lists all known inherited human disorders. It currently contains entries for approximately 9000 distinct genetic loci. OMIM is also linked to the genome database (GDB), **http://gdbwww.gdb.org/,** which contains a wealth of information about genetic markers and the position of known genes on the genetic map.

Mapping Genes for Complex Human Diseases

Most of this chapter and much of the entire book has focused on the molecular genetics of classic Mendelian disorders. However, as discussed in chapter 4, many human diseases have genetic components that cannot be ascribed to the affect of a single gene, but rather represent complex interactions between multiple genes, as well as environmental factors. With the remarkable success of genetic linkage methods for single gene disorders and the powerful tools generated by the Human Genome Project, the study of complex genetic diseases has become a major focus for current genetic research. A number of common human diseases are being approached in this way, including Alzheimer's disease, common forms of cancer, atherosclerosis, hypertension, asthma, and diabetes.

How does one go about identifying genes contributing to a complex genetic trait without any prior knowledge of the genes' locations or functions? This is a much more difficult problem than the standard linkage approaches to classic Mendelian disorders that we have been discussing so far. Generally a much larger number of pedigrees must be studied with a more extensive collection of DNA markers, since the contribution of any one gene may be subtle.

As reviewed in chapter 4, candidate genes can be analyzed for association between a specific allele and a disease in a large population. Alternatively, whole genome scan approaches can be applied, often using sib-pair analysis, as discussed in chapter 4 for insulin-dependent diabetes mellitus. The mathematical and computational problems inherent in these analyses and the interpretation of the results are formidable. Though studies of this type have identified potential susceptibility loci for a number of common diseases, such as schizophrenia and multiple sclerosis, initial observations have often proved disappointingly difficult to replicate.

Even after such a potential susceptibility locus has been successfully mapped, the next step of identifying the specific gene itself is a very difficult task for which most of the positional cloning strategies described in this chapter do not directly apply. Chromosomal rearrangements or large deletions are unlikely to be encountered, and the responsible sequence changes may result in only subtle alterations in gene function, which may be difficult to demonstrate. In the positional cloning of single gene disorders, the identification of recombination events between marker loci and the disease gene is usually a critical step in narrowing the gene search to a manageable segment of the genome. However, for complex diseases it is generally not possible to identify such clear-cut recombinants, as any single susceptibility allele would only be expected to be present in a subset of affected individuals. Thus, even after a candidate locus for a complex disease has been mapped, the interval defining its potential chromosomal location often remains quite large.

As an alternative approach, many investigators have begun to focus their studies on genetically homogeneous populations in the hope that the major susceptibility loci in any one such group will be smaller in number and easier to identify. In addition, specific alleles contributed from a limited number of founders may be identified by the existence of linkage disequilibrium.

Finally, animal models provide a potentially powerful tool for the dissection of complex human diseases. The Human Genome Project (see chapter 10) has provided genetic and physical mapping tools for a number of model organisms. For the mouse, these tools are almost as extensive as those available for humans. Because of the ability to perform selective crossbreeding experiments, it is often much easier to precisely map modifying or susceptibility genes in mice. In addition, the mouse offers the possibility of genetic manipulation of potential candidate genes through knockout or standard transgenic techniques, as described in chapter 5. Genetically modified mice can also be crossbred to test potential interactions among susceptibility genes. This approach is exemplified by studies of atherosclerosis in the mouse, which are examining interactions between a number of genes involved in lipid metabolism, inflammation, and blood coagulation.

It must always be kept in mind that susceptibility genes identified in other mammalian species may not be directly relevant to humans. Mouse models may prove to be particularly useful when preliminary human linkage or association studies suggest a susceptibility locus in a region of the human genome that is evolutionarily related to the chromosomal segment containing the mouse gene under study. The occurrence of genes together on the same chromosome, referred to as **synteny,** is often highly conserved in homologous blocks among the genomes of related species. Subchromosomal regions showing conservation of synteny between two species are termed "syntenic." For example, large segments of human chromosome 17 are syntenic to corresponding regions on mouse chromosome 11. Conservation of synteny has proved to be a powerful tool in the application of animal model systems to the study of human genetic diseases.

Genetic studies of complex human diseases are likely to be an important area of research for many years to come. The identification of susceptibility genes may lead to more accurate predictions of risk for many common human diseases. These analyses could permit sophisticated tailoring of treatment for high-risk individuals. In addition, basic biologic studies of the functions of these genes may eventually lead to the development of novel approaches to therapy.

SUGGESTED READINGS

Scriver CR, Beaudet AL, Sly WS, Valle D, eds. The metabolic basis of inherited disease. 7th ed. New York: McGraw-Hill, 1995. *Also available in an updated CD version. This outstanding text is also cited in several other chapters. The introductory section provides additional information concerning mapping and positional cloning methods. There are also authoritative reviews providing more detail for each of the specific disease examples covered in this chapter.*

Ott J. Analysis of human genetic linkage. Baltimore: Johns Hopkins University Press, 1991. *Textbook providing detailed mathematical consideration of genetic linkage analysis.*

Collins FS. Positional cloning moves from perditional to traditional. Nat Genet 1995; 9:347–350. *Review of recent progress in positional cloning.*

Lander ES, Schork NJ. Genetic dissection of complex traits. Science 1994;265:2037–2048. *Overview of the challenge of genetic approaches to the analysis of complex human diseases.*

Collins FS. Sequencing the human genome. Hosp Pract Off Ed 1997;32:35–43,46–49,53–54. *General review of genetic mapping and positional cloning and the role of the Human Genome Project.*

Appendix A: LOD Score Calculation

As discussed above, a LOD score is calculated from the ratio of the likelihood of observing a set of data if the two test loci are linked and separated by a distance of θ, to the likelihood of obtaining the same data if the two loci are unlinked. The LOD score is the $\log_{10}$ of this odds ratio.

$$LOD = \log_{10}\left(\frac{\text{likelihood of data if loci linked at } \theta}{\text{likelihood of data if loci unlinked}}\right)$$

Using the pedigree data shown in Figure 9.5, we will determine the LOD score for linkage between the *Eco*RI RFLP and NF1. As covered earlier in the text, the LOD score for this data at $\theta = 0$ is $-\infty$ because of the single recombination in individual III-7, which could not occur if the disease gene and marker are inseparable ($\theta = 0$).

Let us now calculate the LOD score at $\theta = 0.05$, or a recombination fraction of 5%. Individual I-1 has one mutated and one normal copy of the NF1 gene and also both a 4.7-kb and a 3-kb *Eco*RI RFLP allele. Identifying which RFLP allele goes with which copy of the *NF1* gene is referred to as determining the phase. Since there are two possible phases, the chance of either being correct is 50% or 0.5. The total likelihood of linkage between the RFLP and the *NF1* gene equals 1/2 times the likelihood for phase 1 (the mutated *NF1* gene on the same chromosome as the 4.7-kb allele) plus 1/2 times the likelihood for phase 2 (the *NF1* gene mutation on the same chromosome as the 3-kb allele).

Let's first calculate the likelihood for phase 1. Under this condition, the *NF1* mutation should be inherited along with the 4.7-kb allele 95% of the time and with the 3.0-kb allele for the 5% of chromosomes in which a recombination has occurred between the marker and the *NF1* gene. Similarly, the father's normal copy of the *NF1* gene should be inherited with the 3.0-kb allele 95% of the time and with the 4.7-kb allele 5% of the time. Since there is an equal chance (50% or 0.5) for each offspring of inheriting either the normal or mutated copy of the *NF1* gene from the father, the overall chance of inheriting the mutation with the 4.7-kb band from the father is $0.5 \times 0.95 = 0.475$ and with the 3.0-kb band is $0.5 \times 0.05 = 0.025$. Similarly, the chance of inheriting the normal copy of the *NF1* gene with the 3.0-kb band is also 0.475 and with the 4.7-kb band, 0.025. Four of the children in generation II inherited the *NF1* mutation and the 4.7-kb marker allele from I-1. The likelihood for this occurring is $0.475 \times 0.475 \times 0.475 \times 0.475$. Four inherited the father's normal *NF1* gene and the 3.0-kb allele $(0.475 \times 0.475 \times 0.475 \times 0.475)$. In generation III, three individuals inherited the NF1 mutation with the 4.7-kb allele from II-8 (0.475^3) and 5 individuals inherited the normal gene and the 3.0-kb allele (0.475^5). One individual (III-7) demonstrates a recombination, inheriting II-8's 3.0-kb marker allele with the *NF1* mutation (0.025). Thus, the likelihood for phase 1 (*NF1*/4.7-kb allele) and observing the data in this pedigree at $\theta = 0.05$, is $0.5 \times 0.475^{16} \times 0.025$.

Let's now examine the term of the likelihood for phase 2 (*NF1* mutation/3-kb allele). Again, the chance of this phase is 1/2. However, now all of the other calculations are essentially reversed from those we have just performed. All of the children inheriting NF1 with the 4.7-kb allele or the normal gene with the 3-kb allele would now represent recombinations (0.025) and the single individual who was recombinant for phase 1 (individual III-7) would now be the only nonrecombinant chromosome (0.475). Thus, the term for the likelihood from phase 2 would be $0.5 \times 0.025^{16} \times 0.475$ (a negligibly small number compared with phase 1).

Remember that the denominator in the likelihood ratio is the likelihood of observing this particular pattern of inheritance among the 17 at-risk individuals in generations 2 and 3, assuming that the *NF1* gene and the RFLP marker are completely unlinked. In this case, the *NF1* gene and RFLP are independently inherited and all four combinations (the normal or mutated *NF1* gene with either the 4.7-kb or 3.0-kb alleles) would occur with equal probability (0.25). Thus, the likelihood for the specific pattern observed in these 17 individuals would equal 0.25^{17}.

Combining all of these calculations together:

$$\text{LOD} = \log_{10}$$

$$\left(\frac{\text{likelihood of data if loci linked at } \theta = 0.05 \; [\frac{1}{2}(\text{phase 1}) + \frac{1}{2}(\text{phase 2})]}{\text{likelihood of data if loci unlinked}} \right) = \log_{10}$$

$$\left(\frac{1/2(0.475^{16} \times 0.025) + 1/2(0.025^{16} \times 0.475)}{0.25^{17}} \right) = \log_{10}(1442.2) = 3.16$$

This value is identical to the LOD score at $\theta = 0.05$ that was calculated by the MLINK computer program, as shown in Figure 9.6.

Let's now calculate the LOD score at $\theta = 0.1$. The calculation is very similar to that which we have just performed except now the chance of inheriting either of the nonrecombinant alleles is 0.45 (0.5×0.9) and the chance of inheriting a recombinant allele is 0.05 (0.5×0.1). Substituting these values in the likelihood equation we have just calculated:

$$ \text{LOD} = \log_{10} \left(\frac{\frac{1}{2}(0.45^{16} \times 0.05) + \frac{1}{2}(0.05^{16} \times 0.45)}{0.25^{17}} \right) = \log_{10}(607) = 3.08 $$

Again note that this value is in perfect agreement with the computer calculation in Figure 9.6.

For comparison, it is instructive to consider the LOD score for this pedigree at $\theta = 0$ if there had been *no recombinants*. In this case, the probability for each individual inheriting either the normal or mutated chromosome and the corresponding marker allele would be simply 0.5 and the equation would become:

$$ \text{LOD} = \log_{10} \left(\frac{\frac{1}{2}(0.5^{17}) + \frac{1}{2}(0^{17})}{0.25^{17}} \right) = \log_{10}(65,536) = 4.82 $$

This example illustrates the greater power to detect linkage of a marker very close to or within the gene, compared with a marker at a distance of only 6 cM. Similarly, the LOD scores observed in the initial genome scanning phase of a positional cloning experiment generally increase considerably, as additional markers progressively closer to the gene are analyzed.

10

The Human Genome Project

Make no little plans; they have no magic to stir men's blood and probably themselves will not be realized. Make big plans; aim high in hope and work, remembering that a noble, logical diagram once recorded will never die, but long after we are gone will be a living thing, asserting itself with evergrowing insistency.

—DANIEL H. BURNHAM

The above quotation, written by a Chicago architect, might have seemed foreign to the field of biomedical research as recently as 10 years ago. Biology and medicine have flourished throughout much of the 20th century as a consequence of the creativity of individual research investigators, each pursuing their own hypotheses and ideas, creating a fabric of research observations that moved medicine from a largely descriptive art in the early years of this century to its current complex, highly technical, and highly information-based state. Physics and engineering may have had their "big science" projects, such as high energy colliders and space exploration, but biology has largely remained the province of the "small science" individual investigator. A modest shift in this paradigm, with major implications for the future of genetics and medicine, has been the emergence of the Human Genome Project, an organized and coordinated effort to map and sequence all of the human DNA by the year 2005. A project of this sort, with specific scientific goals and milestones, therefore differs substantially from the traditional biomedical research format. In reality, however, this project is being carried out by a very large number of laboratories and institutions worldwide, and in a collaborative and creative spirit. Its consequences are likely to be profound, and therefore it is appropriate to devote a chapter of this text to the goals and consequences of this historic effort.

History of the Human Genome Project

In the early 1970s obtaining sequence information on DNA or RNA was an arduous procedure, and an entire year of work might be required to deduce 15 or 20 nucleotides. The development of efficient methods for DNA sequencing by Sanger and by Maxam and Gilbert (for which Sanger and Gilbert received the Nobel Prize in Chemistry in 1980) opened the door to efficient and accurate sequencing of stretches of DNA as long as a few thousand base pairs (Fig 5.17). In the mid 1980s, a few scientists began to discuss the possibilities of a massive scale-up: instead of sequencing small bits of the genome one by one in a "cottage industry" fashion, with all of the attendant inefficiencies, lack of quality control, and potential for slow progress in many areas and no progress at all in others, why not organize a "crash program" to determine the entire 3 billion base-pair sequence once and for all?

Virtually anyone working in the field of genetics agreed that if the entire human genome sequence were handed to them it would benefit the way in which research is carried out and greatly accelerate the pace of disease gene discovery, with considerable potential benefit to human health. But se-

231

rious objections were raised. Many researchers in the mid to late 1980s simply did not believe that adequate technology existed to accomplish this goal or anything approaching it at a reasonable cost. Concern was raised that such an expensive project would be likely to divert resources away from other research efforts, with potential damage to the entire biomedical enterprise. Still others felt that the work would be so boring and unchallenging that no creative scientist would want to be involved. Others raised philosophical objections to obtaining this information in such a wholesale fashion, fearing that the consequences for our species would be dire.

This debate was carried out vigorously and publicly in many countries of the world during the late 1980s. In the United States, a blue-ribbon panel was convened by the National Academy of Sciences, and another by the Office of Technology Assessment. Both panels concluded that such a project could be successful if it was carefully organized with a clear set of milestones. In particular, it was felt essential that initial efforts should be focused on developing better maps, and that sequencing should be undertaken only when the technology had improved to the point at which it could be accomplished on a cost-effective basis.

In October 1990, the Human Genome Project was officially launched in the United States. A number of other countries, particularly the United Kingdom, France, Japan, Canada, and Germany also have significant investments in the Human Genome Project. Thus this effort has been from the outset an international partnership, which seems highly appropriate as the genome itself is certainly international. The Human Genome Organization (HUGO) was founded by an international group of scientists to coordinate efforts on this project among different countries.

Goals of the Human Genome Project

From the outset, the goals and milestones have been very explicit. Figure 10.1 shows in schematic form the three major scientific goals for the human genome. An overarching requirement for the successful achievement of all of these goals is the development of better technologies, which must be capable of handling the very large amount of information that will be accumulated given the size of the human genome. For this purpose, much effort is being devoted to automation of all of the steps necessary for mapping and sequencing. This has required the input of physicists, chemists, engineers, and computer scientists, making the Human Genome Project a highly interdisciplinary effort. This aspect has essentially laid to rest concerns about the potential tedium of the project. Repetitive tasks are generally automated, leaving the scientists free to explore creative solutions to the challenges of dealing with a 3-gigabp genome.

GENETIC MAPS

The information presented in chapter 9 outlined the power of linkage analysis and positional cloning for identification of genes that predispose to human disease, even without prior knowledge of the function of those genes. These methods, initially developed for Mendelian single-gene disorders, and more recently extended to polygenic conditions, can only be successful if a robust genetic map of the human genome is available, because that is the first step in any positional cloning project. A genetic map with highly informative markers spaced on the average 2–5 centimorgans apart was thus felt to be a very high priority for the Human Genome Project. The technology of marker production shifted rapidly from restriction

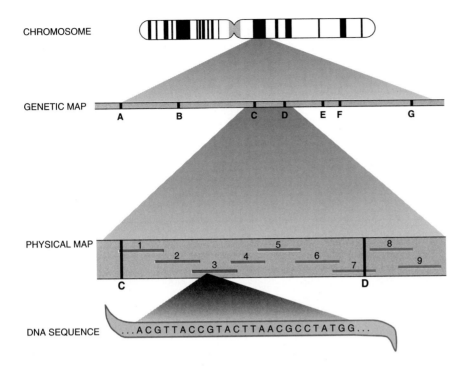

Figure 10.1. **The three major scientific goals of the Human Genome Project are to develop genetic maps, physical maps, and DNA sequence.**   In the process, the entire 3 billion bp of the human genome, containing approximately 80,000 genes, will be determined by the year 2005.

fragment length polymorphisms (RFLPs) to simple sequence repeat (SSR) microsatellites (see chapter 5) because of the highly informative nature of the latter, and their easy adaptation to the polymerase chain reaction. By 1994, more than 5000 highly informative markers had been placed on the map, resulting in an average density four to eight times better than that originally planned for, and achieved more than a year ahead of schedule. Figure 10.2 charts the rate of growth of the genetic map, as well as a number of other parameters of progress (described below). Figure 10.3 shows an example of marker distribution for chromosome 4, indicating the high density now available. With this large array of genetic markers, nearly any human phenotype that has a hereditary component should be mappable, provided a sufficient number of families are available for analysis.

PHYSICAL MAPS

Successful linkage analysis results in a general map location for a particular disease gene, but invariably the positional cloner then will wish to hunt for the gene itself. As described in chapter 9, the next step is therefore to "possess" all of the DNA in the candidate interval and search through it for potential genes that may be involved in the phenotype. Generating a set of overlapping cloned fragments of DNA for a region 1–10 million bp in size (which often must be dealt with in a positional cloning project) is a daunting task if it has to be done from scratch. Here again, there is an economy of scale: producing such physical maps of the entire human genome ahead of time is much more efficient than generating short segments each time a

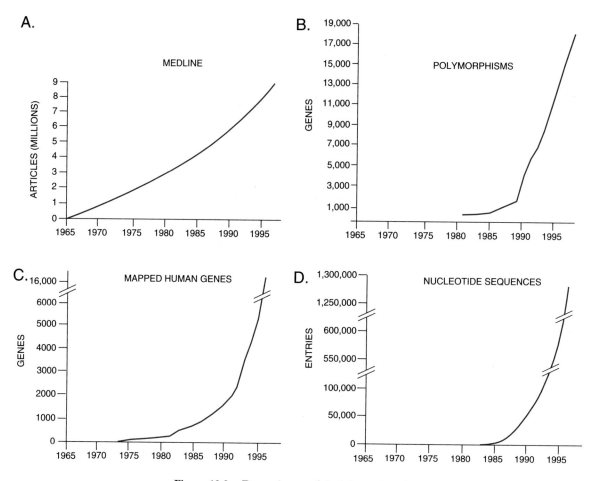

Figure 10.2.   Dramatic growth in information about genetics has occurred in the last 30 years.   Medical information in general is expanding rapidly-note that the number of papers indexed in MedLine (initiated in 1965) is growing at a more than linear rate. Information about genetics is moving even more rapidly, however, as exemplified by the essentially exponential growth in polymorphisms, mapped human genes, and DNA sequence information. (Figure modified from original kindly provided by Mark Boguski, National Center for Biotechnology Information.)

region becomes interesting. After all, in due time, the entire genome will probably be found to contain interesting sequences.

It is beneficial to use vector systems that allow the cloning of very large pieces of human DNA in order to generate such physical maps. Yeast artificial chromosomes (YACs, as mentioned in chapter 5) permit the cloning of pieces of DNA from 100,000 up to 1,000,000 bp, and have been the standard currency for physical maps, despite some of their technical problems. However, it is likely that better vector systems will come along in the future, and therefore the physical map has been constructed using reagents that will not be rendered obsolete in the future and that are also immediately available to any investigator who is interested. The sequence-tagged site (STS) has thus become the common currency of physical mapping. At first glance, this may seem an odd way to define a physical map, but after some reflection the elegance of this system should be apparent.

Figure 10.4 diagrams the concept of the STS. Simply put, this is a unique site in the genome, identified by two primers that can be used in a polymerase chain reaction to amplify from one and only one location in human DNA. The sequence of the primers, which will not change with ad-

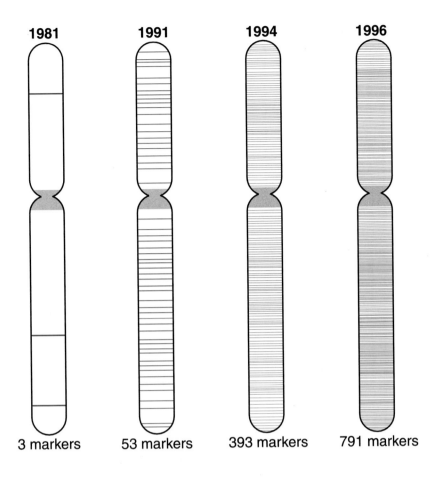

Figure 10.3. Rapid improvements in genetic maps have occurred as a consequence of the Human Genome Project. As an example, this schematic shows the number of genetic markers available during the last 15 years for human chromosome 4. In 1981 there were only 3 restriction fragment length polymorphisms, but by 1996 a total of 791 markers had been derived for this chromosome, the vast majority of which are microsatellites that can be scored by PCR.

vances in vector technology (as the sequence itself is not going to change), defines a landmark at a particular site. Furthermore, such sequences are immediately deposited in public electronic databases, and any investigator interested in obtaining DNA from that region can do so simply by synthesizing the appropriate oligonucleotides.

These STSs can be used to readily construct a set of overlapping clones for any region of interest, provided that the STSs are sufficiently closely spaced. To be more explicit, the spacing of the STSs needs to be on average several fold closer together than the average insert size of the cloned fragments that will be assembled into the map. Figure 10.5 shows how this is car-

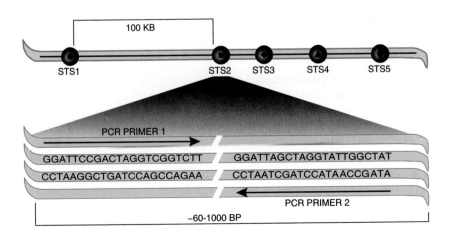

Figure 10.4. The sequence-tagged site (STS) is a unique location in the human genome, defined by two oligonucleotide primers. These primers can be used in the polymerase chain reaction to amplify that specific region of DNA. Although vector systems will change in the future, the sequence defining the STS is a basic property of the genome and thus this "currency" for physical mapping should be quite durable.

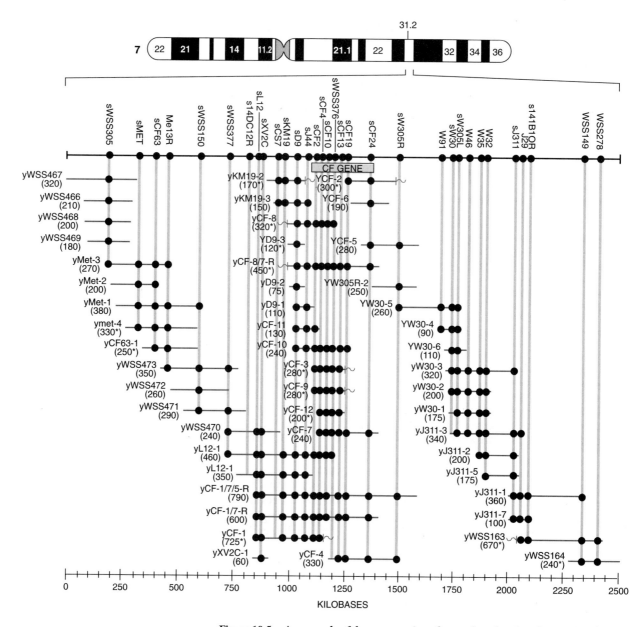

Figure 10.5.   An example of the construction of a set of overlapping clones using the STS concept.   In this instance, the region being represented includes the gene for cystic fibrosis. The STSs (*vertical dashed lines*) were used to screen a library of yeast artificial chromosomes (YACs), and each STS detected several YACs (*horizontal black bars*). The size of each YAC is indicated in kilobases in parentheses, and they range from 60–790 kb in length. YACs that are "chimeric" (that is, they contain more than one piece of human DNA accidentally linked together in the process of YAC construction) have their sizes marked with an asterisk, and a *wavy line* indicates the non-chromosome 7 material. The set of YACs represents a complete overlapping set of clones (referred to as a "contig") of the 2.5-Mb interval.

ried out in practice, in this case for the region of the cystic fibrosis gene. A series of 32 STSs has been used to screen a total human genomic YAC library, and each STS has detected several positive clones. By scoring each of the clones for each of the STSs and noting the pattern of positives and negatives, it is possible to reconstruct the order of the STS markers and the order of the set of overlapping YACs. In the future, if some other library of large insert clones becomes available, the STSs can be readily used to construct a map from those clones as well.

The current goal of the Human Genome Project is to construct a physical map of the human genome consisting of STSs spaced on the average 100,000 bp apart, so that maps such as that shown in Figure 10.5 for the cystic fibrosis gene region can be produced for all regions of all chromosomes. In fact, this is progressing rapidly, with greater than 30,000 STSs having been derived at this writing, placing over 98% of the genome in overlapping sets of ordered yeast artificial chromosomes. This allows an investigator interested in a certain interval to immediately obtain or reconstruct cloned DNA from this region, saving many months or years of work.

SEQUENCING

The ultimate goal of the Human Genome Project is to obtain the sequence of all 3 billion bp of human DNA. When the project was initially begun, there was some concern whether the technology for DNA sequencing would develop rapidly enough to allow such a large volume of data to be generated. However, with appropriate attention to automation, optimization of all of the steps involved, and microscaling, it now appears certain that this effort will succeed. Figure 10.2 shows the exponential rate of growth in numbers of sequences being entered into a public database.

A crucial question remains: once the complete human sequence is in hand, will it be possible to predict the location of genes? Recognizing that less than 5% of the genomic DNA is involved in coding for protein, it is essential to have available computer algorithms that are capable of recognizing the coding information (the exons) from a large stretch of uncharted DNA. Exons do have certain distinguishing characteristics (see chapter 5): they are preceded by a splice acceptor, they in general contain an open reading frame, and they are terminated by a splice donor. However, these characteristics are not sufficiently obvious to pick out coding regions from a large stretch of DNA by simple visual inspection. Recent sophisticated neural net approaches have allowed the development of computer algorithms that appear quite powerful in identifying exons of 100 bp or larger in a region of DNA never previously studied. Figure 10.6 shows an example of the output of a computer algorithm called GRAIL for a sequence of 17,000 bp of DNA from chromosome 16. This region contains part of the gene for polycystic kidney disease, and the agreement between the computer prediction and the actual location of the exons is quite good.

Given that the exons are of particular value, a great deal of interest has also arisen in sequencing cDNAs. A number of groups, originally in the private sector but more recently in the public domain, have determined partial sequences of tens of thousands of cDNAs, and an effort is currently underway to place all of these in their proper location on the physical map, using the 3' untranslated regions of each cDNA (often called ESTs, or expressed sequence tags) as STSs in the physical mapping strategy outlined above. The combination of information from cDNA and genomic sequencing is expected to be very powerful. Some have even argued that the genomic sequence is superfluous, since the cDNAs will contain the coding region. However, this assumes that it will be possible to identify all human cDNAs, which may be difficult for those that are of low abundance or expressed only in tissues that are inaccessible for study. Furthermore, sequencing the cDNAs will not provide crucial information about regulatory sequences that determine which genes are expressed in which tissues.

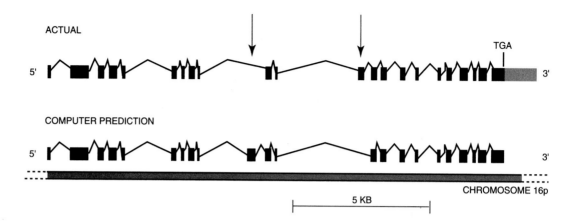

Figure 10.6.   Computer algorithms are now available to scan large regions of genomic sequence and predict the location of coding regions (exons) with reasonable accuracy. In this example, a region of 17 kb on chromosome 16, containing part of the gene for autosomal dominant polycystic kidney disease, has been analyzed. The actual structure of the gene is shown above, as deduced from analysis of cDNAs. Solid boxes represent exons, and the thin lines connect these across the intron sequences. The stop codon (TGA) is shown in the last exon. Below is the computer prediction, by an algorithm called GRAIL, of the location of coding regions based solely on analysis of the genomic sequence. It is apparent that the agreement is quite good, though the computer has predicted one exon that isn't real (*left arrow*) and missed one exon (*right arrow*).

Table 10.1.   Model Organisms Under Investigation Through the Human Genome Project

Organisms	Genome Size	Estimated No. of Genes	Genes/Mb
Mouse	3×10^9 bp	80,000	27
Drosophila (fruitfly)	1.2×10^8 bp	10,000	83
C. elegans (roundworm)	1×10^8 bp	13,000	130
Yeast	1.2×10^7 bp	5,800	483
E. coli (bacteria)	4.6×10^6 bp	4,288	932

Mb, megabase.

MODEL ORGANISMS

As useful as it will be, the complete human genomic sequence will still present many puzzles. Interpretation of the sequence, and the experimental application of that knowledge, will be greatly benefited by a comparison with other model organisms more amenable to research analysis. Accordingly, from the outset the Human Genome Project has also supported the mapping and sequencing of several other organisms, as shown in Table 10.1. These organisms were carefully chosen based on the availability of a large amount of genetic and phenotypic information. Except for the mouse genome, which is the same size as that of the human and therefore every bit as challenging to complete, the genomes of other model organisms have somewhat more manageable size. Their gene density is higher than for humans, so that the sequence is packed with even more information. Much of the sequencing done in the first few years of the Human Genome Project has been devoted to the genomes of these model organisms. The yeast and *E.coli* genome sequences are now complete, and *C.elegans* is expected to be completed in 1998.

Public Databases

The mapping and sequence information produced by the Human Genome Project, which is accumulating at a prodigious rate, is only useful if freely accessible to the scientific community in public databases. Sophisticated electronic resources have been designed and implemented to meet this need, and investigators working in the Human Genome Project with U.S. government support are required to deposit their data in these resources within six months of their experimental derivation, regardless of wheher or not the data has yet been published in a journal. The Appendix to this chapter provides useful electronic addresses to access this valuable information, now freely available to anyone with an internet connection.

Ethical, Legal, and Social Implications

The Human Genome Project proposes to uncover vast amounts of information about the genetic makeup of our species. This will considerably accelerate the rate at which genes responsible for individual predisposition to disease are uncovered. This information has great potential to benefit human health, but also the potential for misuse. Although the Human Genome Project does not actually present any brand new genetic dilemmas, the resulting acceleration of the pace of discovery is sufficient that the planners of the project felt that a major commitment to addressing the ethical, legal, and social implications of this research was justified. This effort, which represents the largest research investment in ethics in the history of humankind, is commonly referred to as the ELSI (Ethical, Legal, and Social Implications) Program.

A number of high-priority ELSI issues have been identified in the early years of the Human Genome Project and targeted for research, deliberation, and, if necessary, legislative initiatives. These include:

1. Fairness in the use of genetic information. Genetic information may carry considerable value for the individual, as for example when one learns that he or she is at risk for a disease that is curable if diagnosed early (such as colon cancer). But this information could also potentially be used to discriminate against individuals. A health insurance system that allows the insurer to discontinue coverage for persons found to have a "preexisting condition," for instance, can be explicitly discriminatory by denying coverage to individuals who have been found to be at increased future risk on the basis of a genetic test. Such individuals may be entirely well, and in fact may have the most to benefit from medical follow-up and preventive care. As none of us have the opportunity to choose the genes we inherit from our parents, it is inherently unjust to have this information used to determine our health care coverage. At the time of this writing, intense efforts are underway, catalyzed by the ELSI Program, to rectify this potential for discrimination through the passage of state and/or federal legislation. Already, the passage of the Health Insurance Portability and Accountability Act of 1996 has provided important protections for individuals in the group health insurance market. But remaining loopholes need to be closed. The urgency of doing this grows with each new gene discovery. After all, all of us carry "preexisting conditions" that will become recognizable in the future, and the potential for discriminatory mischief will be increasingly profound.

Similarly, the potential for genetic discrimination in employment has represented a major concern. But here also some progress has been made: in

1995, the Equal Employment Opportunities Commission (EEOC) issued a formal ruling that such discrimination is prohibited based on the language of the Americans with Disabilities Act. Federal legislation is still needed to provide better protections, however.

2. Privacy. A related issue is the degree to which genetic information about individuals can be passed to others without their consent. Many surveys have indicated that most individuals feel that this kind of information is sensitive, and ought not to be made available without specific permission. However, the medical records system in most parts of the world is not at all secure, and personal genetic information can be far too easily obtained by third parties without the patient's consent. Here again, legislative initiatives are underway to develop a system that better protects individual privacy for sensitive medical information.

3. Safety and efficacy of genetic tests. With increasing numbers of genetic discoveries, each one of which opens the possibility of diagnostic testing to predict future illness in an individual or their offspring, concerns about quality control of the laboratory testing as well as a means for determining when a new test is appropriate for mainstream medicine are increasing. In the United States, a number of groups are extremely interested in these issues. Consumers wish to be reassured that tests are safe and accurate, but also that they are made available in a timely fashion if the information can be of potential value. Professional organizations such as The American College of Medical Genetics, The American Society of Human Genetics, and the National Society of Genetic Counselors have a major investment in seeing that genetic discoveries lead to the greatest benefit with the least risk. Federal agencies in the United States such as the Food and Drug Administration and the Health Care Financing Administration are charged with regulatory responsibility over diagnostic testing. Genetic testing may be even more in need of careful oversight than other forms of laboratory testing. In general, an individual is only tested once, allowing an almost zero tolerance for error. The results of the tests have implications not only for the patient but for relatives. The information can be highly technical and must be connected with accurate genetic counseling for optimum benefits to be achieved. For all these reasons, it is appropriate to consider new genetic tests in the same context that one would consider a new drug. Synthesis of a new drug in the laboratory is followed by careful clinical trials to assess efficacy and toxicity before releasing the drug for general medical practice. Similarly, many individuals feel that a new genetic test should be evaluated on a research basis before making it available in an unrestricted fashion.

These topics represent only the first three major areas of emphasis of the ELSI Program. Many other challenges lie ahead, particularly when it comes to decisions about the proper use of this technology in the prenatal arena. Some of those dilemmas will be addressed in chapter 14.

Future Consequences for Medicine

The scientific goals of the Human Genome Project can be thought of as "building infrastructure" for the entire field of genetics, and have already led to a rapid acceleration in the pace of gene discovery. Figure 10.7 diagrams the flow of molecular medicine discoveries that will be occurring in great abundance as a consequence of this effort. The map and sequence information provided by the Human Genome Project, coupled with the collection

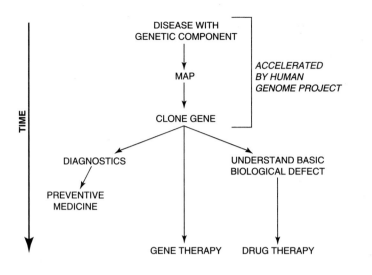

Figure 10.7. Progress in understanding human disease at the molecular level follows a predictable pattern from top to bottom in this diagram, although the time interval involved may be years or even decades. The advent of the Human Genome Project greatly accelerates the ability to identify human disease genes by the positional cloning strategy. After a gene has been identified, preventive medicine strategies can be designed for those individuals found to be at high risk. In the long run, however, the greatest promise of gene discovery will be the development of new and more effective therapies.

of DNA from families in which a particular disorder is occurring at high frequency, should allow the identification of susceptibility genes for almost all possible heritable phenotypes, using the principles of positional cloning. Those gene discoveries will lead quickly to the possibility of presymptomatic testing. In situations in which a single Mendelian gene with high penetrance is present, the testing may predict a high risk of future illness for the individual or their offspring. In polygenic conditions, however, or those with relatively low penetrance, testing will not provide a yes/no answer but rather an increased or decreased relative risk. For many disorders, the information about risk will be useful, as it will allow design of an individual program of medical surveillance and lifestyle planning to reduce that risk. For instance, an individual found to carry a germline mutation in one of the colon cancer mismatch repair genes described in chapter 11 could benefit substantially from annual colonoscopy beginning in the fourth decade, so that a polyp can be detected and removed years before it progresses to a potentially fatal invasive carcinoma.

Not all genetic disorders are associated with the availability of such preventive medicine strategies, however. Huntington disease is the classic paradigm in which precise diagnostic information can now be obtained, but as yet no interventions are available to delay or avoid the eventual onset of symptoms in an individual carrying an expanded triplet repeat. Many other disorders will be of this sort, and it is questionable whether the majority of individuals will wish to know information about their future risk for such conditions.

It is crucial, however, to remember that the ultimate goal of gene discovery is not just the development of better diagnostic information. As shown in Figure 10.7, the long-term promise of the Human Genome Project is that these gene discoveries will also lead to better therapies. In some instances this may come about by using the gene itself to treat the disease (Gene Therapy, see chapter 13). In other instances the discovery of the gene may provide sufficient information about the basic biologic and cellular defect to allow the development of rational drug therapy that will be more successful than existing, often largely empirical, pharmacological approaches. Note, however, in Figure 10.7 that the time between gene discovery and therapeutic advance is an unpredictably long one. In some instances this interval may be traversed in a matter of a few years, whereas for other conditions decades may pass before insights into the precise genetic and molecular biological basis of the disease lead to the development of effective therapies. This window of time between powerful diagnostic abilities and eventual therapeutic successes will present many challenges for the practice of medicine in the coming decades. However, moving forward in the most vigorous way possible seems the greatest hope for the future. To do otherwise would be to delay the eventual understanding and cure of the major diseases that afflict us.

SUGGESTED READINGS

Bishop JE, Waldholz M. Genome. New York: Simon & Schuster, 1990. *An engaging and accessible description of the steps leading up to initiation of the Human Genome Project, by two reporters for the Wall Street Journal.*

Cook-Deegan R. The Gene Wars. New York: Norton, 1994. *An authoritative firsthand account of the scientific and political roots of the Genome Project.*

Collins FS. Ahead of schedule and under budget: The Genome Project passes its fifth birthday. Proc Natl Acad Sci USA 1995;92:10821–10823. *An update (as of November 1995) of progress of the project.*

Hudson KL et al. Genetic discrimination and health insurance: An urgent need for reform. Science 1995;270:391–393. *A call for specific action to prevent the use of genetic information to deny health insurance coverage or set exorbitant premiums.*

Collins FS. Sequencing the human genome. Hospital Practice 1997;32:35–53. *An update on progress and application to the future of medicine.*

Appendix: Databases of Genome Information

For the interested Web browser, here is a partial list of http URLs where a wealth of genome information can be found.

DNA Data Bank of Japan

http://www.ddbj.nig.ac.jp/

European Bioinformatics Institute (EBI)

http://www.ebi.ac.uk/

Genome Data Base

http://gdbwww.gdb.org/

National Center for Biotechnology Information (NCBI)

http://www.ncbi.nlm.nih.gov/
GenBank and other DNA Sequence Databases

Mouse Genome Database

http://www.informatics.jax.org/

Online Mendelian Inheritance in Man (OMIM)

http://www.ncbi.nlm.nih.gov/Omim/

Saccharomyces (yeast) Genome Database

http://genome-www.stanford.edu

Généthon (French genome center)

http://www.genethon.fr

US Department of Energy (DOE) Human Genome Program

http://www.er.doe.gov/production/oher/hug_top.html
General information about the Human Genome Program databases and bioinformation resources and the DOE Human Genome Centers research projects.

National Human Genome Research Institute

http://www.nhgri.nih.gov/
The National Human Genome Research Institute is the component of the National Institutes
of Health with responsibility for the Human Genome Project.

Cancer Genetics

Another possibility is that in every normal cell there is a specific arrangement for inhibiting, which allows the process of division only when the inhibition has been overcome by a special stimulus. To assume the presence of definite chromosomes which inhibit division, would harmonize best with my fundamental idea . . . cells of tumors with unlimited growth would arise if those "inhibiting chromosomes" were eliminated . . . on the other hand, the assumption of the existence of chromosomes which promote division, might (also) satisfy this postulate. On this assumption, cell division would take place when the action of these chromatin parts, which are as a rule too weak, should be strengthened by a stimulus; and the unlimited tendency to rapid proliferation in malignant tumor cells would be deduced from a permanent predominance of the chromosomes which promote division.

—THEODOR BOVERI, 1911

The above quotation, which at first glance may seem densely written and difficult to follow, actually represents an uncannily accurate description of the genetics of human cancer, set down by Boveri 60 years before the tools became available to confirm or refute his ideas. Of all the areas of human molecular genetics, hardly any could be said to have generated more excitement than the investigation of the mechanism of cancer. This story is still incompletely understood and will continue to evolve during the next several decades. Because of its fundamental importance in human disease, however, it seems appropriate to devote an entire chapter to this subject. The story of the effort to understand the molecular basis of cancer is also helpful in underlining principles derived in previous chapters, as it brings together aspects of Mendelian inheritance, cell biology, cytogenetics, virology, and molecular biology.

Most Human Cancer Is Genetically Influenced, but not Mendelian

With the scourges of malnutrition and infectious disease under relatively good control in many parts of the world, cancer has emerged as a major health problem. With continued decreases in mortality rates from heart disease, cancer could soon emerge as the leading cause of death in the developed world. Despite dramatic successes in the treatment for a few specific types of cancer, overall cancer deaths have remained disappointingly high for the past 30 years (though recent reports suggest that these numbers may be beginning to decrease). Of course cancer is not one disease, but a multitude of different diseases, characterized by the site, tissue type, and grade of the malignancy.

The majority of human cancers cannot be explained by single gene inheritance patterns. This is not to say, however, that common cancers have no hereditary component. Decades of research indicate that the first-degree relatives of a person with a particular type of cancer often have a somewhat increased risk of developing the same tumor. Such analyses are complicated by the role played by the environment in many cancers (for example, smok-

Dominant Transforming Genes: "Oncogenes"

The clonality of most tumors suggests that genetic mutations are capable of conferring a malignant phenotype. The identification of the genes responsible for this phenomenon has been a subject of intense research interest. One might hypothesize that evolution would not permit such dangerous genes to be maintained unless they performed important normal functions, and one might further hypothesize that these functions might involve control of cellular growth. Both of these suppositions turn out to be true. Pieces of this puzzle have been provided by diverse and unexpected areas of research and require us to take a brief detour into the world of RNA tumor viruses. Although such viruses are a rare cause of cancer in humans, it turns out that the study of their biology in other organisms provided a critical clue to an understanding of cancer genetics.

TRANSFORMING RETROVIRUSES

Beginning with Peyton Rous's pioneering studies in chickens, a variety of transmissible agents that were capable of inducing cancer were identified in avian and mammalian species. These studies eventually demonstrated that many transmissible agents fell into a class of RNA viruses called **retroviruses**. The genome of such a virus is composed of single-stranded RNA. On entering a cell, as shown in Figure 11.3A, a retrovirus is uncoated and the RNA is copied into DNA, using a unique enzyme called reverse transcriptase. This enzyme is carried along with the retrovirus and encoded by it. The DNA copy is then inserted into the host genome. There it may lie quiescent or may be transcribed to generate multiple RNA copies of itself, which can then be packaged, leading to further rounds of infection. A simple diagram of the usual retrovirus genome is shown in Figure 11.3B and indicates the presence of three genes: the *gag* gene encodes a core protein of the virus, the *pol* gene encodes reverse transcriptase, and the *env* gene encodes a capsule or envelope protein. The packaging sequence (ψ) is necessary for the transcribed RNA molecule to be assembled into a viral particle.

Only a few human retroviruses have been identified, including the AIDS virus (human immunodeficiency virus, or HIV). Intact retroviruses such as HIV can indirectly cause tumors as a result of immunodeficiency, by promoting cell proliferation and increasing the opportunity for somatic mutation, or by activation of nearby genes after insertion into the genome. However, another class of retroviruses, referred to as acute transforming retroviruses, produces tumors much more rapidly through the action of transforming genes carried by the virus itself. These genes replace some or all of the endogenous viral genes, resulting in a virus that is defective in replication and requires the assistance of an intact virus for propagation. The transforming genes were by convention named using a three-letter abbreviation for the virus from which they were originally identified. Thus, for example, the Simian sarcoma virus transforming gene was called *sis*, the avian myelocytomatosis virus transforming gene was called *myc*, and so on. Numerous acute transforming retroviruses have been identified from a variety of avian and mammalian species, though to date such retroviruses have not been directly associated with human tumors.

CLONING HUMAN CANCER GENES BY A TRANSFORMATION ASSAY

Retrovirus researchers continued to identify interesting RNA tumor viruses, though their relevance to human cancer was questioned. In the mid-1970s,

A.

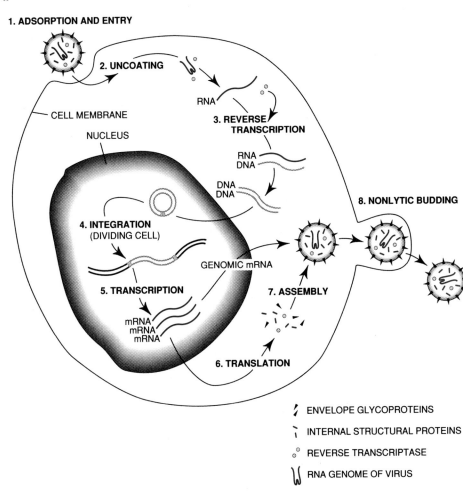

1. ADSORPTION AND ENTRY

2. UNCOATING

RNA

CELL MEMBRANE

3. REVERSE TRANSCRIPTION

NUCLEUS

RNA
DNA

DNA
DNA

8. NONLYTIC BUDDING

4. INTEGRATION
(DIVIDING CELL)

GENOMIC mRNA

5. TRANSCRIPTION

7. ASSEMBLY

mRNA
mRNA
mRNA

6. TRANSLATION

ENVELOPE GLYCOPROTEINS

INTERNAL STRUCTURAL PROTEINS

REVERSE TRANSCRIPTASE

RNA GENOME OF VIRUS

B.

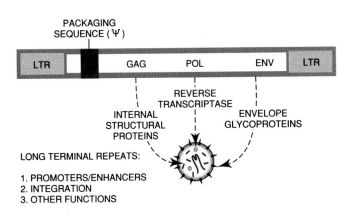

PACKAGING
SEQUENCE (Ψ)

| LTR | | GAG | POL | ENV | LTR |

REVERSE
TRANSCRIPTASE

INTERNAL
STRUCTURAL
PROTEINS

ENVELOPE
GLYCOPROTEINS

LONG TERMINAL REPEATS:

1. PROMOTERS/ENHANCERS
2. INTEGRATION
3. OTHER FUNCTIONS

Figure 11.3. **A.** Life cycle of a retrovirus. **B.** Diagram of the genome of a typical retrovirus.

other researchers began to apply the techniques of molecular biology to a more direct assault on human cancer. If specific mutations in cellular genes are capable of causing a malignant phenotype in human cancers, and if those mutations operate dominantly at the cellular level, then the transfer of DNA sequences from a malignant cell to a normal cell might be expected to result in the transformation into a malignant phenotype. A major advance was accomplished in 1981 when three laboratories simultaneously achieved success in this experiment. The basic principle of the experiment is shown in Figure 11.4. The DNA is prepared from a human tumor cell line; for the initial experiments this was a bladder carcinoma called EJ. This DNA was transfected into the mouse fibroblast cell line called 3T3.

When grown in a culture dish, nonmalignant cells such as 3T3 will stop growing when they touch each other (referred to as "contact inhibition"), whereas malignant cells generally continue to grow, piling up on top of each other to form foci of transformation. When the DNA from the human EJ bladder cancer cell line was introduced into mouse 3T3 cells and the cultures observed, foci of transformed mouse cells appeared. No such foci ap-

Figure 11.4. Transfection assay of human tumor DNA demonstrating its ability to confer malignant transformation on mouse 3T3 cells. DNA was prepared from the human tumor and transfected into 3T3 cells using calcium phosphate. Cells that received the human cancer gene became transformed and piled up on the plate, forming foci. These transformed cells also created tumors in nude mice when injected subcutaneously, whereas the untransfected 3T3 cells did not.

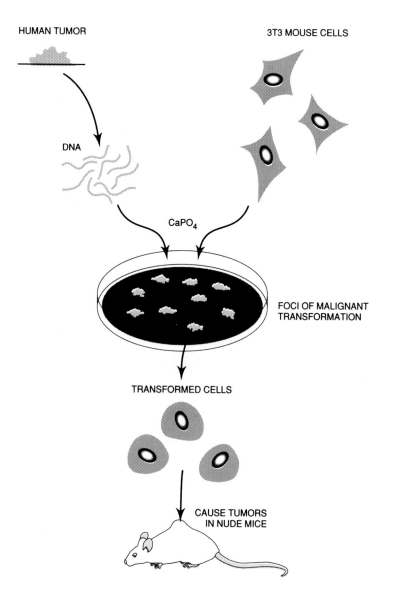

peared when DNA from a nonmalignant source was used. Furthermore, 3T3 cells from transformed foci produced tumor nodules when implanted into immunodeficient mice (called "nude" mice because they have no fur) whereas untransformed 3T3 cells did not. These findings strongly supported the notion that the bladder cancer DNA did contain a dominantly acting cancer gene, which was promptly named an **oncogene.**

To rescue and molecularly clone this oncogene, a clever strategy diagramed in Figure 11.5 was used. This approach depends upon the presence of interspersed repetitive *Alu* sequences in human DNA (chapter 5), which allow its discrimination from mouse DNA. DNA prepared from a primary transformed focus containing many different fragments of human DNA was used to transform 3T3 cells in a second round. At this point, the majority of

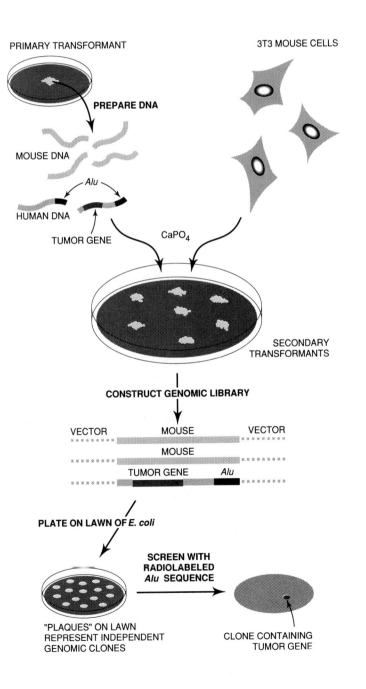

Figure 11.5. Cloning of a dominant oncogene. DNA from a transformed focus (Fig. 11.4) was prepared and mouse 3T3 cells were retransformed with this DNA (a "second round" of transfection, used to limit the amount of human DNA still present in the transformed mouse cells). DNA was then prepared from the resulting foci and cloned into a λ genomic library, as described in chapter 5. The human sequence then was identified by screening the library with a radioactively labeled sequence corresponding to the human-specific *Alu* repeat element.

the DNA in the secondary transformants was mouse in origin, with only a small proportion of human DNA still present, containing the oncogene. A segment of DNA common to all of the secondary transformants was molecularly cloned, using the human *Alu* sequence as a probe. The purified DNA, when transfected back into mouse 3T3 cells, yielded foci at extremely high efficiency, indicating that the responsible oncogene had been cloned. When the sequence of this transforming gene was determined, the research groups found to their surprise that it was extremely similar to the sequence of a retroviral transforming gene called H-*ras*.

How then can the two disparate fields of transforming retroviruses and tumor oncogenes be connected? The answer lies in the life cycle of the retrovirus shown in Figure 11.3A. After integration into the host genome, a rare recombination event can occur, such that the retrovirus is excised, carrying along with it a segment of host DNA. If this segment of DNA happens to contain a growth-promoting gene, and if the retrovirus "activates" this gene by use of the strong promoters in the retroviral flanking sequences (called LTRs, see Fig. 11.3A), the subsequent infection of other cells by this retrovirus will transform them. Such a virus will provide a growth advantage to cells it infects, and thus will be selected for. Endogenous oncogenes found in human tumors like the EJ bladder cancer, on the other hand, apparently represent activation of a normal growth-promoting gene by a somatic event not involving a virus, but with the same outcome, namely, the development of the malignant phenotype. Normal cellular genes that have this potential are referred to as **proto-oncogenes.**

Subsequent experiments showed that even the activated *ras* gene, cloned from the bladder cancer cell line, was not able to transform all cell types. Specifically, cultures of human or rodent fibroblasts derived directly from biopsies, without allowing time for "immortalization" to occur in culture (as with the 3T3 cell line), were not transformed by this gene alone. However, a combination of two oncogenes, such as *ras* plus *myc*, was able to induce transformation in primary fibroblast cells. Thus, the mouse 3T3 cells used for the initial experiments were not entirely normal. These observations are consistent with the hypothesis that the development of malignancy is an event involving two or more steps. We will return to this theme later.

CELLULAR PROTO-ONCOGENES AND THEIR FUNCTIONS

More than 40 proto-oncogenes have been identified, initially by the presence of their activated forms (oncogenes) in acute transforming retroviruses or their isolation from human tumors by DNA transfection. Others were subsequently identified through their activation by DNA amplification or chromosomal translocation, as described below. The prediction that proto-oncogenes would be involved in growth promotion has now been borne out in several specific examples. The *sis* oncogene turns out to be identical to the gene for a subunit of platelet-derived growth factor (*PDGF*), an important substance produced by platelets and other cells that acts as a strong stimulus to cell growth and division and is involved in normal wound healing. Another class of proto-oncogenes turns out to represent the genes for growth factor receptors, structures that are present on the cell membrane and are activated by the presence of a specific growth factor. Binding of the growth factor to its receptor leads to a chain of events that results in the delivery of a mitogenic signal to the nucleus. The *erb*B1 oncogene corresponds to the gene for epidermal growth factor receptor (*EGFR*), and the *fms* oncogene to

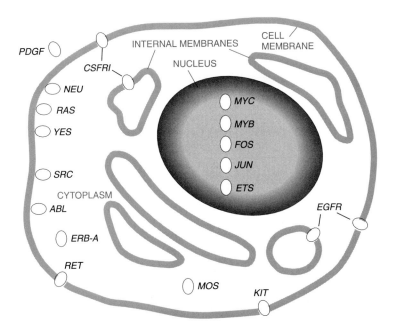

Figure 11.6.   Cellular localization of various proto-oncogene protein products. Some, like platelet-derived growth factor (*PDGF*), are secreted growth factors; others, like epidermal growth factor receptor (*EGFR*), are growth factor receptors residing in the cellular membrane; others, such as *RAS*, are involved in transmission of signals from the membrane to the nucleus, and still others, like *FOS* and *MYC*, are located in the nucleus itself.

the receptor for colony-stimulating factor 1 (*CSFR1*), a growth factor that promotes cell division of a variety of cells in the bone marrow.

Other proto-oncogenes, such as *RAS*, seem to play their role by acting in the signal transduction pathway between transmembrane receptors and the nucleus. Finally, a number of proto-oncogenes, including *MYC* and *FOS*, code for proteins that are located in the nucleus and are likely to be involved directly in the regulation of DNA transcription or replication. A summary of some of these localizations is shown in Figure 11.6.

HOW ARE ONCOGENES ACTIVATED?

If proto-oncogenes represent sequences necessary for normal cell growth, what events are responsible for their activation and subsequent loss of control? Several different mechanisms are possible.

Point Mutation

The *RAS* gene cloned from human bladder carcinoma cells was initially a puzzle. No major rearrangement of this gene was apparent when comparing it to its normal counterpart in nonmalignant cells. Sequencing the gene revealed a surprisingly subtle abnormality, namely a point mutation in codon 12 of the gene, converting a glycine at that position to a valine.

Analysis of a large number of additional lung and colon tumors using the mouse 3T3 cell transformation assay (Figs. 11.4 and 11.5) also resulted in the cloning of activated *HRAS* genes, as well as activated *KRAS* and *NRAS* genes, which are related members of the same gene family. Remarkably, all of these activated genes contained point mutations in codons 12, 13, or 61 of the *RAS* genes, indicating that these positions must be critically important for the normal control of cell proliferation. The RAS protein product can exist in an active form, which binds to GTP, and an inactive form, which binds GDP. Apparently, these point mutations block the conversion of RAS from the active to the inactive form, and thus allow unregulated cell growth (Fig. 11.7).

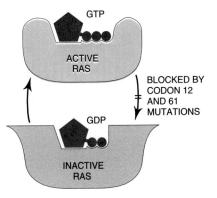

Figure 11.7.   Proposed regulation of activation of the RAS protein. The active form binds GTP, whereas the inactive form binds GDP. Apparently the point mutations in codons 12 and 61, which convert *RAS* to a transforming gene, prevent the conversion from the active to the inactive form, so the protein is left in a "locked-on" position.

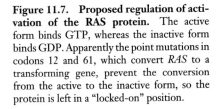

Amplification

Another plausible mechanism for the activation of a proto-oncogene is marked overexpression of its protein product. In some instances this occurs in a cancer cell by actual amplification of the DNA sequences encoding the proto-oncogene. The amplified block of DNA is generally several hundred kilobases in length, often including a number of other genes located near the oncogene. These amplified segments of DNA are sometimes visible on a chromosome spread as separate small fragments, referred to as "double minutes" (Figure 11.8A). When the amplified DNA is inserted into one of the chromosomes, it is termed a **homogeneously staining region**, or HSR (Figure 11.8B). Although HSRs and double minutes are encountered in a number of different cancers, the associated oncogene, which has been amplified, has only been identified in a limited number of cases. One example is a characteristic amplification of the *NMYC* gene that is observed in some neuroblastomas, one of the more common tumors of childhood. This *NMYC* amplification is associated with a relatively poor prognosis.

Figure 11.8. Activation of proto-oncogenes by amplification. A. Multiple copies of "double minutes" (*arrows*) are seen in this tumor cell metaphase stained with Giemsa. **B.** An HSR (*arrow*) is seen here on the short arm of chromosome 7 in this G-banded tumor cell metaphase. (Reprinted with permission from Beaudet AL, Scriver CR, Sly WS, Valle D, (eds.) The metabolic and molecular bases of inherited disease. CD version. New York: Mgraw-Hill, 1997.)

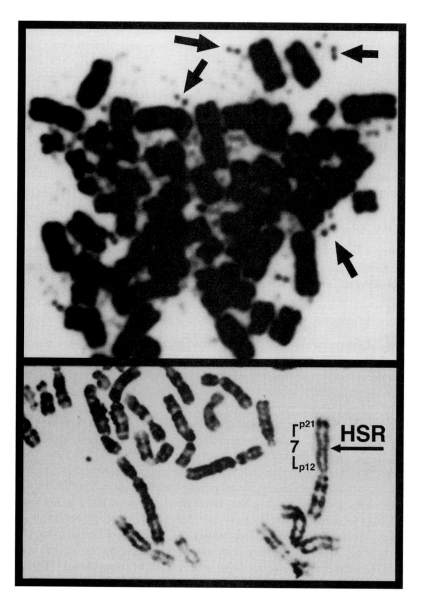

Chromosome Translocation

In some dramatic instances, chromosome translocations occurring at or near a proto-oncogene locus have resulted in activation of the gene. The first such example was found in Burkitt lymphoma, a B-cell tumor, which is rare in the United States but common in parts of Africa. Previous cytogenetic analyses had shown that a high proportion of Burkitt lymphomas are characterized by the appearance of a balanced translocation between chromosomes 8 and 14. Gene mapping efforts carried out in the early 1980s yielded an interesting finding: the *MYC* proto-oncogene maps to 8q24, and the immunoglobulin heavy-chain locus maps to 14q32. These are the bands involved in the Burkitt lymphoma translocation (see Fig. 11.9). Subsequent molecular analysis of multiple Burkitt lymphomas has demonstrated that the breakpoints do occur within or near the *MYC* locus, and within the immunoglobulin locus. As a result, the *MYC* locus is placed close to a gene that is being actively transcribed in a B cell, namely the heavy-chain immunoglobulin gene. Although the exact mechanism of *MYC* activation is not clear, it appears that the *MYC* gene is deregulated in an important way by this event, allowing this nuclear oncogene to run amok, resulting in the lymphomatous transformation.

Another example of oncogene activation by chromosome translocation is the Philadelphia chromosome, for which a karyotype is shown in Figure 11.2. This characteristic chromosomal translocation results in the creation of a unique, chimeric gene that appears to play an important role in the pathogenesis of CML. As illustrated in Figure 11.10, the translocation fuses the *ABL* proto-oncogene, located at 9q, to the *BCR* gene on chromosome 22q. The resulting chimeric BCR-ABL protein retains the protein kinase activity of the *ABL* gene, although its normal function and pattern of expression is now altered by the BCR gene to which it is fused. Aberrant expression of this altered *ABL* protein appears to be a causative factor in the development of CML.

The study of specific chromosomal translocations associated with particular tumor types has identified a number of novel proto-oncogenes and mech-

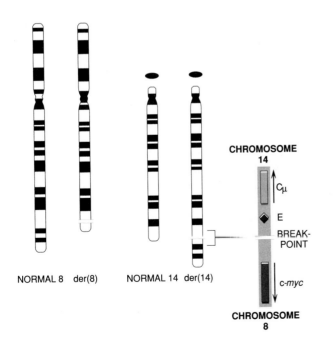

NORMAL 8   der(8)   NORMAL 14   der(14)

CHROMOSOME 14

Cμ

E

BREAK-POINT

c-myc

CHROMOSOME 8

Figure 11.9. Specific translocation seen in Burkitt lymphoma. Most tumors of this sort show a translocation with breakpoints at 8q24 and 14q32. Molecular analysis of these translocations shows that the breakpoint on chromosome 8 is adjacent to or within the *MYC* proto-oncogene, whereas the breakpoint on chromosome 14 is in the heavy chain immunoglobulin locus. The exact nature of the rearrangement varies from tumor to tumor, but a typical example is shown in the right-hand part of the figure. In some instances, it appears that the enhancer (*E*) of the heavy chain gene (Cμ) may play a role in activating overexpression of the *MYC* gene.

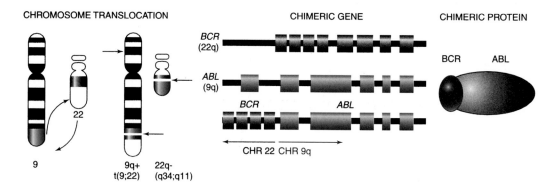

Figure 11.10.   The Philadelphia chromosome translocation fuses the 5′ end of the *BCR* gene (on chromosome 22q) to the 3′ portion of the *ABL* gene (on chromosome 9q).   The resulting chimeric gene directs the expression of a chimeric fusion protein containing the N-terminal portion of the *BCR* gene joined to the active protein kinase portion of the *ABL* gene (Adapted from Fearon ER. Oncogenes and tumor suppressor genes. In: Abeloff MD, Armitage JO, Lichter AS, Niederhuber JE, eds. Clinical oncology. New York: Churchill Livingstone, 1995.)

anisms for their activation. The association between an oncogene and a specific tumor may also provide important clues about the origin of that cancer. In addition to the unique Philadelphia chromosome translocation characteristic of virtually all cases of CML, a number of other specific associations have been identified. The unique translocation between chromosomes 15 and 17, fusing the gene for the retinoic acid receptor with a previously unknown gene termed *PMR*, is identified in nearly all cases of acute promyelocytic leukemia. Analysis of the specific translocation between chromosomes 14 and 18, characteristic of follicular lymphomas, led to the identification of the *BCL-2* gene, a critical protein in the regulation of programmed cell death (**apoptosis**).

DO ACTIVATED ONCOGENES CAUSE FAMILIAL CANCER?

All of the mutations described above, which lead to activation of cellular proto-oncogenes, are acquired (somatic) mutations in cancer cells. That is, when the constitutional DNA from patients with these cancers is examined, these mutations are not found, indicating that they were acquired during the process of the development of malignancy. However, as noted above, it seems very likely that more than one such mutational event is required before a transformation to true malignancy occurs. This raises the question as to whether some familial cancer syndromes are due to the germline inheritance of an activated oncogene. Such individuals would be highly predisposed to the development of malignancy should an additional somatic mutation occur. Indeed, tumors have been produced in transgenic mice by expressing a variety of oncogenes in appropriate target tissues. However, this appears to be a very rare mechanism for inherited cancer in humans. Though there are a number of important human genetic cancer predisposition syndromes, they generally involve inherited mutations in a second class of genes termed tumor suppressor genes, which we will discuss in the next section. The general absence of germline proto-oncogene mutations in familial cancers, despite their prominent role in the somatic mutations of sporadic cancers, remains a puzzle. One exception (the *RET* proto-oncogene) will be considered later. Perhaps the phenotypes resulting from such mutations are subject to strong negative selection because of the resulting disturbances of central cellular processes, as well as the induction of malignancy.

As indicated in the opening quotation from Boveri, it is reasonable to hypothesize that there may be genes that normally restrain growth. Inactivation of such genes would be predicted to contribute to the progression toward malignancy. This is an extremely important pathway.

RETINOBLASTOMA AND THE KNUDSON HYPOTHESIS

The tumor suppressor gene model was first proposed in the early 1970s by Alfred Knudson as an explanation for hereditary retinoblastoma. An elegant series of experiments beginning in the mid 1980s proved Knudson's hypothesis to be remarkably accurate.

Retinoblastoma is a tumor of retinal cells, which develops in children between birth and about 4 years of age. It has been known for some time that approximately half of cases of retinoblastoma are sporadic; these usually involve only one tumor in one eye. The other half of cases, however, occur in an autosomal dominant fashion, often involve both eyes, frequently occur at young ages, and often result in more than one tumor in each eye. Treatment is surgical and often involves removal of the affected eye or eyes. Interestingly, those affected with familial retinoblastoma have an increased incidence of later developing other malignancies, especially osteosarcoma, a malignant tumor of bone. Figure 11.11 shows typical pedigrees contrasting the familial and sporadic forms.

In Figure 11.12 is shown a section of an eye of an individual affected with the familial form of retinoblastoma. There are two sites of tumor formation visible. However, the entire globe is lined with a layer of retinal cells, and inspection reveals that the vast majority of these retinal cells are behaving in a normal fashion. Nonetheless, all of these cells must carry the retinoblastoma mutation, because this was inherited through the germline from an affected parent. Those cells that have developed into tumors, therefore, must have acquired at least one additional genetic abnormality, which led to their clonal expansion. Because a large number of cells of the retina are at risk, an additional mutation ("second hit") of low frequency would still be sufficient to convert a few of these cells to tumorigenic behavior.

In 1971, Alfred Knudson carried this observation one step further by proposing a specific hypothesis, illustrated in Figure 11.13. He proposed that the germline event in familial retinoblastoma is inactivation of one al-

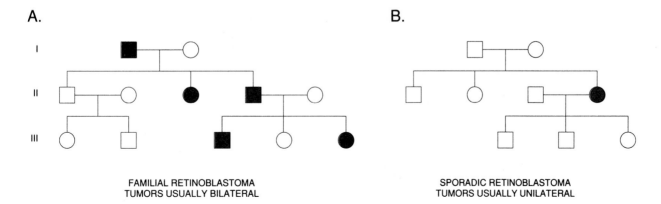

A.

B.

FAMILIAL RETINOBLASTOMA
TUMORS USUALLY BILATERAL

SPORADIC RETINOBLASTOMA
TUMORS USUALLY UNILATERAL

Figure 11.11. Typical pedigrees of retinoblastoma. A. Familial dominantly inherited pattern. In this situation, tumors are usually bilateral and occur at an early age. **B.** Sporadic retinoblastoma. In this situation only one individual in a family is affected, and the tumor is somewhat later in onset and usually unilateral.

Figure 11.12.   Section of an eye of an individual with familial retinoblastoma. Note that, although two independent tumors are apparent, the majority of the thin layer of retina (here artifactually separated from the back of the eye in the preparation) is normal. This suggests that tumor formation requires an additional somatic event on top of the germline mutation. (Used with permission from Willis RA, ed. Pathology of tumours. 3rd ed. Butterworth, 1960;894.)

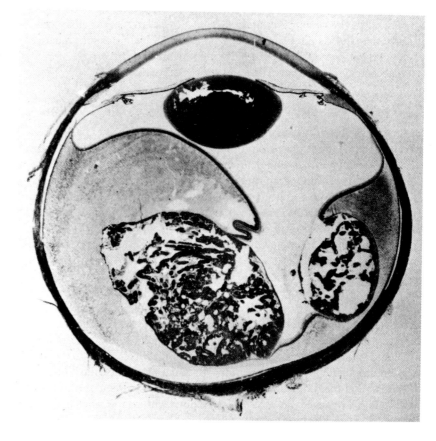

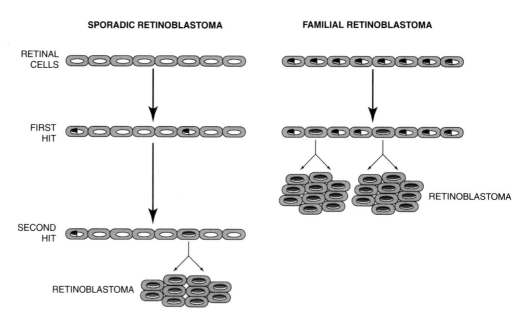

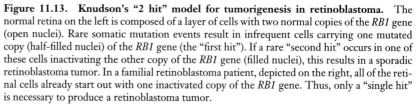

Figure 11.13.   Knudson's "2 hit" model for tumorigenesis in retinoblastoma.   The normal retina on the left is composed of a layer of cells with two normal copies of the *RB1* gene (open nuclei). Rare somatic mutation events result in infrequent cells carrying one mutated copy (half-filled nuclei) of the *RB1* gene (the "first hit"). If a rare "second hit" occurs in one of these cells inactivating the other copy of the *RB1* gene (filled nuclei), this results in a sporadic retinoblastoma tumor. In a familial retinoblastoma patient, depicted on the right, all of the retinal cells already start out with one inactivated copy of the *RB1* gene. Thus, only a "single hit" is necessary to produce a retinoblastoma tumor.

lele of an autosomal tumor suppressor gene. Because the other allele would remain active, only a 50% reduction in the amount of the protein product would occur, which would be expected to have negligible effects. He then proposed that the somatic second hit in retinoblastoma is the loss of the other allele. In a cell in which this had occurred, production of this tumor suppressor protein would be completely abolished, and the result would be unregulated growth. This model leads to a paradoxical conclusion: although inheritance of the tendency to retinoblastoma is dominant, the actual mechanism of tumor development in a specific cell is recessive, because tumors appear only when *both* copies of the retinoblastoma gene are inactivated. Thus, tumor suppressor genes are also sometimes called recessive tumor genes. The sporadic cases in this model are proposed to be due to somatic inactivation of *both* alleles in a single retinal cell, without the presence of a germline mutation.

EVIDENCE FOR THE TUMOR SUPPRESSOR GENE HYPOTHESIS

One of the observations that supported Knudson's hypothesis was the identification of rare children with retinoblastoma who also had a variety of birth defects and mental retardation. These were sporadic cases of retinoblastoma, but tumors occurred bilaterally. Careful cytogenetic analysis of most of these patients revealed an interstitial deletion of the long arm of chromosome 13. Figure 11.14 shows some of the deletions identified. Whereas the precise portion of chromosome 13 which is absent varies from patient to patient, a region of 13q14 is common to all of them. This region thus seemed to be a likely candidate for the location of the retinoblastoma gene. These unusual patients with cytogenetic deletions had probably obliterated one copy of the retinoblastoma gene by chromosomal deletion; the deletion was large enough to involve many other genes as well, presumably explaining the other birth defects and mental retardation of these patients (an example of a contiguous gene syndrome, see chapter 8).

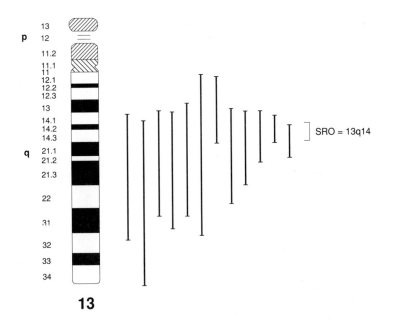

Figure 11.14. Representative examples of chromosome 13 deletions identified in patients with retinoblastoma, birth defects, and mental retardation. Although the exact region of chromosome 13 that is deleted varies from patient to patient, all of these have in common a deletion of 13q14, which is therefore likely to contain the retinoblastoma gene.

If the retinoblastoma gene is on 13q14, then one would expect to find linkage to this region in patients with the inherited form of the disease. Analyses of a large number of families with retinoblastoma indeed identified such linkage, supporting the notion that the same gene (called *RB1*) is mutated in familial retinoblastoma and is completely deleted in the rarer patients with 13q14 deletions.

Genetic Analysis of Retinoblastoma Tumors

Although the above data supported the localization of the retinoblastoma gene to chromosome 13, analysis of tumor tissue itself was necessary to demonstrate that the mechanism of tumor formation involves loss of the normal allele of this gene. There are several mechanisms by which this loss might occur, as shown in Figure 11.15. The simplest would be the loss of the normal chromosome 13 in its entirety. Alternatively, the normal chromosome 13 might be lost, and then the abnormal chromosome 13 duplicated. A more complex mechanism involves mitotic recombination, in which an exchange occurs between homologous chromosomes during mitosis. (Note that, although this is an essential event in meiosis, its occurrence in mitosis was not clearly shown until the investigation of this tumor type.) Finally, the normal chromosome could independently acquire a different mutation in the retinoblastoma gene. The outcome of these events, as well as the effect on a polymorphic DNA marker located close to *RB1*, is diagramed in Figure 11.15. Note that all of these occurrences except independent mutation would lead to loss of one allele for a closely linked DNA marker in the

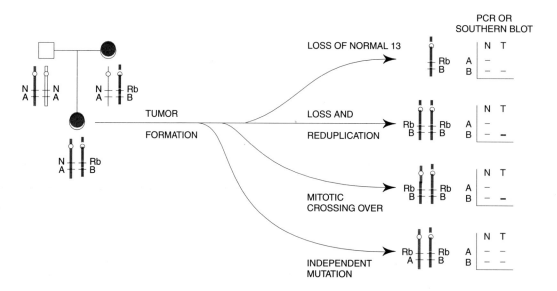

Figure 11.15.   Diagram of possible mechanisms for tumor formation in an individual with familial retinoblastoma.   On the *left* is shown the pedigree of an affected individual, who has inherited the abnormal (Rb) gene from her affected mother. The four chromosomes of her two parents are drawn to indicate their origin. Just below the retinoblastoma locus a polymorphic marker is also analyzed in this family. The patient is AB at this locus, like her mother, whereas her father is AA. Thus the B allele must be on the chromosome carrying the retinoblastoma disease gene. Tumor formation results when the normal allele (N), which this patient inherited from her father, is inactivated. On the *right* are shown four possible ways in which this could occur. In each case, the resulting chromosome 13 arrangement is shown, as well as analysis of the polymorphic marker by PCR or Southern blotting, comparing normal tissue with tumor tissue. Note that in the first three situations the normal allele (A) has been lost in the tumor tissue, which is referred to as loss of heterozygosity (LOH).

tumor tissue. Specifically, the allele located on the chromosome carrying the normal *RB1* gene would be predicted to disappear in the tumor if one of these mechanisms were operative. This is termed "reduction to homozygosity" or **loss of heterozygosity** (LOH) and can be detected by PCR or a Southern blot, comparing constitutional DNA from a retinoblastoma patient with DNA derived from the tumor.

For complete loss of the normal chromosome, with or without duplication of the abnormal chromosome, note that all DNA markers on that chromosome will show LOH. A mitotic recombination, however, will lead to LOH for all markers distal to the site of recombination. If several such events can be detected in independent tumors, it is even possible to obtain a rough idea of where the tumor gene is located, because it must always be reduced to homozygosity in the recombination event.

Careful analysis of retinoblastoma tumors revealed the occurrence of all of these possibilities. By studying families, it was possible to prove that it was always the normal chromosome 13 that was lost in tumor formation. Thus, the data agree precisely with the predictions of the Knudson hypothesis and therefore strongly support the presence of a tumor suppressor gene on chromosome 13q14. Analysis of other tumors often occurring later in retinoblastoma patients, such as osteosarcomas, generally revealed the same pattern with consistent loss of the normal chromosome 13 allele by one of these same mechanisms.

CLONING OF THE RETINOBLASTOMA GENE

Taking advantage of genetic analysis of families and LOH studies of large numbers of tumors, the *RB1* gene was cloned in 1986, one of the first successes of the positional cloning approach (chapter 9). As predicted by the Knudson hypothesis, analysis of retinoblastoma tumors using this cDNA as a probe on Northern blots indicated that in some tumors the message was completely absent, whereas in others an abnormal sized message was seen (Fig. 11.16). In some tumors the messenger RNA appeared normal by Northern blot, but more detailed sequence analysis revealed point muta-

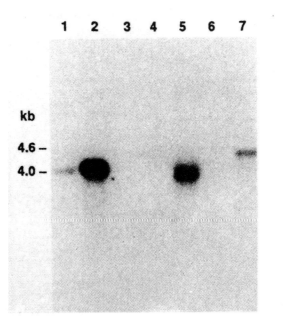

Figure 11.16.   Northern blot of RNA from a variety of retinal tumors.   The probe used on the Northern blot is a cDNA clone representing the *RB1* gene transcript. *Lanes 1–6* represent RNA samples from six different retinoblastoma tumors, whereas *lane 7* is RNA derived from normal fetal retina. Notice that the normal transcript of this gene is 4.6 kb in length, whereas RNA from the retinoblastoma tumors either completely lacks this transcript (*lanes 3, 4, and 6*) or contains a shortened abnormal transcript (*lanes 1, 2, and 5*). Thus, none of the retinoblastoma tumors contain a normal transcript. This indicates that *both* of the alleles of the *RB1* locus are abnormal in these tumors, in accordance with the predictions of the Knudson model. (Used with permission from Lee WH, et al. Human retinoblastoma susceptibility gene: cloning, identification, and sequence. Science 1987;235:1394.)

tions. In no instance where careful analysis was carried out was a normal transcript of the gene found in retinoblastoma tumors.

Since its identification, considerable effort has gone into determining the normal function of the retinoblastoma gene. The specific association of inherited *RB1* gene mutations with tumors in the retina and bone suggested important functions for the *RB1* gene in these tissues. Thus, it was surprising to observe that the *RB1* gene is widely expressed in many tissues throughout the body. The *RB1* protein is localized to the nucleus and appears to play a central regulatory role in the progression of cells through the cell cycle. *RB1* interacts with a number of other regulatory proteins within the cell and is in turn controlled by the activity of a series of cell cycle-specific proteins called cyclins. This process regulates the decision of a cell to undergo cell division and proliferate or to remain quiescent. Why dysfunction of the *RB1* gene should particularly predispose to cancers of the retina and bone remains a mystery. As we shall see, many of the other genes associated with particular tumor types also function in central processes shared by many cells. Despite considerable progress in cancer genetics, the explanation for the association of specific gene defects with particular tumor types remains largely unknown.

The identification of the *RB1* gene is an example of a major advance in fundamental cell biology that resulted from the study of a rare human disease. This is a lesson that has frequently been repeated in the history of medical science.

OTHER RARE FAMILIAL CANCER SYNDROMES

Since the discovery of the retinoblastoma gene, similar approaches have been used to identify the genes responsible for a number of other rare familial cancer syndromes, as listed in Table 11.1. For many but not all of these genes, LOH was identified in the associated tumors, suggesting that the two hit model originally proposed by Knudson is applicable to many tumor suppressor genes. As for *RB1*, a number of these genes have turned out

Table 11.1. Familial Cancer Syndromes and Associated Tumor Suppressor Genes

Familial Cancer Syndrome	Tumor Suppressor Gene	Function	Chromosome Location	Type of Tumors Observed
Familial Retinoblastoma	*RB1*	Cell cycle regulation	13q14	Retinoblastoma, osteogenic sarcoma
Li-Fraumeni Syndrome	*P53*	Regulation of cell cycle and apoptosis	17p13	Brain tumors, sarcomas, leukemia, breast cancer
Familial Adenomatous Polyposis	*APC*	Signaling from cell surface adhesion molecules to nucleus	5q21	Colon cancer
von Hippel-Lindau Syndrome	*VHL*	Regulate transcription elongation	3p25	Renal cancers, hemangioblastomas, pheochromocytoma
Wilms Tumor	*WT1*	Transcriptional regulation	11p13	Pediatric kidney cancer
Familial Melanoma	*CDKN2A*	Regulation of cell cycle	9p21	Melanoma, pancreatic cancer, others
Hereditary Nonpolyposis Colon Cancer	*MSH2*	DNA mismatch repair	2p16	Colon cancer
Hereditary Nonpolyposis Colon Cancer	*MLH1*	DNA mismatch repair	3p21	Colon cancer
Familial Breast Cancer	*BRCA1*	?	17q21	Breast and ovarian cancer
Familial Breast Cancer	*BRCA2*	?	13q12	Breast and ovarian cancer
Gorlin Syndrome	*PTCH*	? early development and cell differentiation	9q22	Basal cell skin cancers
Multiple Endocrine Neoplasia Type 1	*MEN1*	?	11q13	Parathyroid and pituitary adenomas, islet cell tumors, carcinoid
Neurofibromatosis Type I	*NF1*	Catalysis of RAS inactivation	17q11.2	Neurofibromas, sarcomas, gliomas

to be central components of the general cellular machinery. For example, the von Hippel-Lindau (*VHL*) gene on chromosome 3 interacts with several highly conserved transcription elongation factors and appears to play an important role in regulating the normal RNA transcription process. Patients who inherit germline mutation in the *VHL* gene develop multiple kidney cancers as well as unusual vascular tumors (hemangioblastomas) of the retina, cerebellum, and spinal cord. Somatic mutations in the *VHL* gene are also identified in a high percentage of sporadic kidney cancers. Mutations in specific genes involved in regulation of the cell cycle, such as *CDKN2A*, have also been identified in familial melanoma. As another example, the recently identified gene for basal cell nevus syndrome (or Gorlin syndrome), an unusual genetic disease associated with multiple basal cell skin cancers and a variety of birth defects, is closely related to a gene called *patched*, which regulates early embryo development and differentiation in the fruit fly, *Drosophila*.

As is evident from our discussion so far, the genes underlying familial cancer syndromes are generally of the tumor suppressor type, acting in a "recessive" manner at the level of the cell. However, inheritance of the syndrome is autosomal dominant. A rare example of an inherited activating mutation in a proto-oncogene is found in the *RET* gene, leading to multiple endocrine neoplasia type 2 (MEN2). The *RET* proto-oncogene, first identified as an oncogene, by DNA transfection studies, is a member of the large family of transmembrane tyrosine kinase growth factor receptors. The *RET* gene is found to be rearranged in about 30% of papillary thyroid carcinomas and a mouse model for this disease has been generated by targeting a mutant form of *RET* to the thyroid gland. The gene is also found to be amplified in some carcinomas of the breast. Patients with MEN2 are generally found to have inherited germline mutations in the *RET* gene that result in constitutive activation of the receptor. MEN2 patients develop a characteristic type of thyroid cancer called medullary carcinoma, as well as tumors of the adrenal gland and parathyroid. Although LOH is observed at a variety of chromosomes in MEN-related tumors, these sites do not include the *RET* locus itself. Curiously, loss of function mutations in the *RET* gene result in a completely distinct disorder called Hirschsprung disease in which there is absence of the normal autonomic nerve plexi in the colon and rectum, resulting in massive dilatation of the colon. This is a dramatic example of the way in which different mutations of the same gene can produce drastically different phenotypes.

The *P53* gene provides another very instructive example of a gene that can be both a tumor suppressor gene and a dominantly acting oncogene. Transfection studies in NIH 3T3 cells showed that *P53* could function as an oncogene to immortalize cells and could also transform cells in conjunction with a mutant *RAS* gene. Mutations in the *P53* gene were subsequently shown to be one of the most common somatic mutations in a wide variety of tumor types. The *P53* protein is a transcription factor that may play a critical role in regulating progression of cells through the cell cycle, as well as entry of cells into the apoptosis (programed cell death) pathway.

It now appears that the normal *P53* gene functions predominantly as a tumor suppressor gene. Loss of *P53* function relieves a normal block to cell growth giving mutant cells an advantage. Loss of *P53* function also allows cells to escape apoptosis. Germline mutation in the *P53* gene results in the autosomal dominant cancer predisposition disorder, Li-Fraumeni syndrome. This condition is notable among the inherited cancer syndromes for the pleomorphic assortment of tumors that can be observed. Patients typically develop sarcomas of diverse soft tissues as well as breast cancers, brain cancers, leukemias, and a variety of other cancer types. These tumors also arise early, with 50% of patients developing a first cancer by age 30.

Defects in DNA Repair Genes

All of the genetic cancer predisposition syndromes that we have discussed so far, as well as the recently identified genes for common cancers that we will discuss later in this chapter, are inherited in an autosomal dominant fashion. At this time, there are only a few known recessive cancer predisposition syndromes. The genetic defects for a number of these syndromes reside in genes involved in DNA repair or replication. For example, several different types of xeroderma pigmentosum are caused by mutations in genes that repair ultraviolet damage to DNA. Not surprisingly, these patients develop multiple cancers of the skin, particularly in sun (ultraviolet) exposed areas. The genetic defects in Fanconi anemia and Bloom syndrome result in general instability of the genome and frequent chromosome breakage. In addition to the high frequencies of cancer in these syndromes, these patients also have a number of characteristic skeletal and other developmental abnormalities.

Recently, a new class of genes involved in the repair of DNA mismatches has been identified through the study of inherited colon cancer. Together, this group of "mutator genes," which we will discuss below, defines a novel mechanism in the cancer pathway.

Genetic Predisposition for Common Cancers

Until recently, inherited forms of cancer were thought to be restricted to a few rare syndromes. Though the same genes may participate in the development of sporadic cancers by chance somatic mutation events, it was generally thought that germline mutations would be of limited direct relevance to the routine practice of medicine. This situation has changed dramatically during the past few years with the identification of specific germline mutations in significant subsets of patients with two very common types of cancer, breast cancer and colon cancer. A susceptibility gene for prostate cancer has also recently been mapped. Though inherited predisposition has not yet been demonstrated for some other common cancers, such as lung cancer (the number one cause of cancer death), this situation is likely to change in the coming years.

A number of general observations taken from the rare familial cancer syndromes provided helpful clues for the identification of inherited forms for common cancers. Cancers caused by germline mutation generally develop at younger ages than sporadic cancers and more often result in multiple tumors in the same individual. Association with other less common cancer types may also provide a useful clue. However, identification of predisposition genes for common cancers is made considerably more difficult by the large background of unrelated sporadic cancers in the general population. For example, breast cancer is the most common cancer in females, affecting 11% of women during their lifetime. Though it now appears that 5–10% of breast cancers may be related to the inheritance of a germline mutation in one of several specific predisposition genes, the vast majority of cases (~95%) are sporadic, presumably arising through interactions between chance somatic mutations, contributions from environmental factors, and multiple minor predisposing genes (see discussion of multifactorial disorders in chapter 4). By chance, 11% of the sisters of a sporadic breast cancer proband would be expected to develop a sporadic breast cancer. Similarly, there would be an approximately

1% chance of sporadic breast cancer developing independently in both the sister and mother of a sporadic breast cancer patient. For this reason, it can be very difficult to distinguish between breast cancer caused by the inheritance of a cancer gene and that resulting from chance clustering of sporadic breast cancer cases in a family. This problem also provides a major challenge to the clinical management of cancer families. This situation should be contrasted with a familial cancer syndrome associated with rare tumors, such as MEN2. The occurrence of an uncommon medullary carcinoma of the thyroid and pheochromocytoma in several individuals in the same family is extremely unlikely to have arisen by chance. Similarly, the occurrence of renal cell carcinoma in von Hippel-Lindau syndrome in association with retinal hemangioblastomas, a tumor that rarely occurs in any other setting, allows sporadic renal cell cancers to be easily distinguished from those associated with the syndrome.

Familial Breast Cancer

Family history has long been recognized as the most important risk factor for the development of breast cancer. However, for the reasons we have just outlined, it was very difficult to distinguish a clear-cut autosomal dominant inherited form of breast cancer from the very frequent, sporadic form of this disease. As a result, it was not until the late 1980s that a distinct autosomal dominant breast cancer susceptibility gene was proposed. Two such breast cancer susceptibility genes, termed *BRCA1* and *BRCA2*, have now been identified by positional cloning approaches. Together, these two genes may account for as many as 5–10% of all breast cancers, though it is likely that at least one other major BRCA gene remains to be identified. Though LOH evidence in affected families suggests that the *BRCA1* and *BRCA2* genes are tumor suppressors, their functions within the cell are still largely unknown. Women inheriting germline mutations in the *BRCA1* or *BRCA2* genes have a 60–90% lifetime risk of developing breast cancer as well as a 20–60% risk for ovarian cancer. There also appears to be a modest increase in the risk for other cancers in BRCA families, including prostate cancer in *BRCA1* and male breast cancer in *BRCA2*. The identification of the BRCA genes has raised difficult questions for the role of DNA testing and mutation screening in the clinical management of patients. This problem will be discussed later in this chapter.

Familial Colon Cancer

Familial polyposis coli is a rare autosomal dominant form of colon cancer (prevalence approximately 1:10,000) that can usually be readily distinguished from sporadic colon cancer. Though the colon is normal at birth in familial polyposis patients, during the first 20 years of life hundreds of small polyps appear in the colon and occasionally elsewhere in the intestinal tract. Although these polyps are asymptomatic, their major significance is the risk of progression to colon cancer, which approaches 100% by age 50 years in a patient with this disease. A total colectomy in early adulthood completely prevents this outcome. Figure 11.17 shows an x-ray film and a pathologic specimen from a patient with this condition, illustrating the innumerable polyps. Because this is an autosomal dominant disorder, making the diagnosis in one individual obligates the physician to investigate the rest of the family, as there may be no other warning signs of the presence of the disease until the appearance of malignancy. Because surgical therapy is so successful, individuals at risk should be evaluated with DNA testing, and colonoscopy if indicated, by the age of 20 years.

of this initiation process and develop multiple foci of dysplastic epithelium, many of which progress to early adenomas or polyps. The stepwise progression of this benign tumor to a full-blown cancer is the result of a number of somatic mutation events, including activation of the *RAS* proto-oncogene and progressive loss of tumor suppressor genes such as *DCC* and *P53*. Mutation in mismatch repair genes accelerate this somatic mutation process. There are undoubtedly other genetic alterations along the way that remain to be identified. In general, the more malignant tumors have acquired a larger number of mutational events along this pathway. It is often possible to see histologically that a carcinoma is arising out of an area of epithelium with a lower grade neoplasm, and to show that the more malignant area has acquired an additional genetic event. (Adapted from Weinberg RA, Hanahan D. The molecular pathogenesis of cancer. In: Bishop JM, Weinberg RA, eds. Scientific American molecular oncology. New York: Scientific American, Inc, 1996:187.)

somes 5q, 17p, and 18q (see Figure 11.18A). The earliest event appeared to involve the chromosome 5q gene, which turned out to be the *APC* gene. The gene on 17p is the *P53* gene that we have already discussed. The 18q gene, named *DCC* for "deleted in colon cancer" is still of unknown function and germline mutations in this gene have not yet been identified. Colon cancer cells undergo other types of changes or modifications to DNA, such as DNA methylation, that may also contribute to the malignant phenotype. Most recently, studies of familial colon cancer not associated with polyposis have identified a novel set of mutator genes that may also contribute to the development of sporadic colon cancer and other cancer types.

Hereditary Nonpolyposis Colon Cancer (HNPCC)

Although familial polyposis accounts for less than 1% of colon cancer, familial clustering of colon cancer without polyps is frequently observed. These families often also have features associated with familial cancer syndromes, such as young age of onset and association with other specific tumors such as ovarian and endometrial cancer. This syndrome is referred to as hereditary nonpolyposis colon cancer (HNPCC) or Lynch syndrome. Using the now familiar methods of positional cloning, the first gene responsible for a subset of HNPCC families, termed *MSH2*, was identified in 1993. This gene is closely related to a family of genes in bacteria and yeast involved in the repair of DNA sequence mismatches. Three other genes subsequently identified in HNPCC families also appear to be involved in the same DNA repair pathway. Consistent with this function, colon cancer cells from HNPCC patients are particularly susceptible to spontaneous mutations. This alteration presumably increases the occurrence of additional somatic mutations in other genes, thereby contributing to the multistep progression from normal to cancer cell (Figure 11.18B). The specific target genes for these additional somatic mutations are currently a subject of intense investigation.

Though the DNA mismatch repair genes appear to account for the majority of HNPCC families, additional genes probably remain to be identified. The prevalence in the general population of germline mutations in the HNPCC genes may be as high as 1:200, perhaps accounting for as many as 10–15% of all colon cancers. The similar phenotype among HNPCC families, regardless of which gene is involved, provides an excellent example of locus heterogeneity (see chapter 3).

A General Mechanism for Cancer

Several principles can be derived from the information presented in this chapter. Two major mechanisms for genetically altering a cell in such a way that its growth is increased were proposed by Boveri in the opening quota-

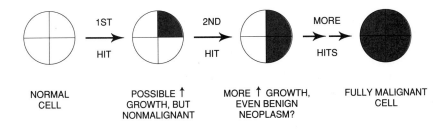

NORMAL CELL → 1ST HIT → POSSIBLE ↑ GROWTH, BUT NONMALIGNANT → 2ND HIT → MORE ↑ GROWTH, EVEN BENIGN NEOPLASM? → MORE HITS → FULLY MALIGNANT CELL

Figure 11.19. Diagram of the multistep origin of cancer. At least two genetic events appear to be necessary to convert a cell to a neoplastic phenotype, and for some tissues more than two events may be required. A germline predisposition to cancer can be thought of as shifting this diagram one step to the right.

tion. In fact, if the word "gene" is substituted for "chromosome" in his usage, then that paragraph accurately describes both oncogenes and tumor suppressor genes.

We have seen that the activation of proto-oncogenes is a frequent somatic event in the progression from normal cell to malignant cell. Tumor suppressor genes generally require two "hits" to be inactivated. Though both alleles can be inactivated by somatic events, individuals inheriting one allele that is already inactive can exhibit a marked predisposition to cancer. A third class of mutator genes directly interferes with the process of DNA repair, leading to more general genetic instability.

A recurring theme in these discussions is the fact that more than one mutational event is required to convert a normal cell to a malignant cell. Figure 11.18B depicts the multiple distinct mutation events required for the gradual progression of a normal epithelial cell to a full-blown colon cancer.

This multistep model as a general paradigm for the origin of cancer is shown in Figure 11.19. Beginning on the *left* is a normal cell, which possesses the necessary mechanism to inhibit its own growth when that is appropriate. A single mutation may somewhat increase the ability of that cell to proliferate, but appears insufficient to escape the normal control mechanisms completely. There are, in fact, compelling reasons why this must be so. Given the fact that there are an estimated 10^{14} cells in the body, and during replication a mutation rate of 10^{-6} per gene is estimated to occur, cancer would be an everyday event if a single mutation were sufficient. The single mutated cell may have a completely normal phenotype or may possess a slight growth advantage allowing it to survive, propagate, and eventually acquire another mutation. With each step along the way, the cell acquires somewhat more autonomy and is therefore able to propagate better than its neighbors. Eventually a point is reached at which the cell is able to grow in spite of signals that would normally arrest its proliferation, and it can then go on to destroy neighboring tissues and spread to other parts of the body.

Familial cancer syndromes, representing germline predisposition to cancer, can be thought of as shifting this diagram one step to the right. The individual with such a germline mutation still is made up of cells that behave essentially normally. However, they are one step closer to malignancy than in the normal situation, and hence a higher risk applies.

Genetic Diagnosis for Cancer Predisposition

The remarkable progress in cancer genetics that we have briefly reviewed in this chapter has occurred almost entirely during the last 10–15 years. Though dramatic discoveries in the research laboratory have revolutionized our basic understanding of the cancer problem and opened up many exciting new avenues for research, a direct impact on patient care is just beginning to emerge. It was generally hoped that this scientific progress would be rapidly translated into new treatment approaches, including gene therapy targeted at many of the cancer genes described in this chapter. However, it is important to acknowledge that such new therapies are still at this time more dream than reality. Current cancer treatment still relies on the basic principles of surgery, chemotherapy, and radiation therapy that were largely developed in the 1960s and 70s. In the short term, the major impact of cancer genetics may be primarily in the realm of the identification of individuals at increased risk for cancer.

The identification of numerous familial cancer syndromes and cancer predisposition genes opens up the possibility of predictive DNA testing, using the same general approaches as those described in chapter 5 for other genetic diseases. The prospect of large-scale population screening for BRCA and HNPCC mutations has generated strong interest in both the academic and commercial sectors for the development of new testing technologies. However, there are a number of obstacles to widespread DNA testing for cancer susceptibility genes, as outlined in Table 11.2. The specific mutation in a given family is often unique, requiring detailed sequence analysis of the entire gene for identification, an approach that is lengthy and expensive and not yet practical for large-scale testing.

Even when a novel mutation is identified in a specific family, it can sometimes be difficult to determine whether the mutation is causative of the cancer syndrome. This is particularly a problem for subtle mutations that result in only a single amino acid substitution in the coding sequence of the cancer gene. In the case of the *P53* gene, a functional screening test has been developed that relies on the capacity of the wild-type *P53* gene to complement a molecular defect engineered into yeast. Failure of a mutant *P53* sequence to function in this assay provides strong evidence that the corresponding mutation was responsible for the cancer phenotype in the patient.

In the case of the *APC* gene, approximately 80% of mutations identified to date are either nonsense mutations or insertions or deletions that prevent translation of the full-length APC protein. Based on this observation, a screening test (called the protein truncation test) has been developed that amplifies the mRNA from a patient blood sample by PCR and then translates it into protein in vitro. The production of an aberrant, truncated protein product in this assay provides a sensitive screen for disease-causing APC gene mutations.

These genes, along with a number of other cancer predisposition genes such as the clinically important HNPCC and BRCA genes, are also currently analyzed by a variety of DNA sequence screening approaches outlined in chapter 5. As sequencing technology continues to improve, perhaps with the development of automated DNA "chips" for rapid screening of an entire gene by hybridization, mutation analysis in large numbers of patients may become increasingly efficient and affordable.

IMPLICATIONS OF PRESYMPTOMATIC DNA TESTING FOR CANCER SYNDROMES

Recent studies have identified a limited number of cancer predisposition mutations present at high frequency in particular restricted populations. For example, two specific *BRCA1* and one *BRCA2* gene mutations together account for approximately 90% of BRCA gene-related breast cancer in Ashkenazi Jewish women. This striking association is apparently because of a founder effect in this population. Approximately 1% of Ashkenazi Jewish women carry the 185delAG (del of an A and G nucleotide at position 185) *BRCA1* mutation and about 1.4% carry the 6174delT *BRCA2* gene mutation. Together with a third mutation (5382insC), the prevalence of BRCA gene mutations in this population is estimated to be about 1:40. In contrast, more than 100 different *BRCA1* mutations have been identified in the general population, with the overall population frequency of BRCA gene mutations in this group estimated to be close to 1:500. Given the limited number of BRCA gene mutations among Ashkenazi Jews, screening for breast cancer susceptibility in this population is technically simple and direct. However, the availability of this simple screening test raises a number of difficult and complex ethical issues (Table 11.2).

A major concern for many patients is the potential impact of DNA test results on their ability to obtain or maintain health insurance, as well as the effect of this information on future employment. These are issues that are receiving considerable public and political attention, and that should soon lead to appropriate legal safeguards for patients.

The impact of a DNA test result on medical management varies considerably among patients with different cancer predisposition syndromes. For example, for patients with familial colon cancer, a negative test result might obviate the need for costly and uncomfortable yearly colonoscopies. Similarly, in the case of von Hippel-Lindau syndrome, DNA testing could potentially save 50% of at-risk patients from the inconvenience of the yearly surveillance computed tomography and magnetic resonance imaging scans that are generally recommended for these individuals. Unfortunately, the impact of DNA testing on medical management is not always this straightforward. Despite the grave risk of cancer in patients with germline mutations of the *P53* gene (Li-Fraumeni syndrome), the multiple potential organs affected by these cancers make it difficult to recommend any standard surveillance program that is likely to be of benefit. The ethical issues involved in testing for this condition thus begin to resemble those of presymptomatic testing for Huntington disease, another disorder for which no specific treatment is available (see chapter 14).

Because of the considerable uncertainty surrounding clinical guidelines for management of patients with familial breast cancer, routine screening for BRCA gene mutations is currently controversial. Mammograms are a useful screening procedure for breast cancer and can be initiated at an earlier age for those at high risk, but are not universally successful in preventing deaths from breast cancer. Though prophylactic mastectomy and oophorectomy reduce the risk for breast and ovarian cancer in these patients, these procedures also do not completely prevent these cancers. Thus, no clear rec-

---

Table 11.2.   Obstacles to Widespread DNA Testing for Familial Cancer Syndromes

Technical
- Size and complexity of many tumor suppressor genes
- Multiple different mutations in the population
- Distinguishing neutral missense substitutions from true disease-causing mutations
- High cost of testing

Medical
- Thorough patient education required to obtain truly informed consent
- Complexity of genetic counselling about test results on a large scale
- Uncertainty about optimum medical management for mutation carriers

Ethical and social
- Potential impact of DNA testing on availability and cost of health insurance
- Potential for loss of employability
- Inability to ensure confidentiality of testing results
- Effect of testing on other family members

ommendations for medical management can yet be given to women who test positive for a BRCA gene mutation. In families with a known BRCA mutation, women who test negative are still left with the 11% sporadic breast cancer risk of the general population. With the considerable uncertainty currently surrounding DNA testing for cancer predisposition, the duties of the physician to educate the patient and to obtain fully informed consent are of paramount importance.

SUGGESTED READINGS

Fearon ER, Cho KR. The molecular biology of cancer. In: Rimoin DL, Connor JM, Pyeritz RE, eds. Emery and Rimoin's principles and practice of medical genetics, 3rd ed. New York: Churchill Livingstone, 1996;405–438. *Excellent overview of oncogenes and tumor suppressor genes.*

Bishop JM, Weinberg RA, eds. Scientific American molecular oncology. New York: Scientific American, Inc, 1996. *Nicely illustrated, multi-author review of many aspects of cancer molecular biology and genetics.*

Beaudet AL, Scriver CR, Sly WS, Valle D, eds. The metabolic and molecular bases of inherited disease. CD version. New York: McGraw-Hill, 1997. *This is an outstanding text that covers many aspects of medical genetics and is cited in several other chapters. The recently released CD version contains a new section, edited by KW Kinzler and B Vogelstein, with authoritative reviews of many topics in cancer genetics.*

Kinzler KW, Vogelstein B. Lessons from hereditary colorectal cancer. Cell 1996;87:159–170. *Excellent review of the current understanding of colon cancer biology by the leaders in the field.*

Tonin P, Weber B, Offit K, et al. Frequency of recurrent *BRCA1* and *BRCA2* mutations in Ashkenazi Jewish breast cancer families. Nat Med 1996;2:1179–1183. *Review of the complex issues of DNA screening for the common breast cancer gene mutations in the Ashkenazi Jewish population.*

Burke W, Petersen G, Lynch P, et al. Recommendations for follow-up care of individuals with an inherited predisposition to cancer I. Hereditary nonpolyposis colon cancer. JAMA 1997;277:915–919. Burke W, Daly M, Garber J, et al. Recommendations for follow-up care of individuals with an inherited predisposition to cancer II. BRCA1 and BRCA2. JAMA 1997;277:997–1003. *Recommendations for management of patients with hereditary nonpolyposis colon cancer and familial breast cancer from a consensus panel of experts.*

12

Clinical Genetics

Previously the geneticist was like a "bookie" offering odds for any given event to happen. Now that the geneticist is involved in the "action," i.e., diagnosis and therapy, he has changed from a bookie to a fixer.

ROY D. SCHMICKEL (FROM GENETIC COUNSELING AS A FORM OF MEDICAL COUNSELING. UNIV MICHIGAN MED CTR J 1974;40:38–43.)

With the explosion in knowledge about mutational mechanisms and the molecular pathophysiology of genetic diseases, and the rapid progress in mapping human disease genes, the geneticist has indeed become a central part of the action. The American Board of Medical Genetics (ABMG), established in 1979, began to certify medical geneticists and genetic counselors in 1981. The important role of medical genetics as a full-fledged medical specialty was recognized in 1991, when the American Board of Medical Specialties (ABMS) recognized the ABMG as a member board, the first new certification board recognized by the ABMS in 12 years. The American College of Medical Genetics was established in 1991 to represent the medical genetics professional community and was admitted to the American Medical Association's House of Delegates in 1996. A separate American Board of Genetic Counselors was established in 1993 for the certification of genetic counselors.

The clinical management of patients with genetic diseases involves many of the same techniques of diagnosis and treatment that are used in other medical specialties. A major emphasis of medical genetics, however, is its focus on the prevention and/or avoidance of disease. Central to this approach are the concept of presymptomatic diagnosis, the provision of genetic counseling, the use of genetic screening programs, and prenatal diagnosis. Each of these topics will be covered in this chapter.

How To Take a Family History—And Why

The family history plays a central role in clinical genetics. Properly obtained and interpreted, it is one of the most useful and accessible tools available to physicians caring for patients with genetic diseases.

Before considering how to take a family history, it is worth considering why. First, the family history provides an aid to reaching a correct *diagnosis*. W.H., discussed in chapter 3 (Fig. 3.3), began to develop chest pain typical of angina pectoris at the age of 25 years, but the diagnosis of coronary artery disease was dismissed because of his age. At age 30 when W.H. experienced his first heart attack, the diagnosis was again missed because it was felt he was too young to have a heart attack. Had his physician obtained the family history of early coronary artery disease in his father and paternal uncle, it should have led to the correct diagnosis of familial hypercholesterolemia and to the early institution of appropriate therapy.

Another illustrative case is that of a 26-year-old woman who sought medical attention because of a breast lump. Her physician recommended that she return in 6 months for a follow-up examination; the physician did not seriously consider breast cancer because of her young age. Four months later, she again sought medical attention because of severe back pain, which proved to be the result of bone metastases from her breast cancer. Family history, subsequently obtained, revealed that one sister had died at age 26 years of metastatic breast cancer and another sister had undergone bilateral mastectomy for breast cancer at age 28 years. Obtaining this simple family history would have alerted the physician to consider seriously the diagnosis of breast cancer and to pursue appropriate studies.

The second reason for obtaining the family history is to help determine an accurate *prognosis*. The case of R.B. illustrates the usefulness of the family history in both making a correct diagnosis and providing appropriate prognosis, or information about the future course of the disease. She was referred to the Medical Genetics Clinic at the age of 52 years because of a 5-year history of involuntary movements (chorea) thought to represent Huntington disease. Her movement disorder did indeed resemble Huntington disease, but she did not show any signs of dementia or mental deterioration. A family history, shown in Figure 12.1, revealed that several relatives on her mother's side of the family suffered from a similar illness, suggesting that her disorder was inherited in an autosomal dominant fashion. Strikingly, however, none of these affected individuals developed any signs of dementia, nor did they have a shortened life span. Both of these latter observations are incompatible with the diagnosis of Huntington disease and would suggest that in this family there is a benign form of chorea quite different from Huntington disease in its clinical severity and prognosis. With the discovery of the CAG triplet-repeat expansion in Huntington disease, this diagnosis can now be confirmed or excluded by DNA tests. The family history also suggests that in this family this particular neurologic movement disorder was fairly constant in its expression in various affected family members, providing useful prognostic information for the patient. It should be remembered, however, that many autosomal dominant diseases, such as Marfan syndrome or neurofibromatosis, show a great deal of variability.

The third and most important use of the family history is for the *presymptomatic diagnosis of genetic disease and the prevention or avoidance of clinical disease*. Correct interpretation of family history information allows one to offer genetic counseling to individuals or families at risk, and it allows the early diagnosis and therapy of genetic diseases. Specifically, it allows the physician to concentrate intervention in a small, defined population at high risk. It should be clear that this opportunity also involves a responsibility to

Figure 12.1. Pedigree of a family with benign autosomal dominant chorea. Affected individuals are indicated by the *red symbols*. See text for discussion.

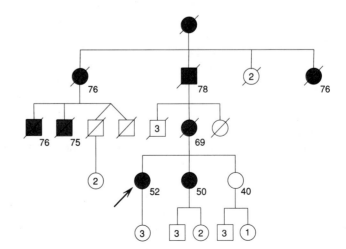

extend medical services beyond the individual patient to other family members at risk of disease. Several examples will illustrate these principles.

After the diagnosis of familial hypercholesterolemia was made in W.H., all of his living first-degree relatives could be identified as being at high (50%) risk of this same disease. Although the disease is common (1/500), the risk among W.H.'s first-degree relatives is 250 times higher than in the general population. Because early intervention may retard the progress of atherosclerosis, children of affected individuals are the ones in whom we should focus preventive measures. All three of W.H.'s children, although entirely healthy, were affected with familial hypercholesterolemia on the basis of blood lipid measurements. Dietary and subsequently drug therapy was instituted at ages 2, 6, and 9 years with normalization of serum cholesterol levels in all three children. Hopefully, such early intervention should slow the progress of their disease.

Familial adenomatous polyposis of the colon (FAP) provides another unique opportunity to apply the results of the family history to early intervention (Fig. 12.2). The proband had a massive hemorrhage from her large bowel at age 42 years and was discovered to have multiple polyps and cancer of the colon; she died 18 months later of metastases. Her father had undergone removal of the colon for colon cancer and was alive at age 66 years; his father had died of colon cancer. The surgeon caring for this family obtained radiographic and endoscopic studies on the three daughters of the proband. The eldest underwent colectomy at age 18 with the discovery of multiple polyps in her colon. The middle daughter appeared to be normal when examined at age 16, but was found to have multiple polyps when re-examined at age 18 and underwent total colectomy. The youngest daughter was found to be affected at the age of 16 and underwent colectomy. Although the removal of the colon is a fairly drastic surgical procedure in an adolescent, it prevented the virtual certainty of colon cancer in these young women at risk. The mapping and cloning of the adenomatous polyposis coli (*APC*) gene on chromosome 5q now provides molecular diagnostic techniques to identify family members at risk before they are symptomatic, as discussed in chapter 11.

Familial polyposis is usually diagnosed in the second decade of life and cancer of the colon or rectum usually develops in the third and fourth decades, approximately 30 years earlier than this cancer develops in the general population (Fig. 12.3). However, some families show an earlier age of onset and, once again, a careful family history may prove very useful in prevention of disease. F.H. was diagnosed as having multiple polyposis at the age of 17 years, was found to have cancer of the colon at age 23, and died shortly thereafter of metastatic disease. Among his three children, two had rectal bleeding before the age of 10 years and were shown to have multiple polyps in their colon. Their primary physician was planning to evaluate them further in their late teens. However, because of the very early age of onset of multiple polyposis in this family and of colon cancer in the proband, it was felt that these two children were at high risk of having colon cancer in their teens as did their father. Therefore, both underwent total colectomy at age 10 years; fortunately, no cancers were found in the colon at the time of surgery. Applying information obtained from the family history led to more aggressive therapy and earlier intervention in this particular family than would be true in the average family with familial polyposis.

The pedigree shown in Figure 12.4 illustrates the application of family history information to the prevention of a common cancer. C.R. was referred to the Medical Genetics Clinic for genetic counseling regarding α_1-

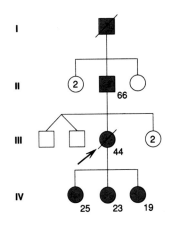

Figure 12.2.   Pedigree of a family with familial polyposis of the colon.   See text for discussion.

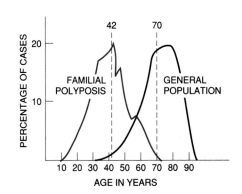

Figure 12.3.   Age distribution of cancer of the colon in individuals with familial polyposis of the colon and in the general population.   (From Bussey HJR. Familial polyposis coli. Baltimore: Johns Hopkins University Press, 1975.)

Figure 12.4. Pedigree of a woman with α_1-antitrypsin deficiency. Note, however, that the probands' mother, maternal grandmother, and a maternal first cousin (indicated by the *red circles*) had early-onset breast cancer.

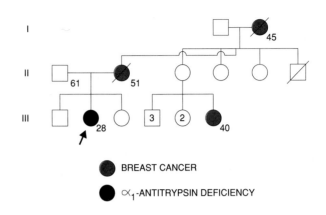

⬤ BREAST CANCER

⬤ α_1-ANTITRYPSIN DEFICIENCY

antitrypsin deficiency. However, family history also revealed that her mother had died of breast cancer at the age of 51 years, 11 years after the cancer had been diagnosed. Her maternal grandmother was diagnosed with breast cancer at age 41 and a maternal cousin had recently been discovered to have breast cancer at the age of 40. These three close relatives with premenopausal onset of breast cancer suggest that in this family the risk of developing breast cancer is at least several times higher than in the general population (chapter 11). Therefore, it would be prudent for C.R. to obtain earlier, more frequent, and more thorough follow-up for the detection of breast cancer than would be advised for a young woman without this family history. As discussed in chapter 11, the possibility of a *BRCA1* or *BRCA2* mutation must also be considered given this striking family history.

HOW TO TAKE A FAMILY HISTORY

The salient points of the family history are listed in Table 12.1. The family history need not be lengthy, but it must be thoughtful. Most importantly, it must be relevant to the clinical problem at hand. Although the family history is usually included among that miscellany of items including "Past Medical History," "Social History," and "Review of Systems," it is most relevant and most useful when it is a part of the "Present Illness." Thus, in obtaining the family history one should ask first about the same or related diseases found in the index case or patient, rather than about a list of diseases of "familial tendency." If the patient has suspected heart disease, then one should ask whether any other family members have heart disease or have related conditions known to be associated with heart disease such as diabetes mellitus and hypertension. The rote inquiry about any family history of diseases ranging from allergy and asthma to tuberculosis may impress the patient with the physician's memory for a list of diseases, or worse, lull the physician into thinking he or she has obtained a family history, but it rarely yields useful information. An exception to the above dictum is asking about pre-

Table 12.1.   Taking the Family History
1. Make it relevant to the "Present Illness"
2. Ask about early-onset preventable diseases
3. Specifically ask about all first-degree relatives
4. Ask about informative relatives
5. Record racial and ethnic background
6. Inquire about consanguinity
7. Keep it up-to-date

ventable or treatable diseases. Therefore, in addition to asking about diseases related to the patient's current problem, it is worthwhile asking about hypertension, early coronary artery disease, early onset of cancer or multiple family members affected with cancer (especially breast or colon), or death early in life from any cause. In this way one can detect individuals at greater-than-average risk for common diseases such as hypertension, coronary artery disease, and cancer.

One must ask specifically about first-degree relatives (parents, siblings, and children) who share 50% of their genes with the index case. One should ask about their age and state of health, and if they have died, the age and cause of death. One must ask specifically about infant deaths because these are sometimes not reported. In many cases, information that certain relatives are unaffected can be helpful, as will be discussed below. When one is dealing with a known genetic disease, it is essential to ask about informative relatives. For example, one should inquire about male relatives on the mother's side of the family when dealing with an X-linked recessive disease. In contrast, one should specifically focus on siblings when one is dealing with an autosomal recessive disease, and on all first-degree relatives on the affected side of the family in the case of an autosomal dominant disease. In the course of obtaining such information, the physician is demonstrating his or her responsibility beyond the individual patient. Information obtained on these other relatives may be used to offer them early intervention or prevention of disease.

Because some genetic diseases show striking differences in their frequency in different racial and ethnic groups (e.g., Tay-Sachs disease, sickle cell anemia, thalassemias, cystic fibrosis), it is useful to record the racial and ethnic background of the family. Finally, although consanguinity is uncommon in the United States, one should also ask about this possibility among parents of an individual suspected of having a rare, autosomal recessive disease.

The family history is frequently deferred in an emergency situation. However, when such information could be helpful in diagnosis, it should be remembered that it takes only a minute to ask whether or not the patient has a family history of related illness. The family history is not static. As individuals get older, the chances increase that they will manifest genetic diseases of late onset. As families at risk of having children with genetic diseases have more children, more information can be obtained. Thus, family history information must be updated.

The pedigree shown in Figure 12.5 indicates the importance of reliable negative information. A young physician and his wife (indicated by the *arrows*) sought genetic counseling because the wife's older sister (II-1) had a son who died of Duchenne muscular dystrophy. The *top half* of the figure (*A*) shows the family history information available at the time of their initial contact with our clinic. On the basis of this information, it is impossible to determine whether the affected boy's disease is the result of a new mutation or has been inherited from a carrier mother. If the latter were the case, the physician's wife would be at increased risk of also being a carrier and of having a child with Duchenne muscular dystrophy. The *bottom half* of the figure (*B*) shows the information obtained at the time the couple actually came for counseling and had had an opportunity to obtain more detailed family history. It is intuitive from the larger pedigree that it is now much less likely that the wife's mother (I-2) is a carrier of Duchenne muscular dystrophy because she has five sons who are unaffected. Thus, it is unlikely that either of her two daughters are carriers and much more likely that the affected child's disease is the result of a new mutation. Using Bayes' theorem (discussed be-

Figure 12.5. Pedigree of a family with a sporadic case of Duchenne muscular dystrophy.   The *top half* of the figure (**A**) indicates the information available at the time of initial contact with the clinic and the *bottom half* of the figure (**B**) indicates the family history obtained at the time of the actual genetic counseling. Note the five unaffected males in generation II. The consultands are indicated by the *arrows*.

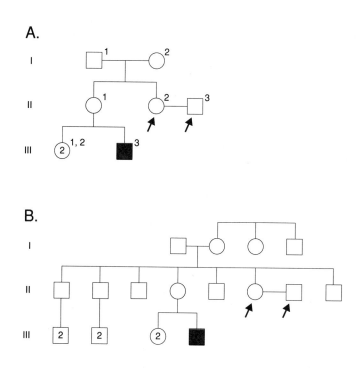

low), such "intuitions" can be translated mathematically into more accurate assessment of risk for couples seeking counseling. With the cloning of the dystrophin gene (see chapter 9), molecular diagnostic tests are available to detect heterozygous carriers of Duchenne muscular dystrophy. In the absence of a living affected male or a definite carrier female, however, such testing is less clear in this family; thus the pedigree information is very helpful in counseling.

As discussed above, the obligations of the physician should extend beyond the individual patient at least to the patient's relatives who might be at risk of a genetic disease and in whom genetic counseling or early intervention might be applicable. This is well illustrated in the cases of familial hypercholesterolemia and familial polyposis of the colon, discussed above, and is shown in Figure 12.6, for a family with Duchenne muscular dystrophy. The man who sought genetic counseling is not at risk of transmitting the disease to his children because he is a healthy 27-year-old and therefore cannot be carrying the mutant allele. However, from the family history it is clear that he has several maternal relatives, aunts, cousins, and nieces, who are at risk and should be informed, through him, that genetic counseling and carrier detection tests are available. With the availability of DNA diagnostic

Figure 12.6. Pedigree of a family with Duchenne muscular dystrophy.   Note the female relatives (indicated by the *shaded symbols*) who are at risk of being carriers of this X-linked disease.

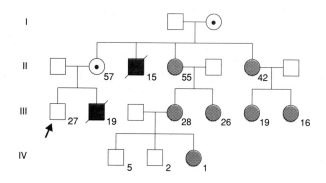

tests, highly accurate carrier detection and prenatal diagnosis for this disease are now available.

Family histories have also been obtained for a variety of nonmedical purposes and have been recorded in unusual ways. Figure 12.7 shows the first of six paintings from William Hogarth's famous series, "Marriage a la Mode." The fathers of the bride and groom are negotiating the financial aspects of the marriage contract. One father has a scroll in which the family tree arises from the umbilicus of a knightly ancestor. Presumably, the quality of this pedigree is worth money. Figure 12.8 shows a portion of the pedigree of Queen Elizabeth I of England. This 33-foot-long parchment scroll modestly traces the queen's ancestry back to Adam and Eve. The pedigree, exhibited at Hatfield House, north of London, where Elizabeth spent her childhood and adolescence, is depicted in artistic heraldic symbols. Finally, genetics, like any other aspect of science and medicine, can be abused for evil ends. Figure 12.9 shows two schematic pedigrees taken from the notorious Nuremberg Racial Laws of 1935 illustrating the Nazis' view of what determined Jewishness or Aryan background and what kind of marriages were allowed, allowed only under special circumstances, or strictly forbidden.

THE PHYSICAL EXAMINATION IN MEDICAL GENETICS

As in other areas of medicine, the physical examination is an essential part of the evaluation of a patient with genetic disease. Despite the rapid advances in DNA mutation analysis, the diagnosis of many genetic diseases, such as neurofibromatosis 1 and the Marfan syndrome, is still based primarily on the results of a careful physical examination. The physical examination is of particular importance in the evaluation of children with congenital anomalies, who comprise a large fraction of the patients seen by clinical geneticists. Congen-

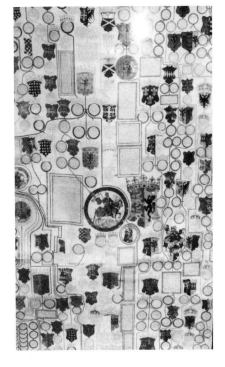

Figure 12.8. Portions of a pedigree of Queen Elizabeth I of England. The large heraldic symbol in the center indicates William the Conqueror. The scroll is displayed at Hatfield House, north of London. (Reproduced with permission of the curator of Hatfield House.)

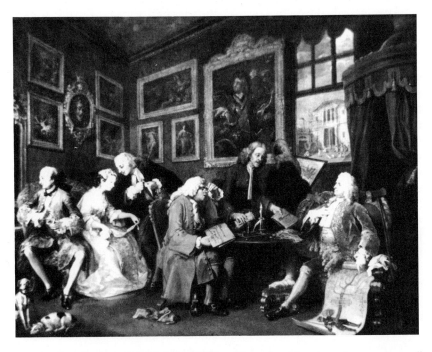

Figure 12.7. "Marriage a la Mode" by William Hogarth. Note the pedigree on the scroll in the *lower right-hand corner* of the painting. This is the first of a series of six paintings that hang in the National Gallery in London.

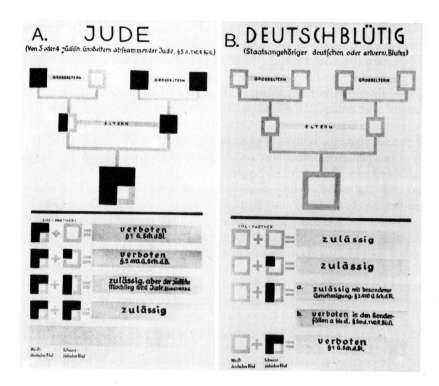

Figure 12.9. Schematic pedigrees from the Nuremberg Racial Laws of 1935 defining Jewishness (A) or German (B) background. (Reprinted with permission from the archives of Yad Vashem in Jerusalem.)

ital anomalies are an important cause of infant mortality and morbidity. Significant congenital malformations are diagnosed in 2 to 3% of newborns, and more than 5% of 2-year-old children are found to have anomalies. In the United States, congenital anomalies, usually believed to be multifactorial in etiology, are the most common cause of death during the first year of life.

DYSMORPHOLOGY

Dysmorphology is the area of clinical genetics concerned with the diagnosis and management of congenital anatomic abnormalities. Congenital anomalies are generally classified according to the definitions given below. A **malformation** is defined as a morphologic defect of an organ, or part of an organ, resulting from an *intrinsically* abnormal developmental process, e.g., cleft lip. In contrast, a **disruption** is a morphologic defect resulting from the *extrinsic* breakdown of, or an interference with, an originally normal developmental process. In contrast to a malformation, the developmental potential of the involved organ was originally normal (Fig. 12.10). The extrinsic factor could be trauma, infection, or a teratogen such as a drug. For example, radial aplasia, or failure of normal development of the radius and associated structures, can occur as a malformation, occurring in association with cardiac abnormalities in the Holt-Oram syndrome. This is an autosomal dominant disorder resulting from a mutation in the *TBX5* gene encoding a transcription factor. Radial aplasia may also occur, however, as a disruption, as part of the embryopathy caused by the drug thalidomide.

A **deformation** is defined as an abnormal form, shape, or position of a part of the body caused by mechanical forces. These forces may be extrinsic to the fetus, such as alterations in the amount of amniotic fluid (see below), or intrinsic, such as diminished fetal movement caused by neurologic or muscular disorders. For example, equinovarus foot, or club foot, can be the result of extrinsic compression of the fetus, caused by oligohydramnios (de-

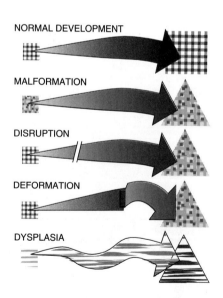

Figure 12.10. Schematic representation of the development of different types of congenital anomalies. Abnormal primordia, processes, or outcomes are indicated in *red*. See text for details. (Redrawn from Spranger J, Benirschke K, Hall JG, et al. Errors of morphogenesis: concepts and terms. J Pediatr 1982;100:160–165.)

ficient amounts of amniotic fluid), or can result from fetal immobility caused by neurologic defects secondary to meningomyelocele or by muscle weakness as in congenital myotonic dystrophy.

Dysplasia refers to an abnormal organization of cells into tissues and its morphologic consequences. Because the defect can involve all anatomic sites in which the affected tissue is found, dysplasias may show widespread involvement. Achondroplasia, discussed in chapter 3, in which there is an abnormality in chondrocytes, is a good example.

Multiple anomalies in a given patient may be causally or pathogenically related. A **sequence** is a pattern of multiple anomalies derived from a single prior anomaly or mechanical factor. The Potter sequence is caused by oligohydramnios, which can result from either diminished fetal urine output, secondary to failure of normal kidney development or to urethral obstruction, or chronic leakage of amniotic fluid. In either case, the oligohydramnios causes fetal compression, resulting in the characteristic flattened face, abnormal position and development of hands and feet, and pulmonary hypoplasia with ensuing respiratory insufficiency and death. In contrast, a **syndrome** is a pattern of multiple anomalies thought to be pathogenically related, but not known to represent a simple single sequence. The Marfan syndrome, also discussed in chapter 3, is a familiar example.

It is important clinically to determine whether a congenital malformation is an isolated anomaly or is a component of a pattern of malformation, such as a sequence or syndrome. For example, a baby with an isolated cleft lip and no other malformations has a good prognosis, and the recurrence risk for siblings is low, as discussed in chapter 4. On the other hand, cleft lip can be a feature of the trisomy 13 syndrome discussed in chapter 8, a serious chromosomal disorder with multiple other life-threatening abnormalities.

Correct classification of congenital anomalies has implications for diagnosis, management, and genetic counseling. Malformation syndromes and dysplasias tend to have a definite cause that is chromosomal, single gene, or multifactorial in origin. A specific diagnosis is necessary in order to provide optimal management and genetic counseling. The recurrence risk for deformations depends on the cause of the mechanical constraint. Disruptions, however, tend to be sporadic occurrences without significantly increased recurrence risks. Helpful information for the diagnosis of congenital anomalies is accessible in two searchable photolibrary databases that are commercially available in CD-ROM format: POSSUM (Pictures of Standard Syndromes and Undiagnosed Malformations) Murdoch Inst. for Research into Birth Defects. PO Box 1100 Parkville 3052, Melbourne, Australia, tel: (613) 345-5045; and the London Dysmorphology Database. Oxford Univ. Press, 200 Madison Ave, New York 10016.

Genetic Counseling

Genetic counseling is a process of communication, the intent of which is to provide individuals and families having a genetic disease or at risk of such a disease with information about their condition, to explore the personal consequences of this information, and to provide information that would allow couples at risk to make informed reproductive decisions. The following definition of genetic counseling was adopted by the American Society of Human Genetics in 1975 (From Ad Hoc Committee on Genetic Counseling (Epstein CJ, Chairman). Genetic counseling. Am J Hum Genet 1975;27: 240–242. Published by The University of Chicago.)

Genetic counseling is a communication process that deals with the human problems associated with the occurrence, or the risk of occurrence, of a genetic disorder in a family. This process involves an attempt by one or more appropriately trained persons to help the individual or family to (a) comprehend the medical facts, including the diagnosis, probable course of the disorder, and the available management; (b) appreciate the way heredity contributes to the disorder, and the risk of recurrence in specified relatives; (c) understand the alternatives for dealing with the risk of recurrence; (d) choose the course of action that seems to them appropriate in view of their risk, their family goals, and their ethical and religious standards, and to act in accordance with that decision; and (e) to make the best possible adjustment to the disorder in an affected family member and/or to the risk of recurrence of that disorder.

INDICATIONS FOR GENETIC COUNSELING

The indications for genetic counseling are listed in Table 12.2. Although the value of genetic counseling for patients and families with known or suspected hereditary diseases is widely recognized by the medical community, the role of genetic counseling in other settings can be equally important. Birth defects and/or mental retardation can occur as part of single gene syndromes or chromosomal disorders, or may result from the interplay of genetic and environmental factors. In every case, accurate diagnostic evaluation and genetic counseling are important parts of patient management and may permit informed reproductive decision-making by other family members. Pregnancy in women older than 35 years of age is associated with an increased risk of Down syndrome (see Fig. 8.18) and other trisomies, and genetic counseling and prenatal diagnosis should be offered to such women. Early onset of certain cancers in multiple family members often suggests strong genetic factors in their etiology, factors that may be amenable to detection by screening tests. Recurrent pregnancy loss is sometimes associated with balanced chromosomal translocations in a parent. Certain viral infections, such as rubella (German measles), and drugs, such as retinoic acid derivatives used for treating cystic acne and anticonvulsants used for treating epilepsies, are known to be teratogenic. Although not strictly genetic, counseling should be provided for women exposed to potential teratogens during their pregnancy. Finally, as described in chapter 4, the offspring of consanguineous matings are at increased risk of being homozygous for rare mutant alleles and thus being affected with rare autosomal recessive diseases. The magnitude of this risk varies considerably among different ethnic, religious, and racial groups. There is also a theoretically increased risk for polygenic disorders. It should be noted that for all pregnancies there is a risk of approximately 3% that the child will be born with a serious genetic disease or birth defect. Empirically, the risk to offspring of first cousin matings has been found to be two to three times as great.

Table 12.2.   Indications for Genetic Counseling

1. Known or suspected hereditary disease in a patient or family.
2. Birth defects.
3. Mental retardation.
4. Advanced maternal age.
5. Family history of early onset cancer.
6. Recurrent pregnancy loss.
7. Teratogen exposure.
8. Consanguinity.

Table 12.3.   Information Conveyed in Genetic Counseling

1. The **magnitude** of the **risk** of **occurrence** or **recurrence**.
2. The **impact** of the **disease** on the patient and the family.
3. The possibility of **modification** of either the impact or the risk.
4. Anticipated **future developments**.

INFORMATION CONVEYED IN GENETIC COUNSELING

Table 12.3 lists the major kinds of information we feel are necessary to provide in genetic counseling. Each will be discussed below.

The Magnitude of the Risk of Occurrence or Recurrence

To provide accurate genetic counseling, it is necessary to make a correct diagnosis of the condition for which the couple or family is at risk. Therefore, it is essential to examine the affected patient whenever possible, to obtain appropriate laboratory analysis where it is helpful, and to obtain all relevant medical records. Genetic heterogeneity, discussed in chapter 3, can create significant problems in reaching an accurate genetic diagnosis. Figure 12.11 shows two infants with similar appearing forms of short-limbed dwarfism. The child on the *left* has achondroplasia, which is inherited as an autosomal dominant condition and is often the result of a new mutation, both parents being entirely normal. In this situation, the recurrence risk to these parents is virtually zero. In contrast, the child on the *right* has diastrophic dwarfism, which is inherited as an autosomal recessive condition. Therefore, the phenotypically normal parents of this child face a 25% risk that each subsequent child will be affected with this form of dwarfism. An inaccurate diagnosis in such a case could result in disastrously inaccurate counseling.

Variable expressivity also creates problems in diagnosis. In the case of neurofibromatosis, manifestations may be so mild in some individuals that they may appear to be normal and an affected child may be thought

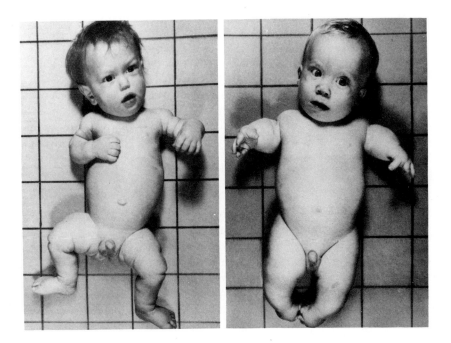

Figure 12.11.   Two infants with short-limbed dwarfism.   The child on the *left* has achondroplasia. Note the large head, scooped out bridge of the nose, and shortening of the proximal portion of the limbs. The infant on the *right* has diastrophic dwarfism. Note the abnormal thumbs and clubbed feet. The head size is not enlarged. (Reprinted with permission from McKusick VA. The nosology of genetic disease. In: McKusick VA, Claiborne R, eds. Medical genetics. New York: HP Publishing, 1973.)

to represent a new mutation. In neurofibromatosis, approximately half of probands have phenotypically normal parents; their disease is thought to result from new mutations. However, a thorough examination of both parents is necessary to ensure that one or the other is not mildly affected. If a parent were affected, then each subsequent child would face a 50% chance of being affected rather than the extremely low risk of a second new mutation.

The inheritance pattern of a condition is often established by careful analysis of the pedigree. When the family history is not informative, but a definite diagnosis can be made, McKusick's *Mendelian Inheritance in Man* is extremely helpful. This catalog provides information on the inheritance patterns of more than 5000 Mendelian traits, as well as useful clinical information on nearly 4000 diseases. This resource is regularly updated and available on-line (OMIM) with valuable links directly to references about the diseases in question. It can be accessed on the World Wide Web (or Internet) at **http://www.ncbi.nlm.nih.gov/Omim/**.

Bayes' Theorem

In order to provide optimal assessment of recurrence risk, it is important to use all available information, especially when the genotype of the individual being counseled (the **consultand**) is unknown. This is commonly accomplished by applying Bayes' theorem, named after an 18th century English scientist-cleric. Before describing Bayes' theorem, it is appropriate at this point to introduce some basic principles of probability. The **additivity principle** states that if two events (A and B) are mutually exclusive, the probability of obtaining *one or the other* is the *sum* of their separate probabilities.

$$\Pr(A \text{ or } B) = \Pr(A) + \Pr(B)$$

For example, the probability of throwing a two *or* a three on a single roll of one die (of a pair of dice) is $1/6 + 1/6$, or $1/3$.

The **independence principle** states that the probability of the *joint* occurrence of two or more *independent* events is the *product* of their separate probabilities.

$$\Pr(A \text{ and } B) = \Pr(A) \cdot \Pr(B)$$

The probability of throwing boxcars (two sixes) on a single roll of a pair of dice is $1/6 \times 1/6$, or $1/36$.

The probability of the joint occurrence of two *nonindependent* events is the *product* of the probability of one event times the probability of the second event *given* that the first event has occurred. The latter is known as **conditional probability**. Note that $\Pr(B|A)$ means the probability of B given A.

$$\Pr(A \text{ and } B) = \Pr(A) \cdot \Pr(B|A)$$

The probability of drawing the ace of spades from a standard 52-card deck of playing cards is $1/52$; but, the probability of drawing the ace of spades, *given* that the card you have drawn is a spade, is $1/13$.

Bayes' theorem states that, given some event (E) that has already occurred and a set of all causes (C_i) that might have caused that event, then the probability of a particular cause C_i, given E (written as $\Pr(C_i|E)$), is equal to the probability of that cause, $\Pr(C_i)$, multiplied by the probability of the event given that cause, $\Pr(E|C_i)$, all divided by the total probability of event E. The probability of event E is equal to the sum of the probabilities of the potential causes multiplied by the probability of event E given each cause. This can be written as an equation:

$$Pr(C_i|E) = \frac{Pr(C_i)Pr(E|C_i)}{Pr(E)}$$

where

$$Pr(E) = \Sigma_i \ Pr(C_i)Pr(E|C_i)$$

As Bayes' theorem is commonly used in medical genetics, E usually refers to an individual who is affected or unaffected with a given disease or who has a certain test result, and C_i refers to a specific genotype.

The application of Bayes' theorem can be appreciated by looking first at a simple example (Table 12.4). What is the probability that a clinically unaffected brother of a child with an autosomal recessive disorder, such as cystic fibrosis, is a carrier for that disorder? In this case, the event E is that the brother is clinically unaffected and the cause C_i is that he is heterozygous for a mutant *CFTR* allele. At conception, before any knowledge of his phenotype, the probability that the brother is a carrier is 1/2, as shown in the mating diagram for autosomal recessive traits (Fig. 3.14). This is called the **prior probability**. The probability that he would be clinically normal, *given* that he is a carrier, is equal to 1; this is called the **conditional probability**. The **joint probability** that he is a carrier *and* that he is clinically normal, given that he is a carrier, is the product of the prior and conditional probabilities, or $1/2 \times 1 = 1/2$. This is the numerator of the equation shown above. The denominator of the equation is the sum of the probabilities of the different ways in which he could be clinically normal, basically the sum of the different joint probabilities. The first of these ways is that defined in the numerator, i.e., he is a carrier. The second possibility is that he is homozygous normal, which has a prior probability of 1/4. If he is homozygous normal, then the conditional probability that he will be clinically normal is of course 1. The joint probability that he would be genotypically homozygous normal *and* clinically normal is $1/4 \times 1 = 1/4$. Therefore, the sum of the joint probabilities by which he could be clinically normal is $1/2 + 1/4$ or 3/4. Now the **posterior probability,** or *relative likelihood*, that he is a carrier, given that he is clinically normal, $Pr(C_i|E)$, is $1/2 \div 3/4$ or 2/3. This conclusion can also be seen graphically by examining the "pie diagram" shown in Figure 12.12. There are three slices of pie corresponding to a clinically normal phenotype; two of these represent the heterozygous carrier genotype Aa. In summary, the unaffected brother had an a priori probability of being a carrier of 1/2. However, by using the additional information that he is clinically normal, the estimate of the probability that

Table 12.4. Bayesian Calculation of Carrier Status for an Autosomal Recessive Trait

	Unaffected Sibling Is a Heterozygous Carrier	Unaffected Sibling Is Homozygous Normal
Prior probability	1/2	1/4
Conditional probability	1	1
Joint probability	$1/2 \times 1 = 1/2$	$1/4 \times 1 = 1/4$
Posterior probability	$\dfrac{1/2}{1/2 + 1/4} = 2/3$	$\dfrac{1/4}{1/4 + 1/2} = 1/3$

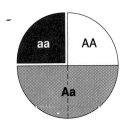

Figure 12.12. Pie diagram showing that the probability that a clinically normal sibling is a carrier (Aa) of an autosomal recessive trait is 2/4 [db] 3/4 or 2/3.

1/100 or 1%). A specific diagnostic test must then be applied to those with positive screening tests to identify carriers with a high degree of accuracy.

Types of genetic screening tests

There are two major types of genetic screening tests. The *first* is aimed at the early recognition of affected individuals in whom medical intervention will have a beneficial effect for the affected individual and/or the patient's family. Within this group are fetal screening, which includes prenatal diagnostic tests for such conditions as Down syndrome, newborn screening, of which the classical example is screening for phenylketonuria (PKU), and now the potential for screening for adult-onset diseases such as colon or breast cancer. A specialized form of prenatal screening is maternal α-fetoprotein screening for pregnant women carrying a fetus with a neural tube defect or with Down syndrome. The *second* major form of genetic screening is the identification of individuals at risk of transmitting a genetic disease. Classic examples of this form of screening are carrier detection tests for diseases such as Tay-Sachs disease, sickle cell anemia, and the thalassemias.

Prenatal diagnosis of genetic diseases is discussed later in this chapter. An indirect type of fetal screening is the measurement of maternal serum α-fetoprotein (MSAFP). It has been shown that women carrying a fetus with an open neural tube defect (meningomyelocele or anencephaly) or an open ventral body wall defect have elevated levels of serum α-fetoprotein (AFP), reflecting elevated levels of AFP in the amniotic fluid. Because serum AFP levels can vary considerably with gestational age and number of fetuses, it is important to determine accurately the stage of gestation by ultrasound examination of the fetus. It is now known that two consecutive elevated AFP levels at 16 to 18 weeks gestation indicate a risk of approximately 1 in 20 that the woman is carrying a fetus with an open neural tube defect. This compares with the frequency of 1 in 1000 in the general population. Therefore, the screening test identifies a group of women at 50-fold higher risk, in whom high-resolution, targeted ultrasonography and/or amniocentesis for measurement of amniotic fluid AFP may be offered for prenatal diagnosis of neural tube defects. It is estimated that 80–85% of open neural tube defects can be detected by elevated MSAFP.

During the course of such screening programs, it was found that low levels of MSAFP were associated with an increased risk of Down syndrome and other chromosomal trisomies, and could, coupled with amniocentesis, detect 15–20% of cases of Down syndrome born to women younger than the age of 35. By combining measurements of MSAFP with human chorionic gonadotropin (hCG) and unconjugated estriol in maternal serum ("multiple marker screening"), as many as 50 to 60% of cases of Down syndrome born to mothers younger than 35 years of age could be detected. Because pregnant women younger than 35 years of age are generally not otherwise offered routine prenatal testing, and because 75% of all Down syndrome babies are born to this age group of women, multiple marker screening is now an important genetic screening test for Down syndrome. The American College of Medical Genetics currently recommends that it should be offered to all pregnant women who are less than 35 years old.

NEWBORN SCREENING FOR TREATABLE AND/OR PREVENTABLE DISEASE: PHENYLKETONURIA

The best example of a newborn screening test is the Guthrie test for the detection of phenylketonuria (PKU). PKU is an autosomal recessive disorder occurring in Northern European populations in about 1/10,000 live births. It is characterized, if untreated, by microcephaly (small head) and profound mental retardation. It is caused by a deficiency of hepatic phenylalanine hydroxylase, which converts phenylalanine to tyrosine, and is characterized biochemically by low plasma tyrosine and high phenylalanine concentrations, and by excretion of phenylalanine metabolites such as phenylketones in the urine, giving it a characteristic "mousy" odor. Strict restriction of dietary phenylalanine, if begun early in infancy, can lower plasma phenylalanine levels and prevent significant mental retardation.

The Guthrie test is based on the observation that β-2-thienylalanine can inhibit the growth of the bacterium *Bacillus subtilis* and this inhibition can be overcome by phenylalanine (Fig. 12.16). A drop of blood collected from a newborn infant (usually at 3 days) is allowed to dry on a piece of filter paper. Disks containing the dried blood are placed on agar containing thienylalanine and *B. subtilis*. In the absence of phenylalanine, bacterial growth is inhibited by the thienylalanine; bacterial growth around a test disk indicates the presence of sufficient phenylalanine in the blood sample to overcome the growth inhibition. The test is standardized by using disks with known amounts of phenylalanine; a positive result is usually set at a phenylalanine concentration greater than 4 mg/dL. Each positive result must be followed up by a quantitative assay of plasma phenylalanine and tyrosine to establish the diagnosis of PKU.

For every 20 positive Guthrie tests, only one infant will be found to have classical PKU with a phenylalanine level greater than 20 mg/dL (normal is less than 2 mg/dL) and a low plasma tyrosine. These children must be placed on strict phenylalanine restriction for as long as possible in order to prevent mental retardation. A somewhat smaller number of infants have been described who have persistent, modest elevations of plasma phenylalanine (usually less than 10 mg/dL) and are characterized as having hyperphenylalaninemia, now known to be secondary to an allelic mutation of phenylalanine hydroxylase, causing a milder deficiency of this enzyme. These children usually do not require severe dietary restriction and most do not

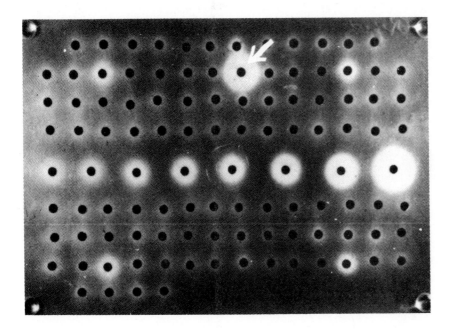

Figure 12.16. Bacterial inhibition assay or Guthrie test. *Row five* shows control discs containing concentrations of phenylalanine from 2 to 50 mg/dL. The *arrow* indicates a positive test in *row two*. (From Levy HL. Genetic screening. Adv Hum Genet 1973;4:1–104.)

become mentally retarded. The most common cause for a false-positive Guthrie test is transient tyrosinemia caused by hepatic immaturity. These babies have high levels of plasma tyrosine as well as phenylalanine and both levels will fall with time; they do not require any specific therapy. Finally, newborn screening for PKU has detected a rare condition associated with high levels of blood phenylalanine and severe mental retardation that is not prevented by restricting dietary phenylalanine. These babies have disorders of pteridine biosynthesis, resulting in deficient levels of an essential cofactor of phenylalanine hydroxylase.

Before the initiation of widespread neonatal screening for PKU in the 1960s, it was estimated that PKU accounted for approximately 1% of severe mental retardation. The nationwide use of the Guthrie test and early institution of dietary therapy has virtually eliminated PKU as a major cause of mental retardation. Because there is a very low but finite false-negative rate, some affected babies are missed, particularly if they are tested very early in the neonatal period (before 3 days) before blood phenylalanine levels have had a chance to increase (the fetus is protected from high blood phenylalanine by the maternal metabolism).

The dramatic success of this genetic screening program has produced an unexpected new problem. Women with PKU, successfully treated with dietary therapy in childhood but off phenylalanine restriction as adults, were found to have babies who were microcephalic and severely retarded. Although all of these babies are at least obligate heterozygotes for PKU, only 1% would be expected to have PKU. The retardation was presumably the result of in utero exposure to high phenylalanine levels from the maternal circulation. It may be possible to prevent this form of mental retardation by continuing dietary restriction throughout life and maintaining blood phenylalanine levels less than 10 mg/dL throughout pregnancy.

Once programs are in place for screening for PKU, it becomes cost-effective to add other newborn screening tests that can be run on spots of dried blood obtained at the same time. The state of Michigan, for example, screens all newborns (approximately 135,000/year) for PKU (a rapid flow fluorimetric assay has now replaced the Guthrie test), congenital hypothyroidism (a usually sporadic disease associated with growth and mental retardation), sickle cell anemia, congenital adrenal hyperplasia (a disorder of steroid hormone biosynthesis associated with virilization of the female fetus and electrolyte imbalance that can cause shock and death), galactosemia (an inborn error of metabolism also associated with mental retardation as well as severe liver failure), and biotinidase deficiency and maple syrup urine disease (inborn errors of metabolism causing physical and mental retardation that can be treated by pharmacologic doses of biotin or a diet restricting branched-chain amino acids, respectively) (Table 12.9). These seven diseases being screened range in frequency from a high of 1 in 2,600 (1 in 400 blacks) for sickle cell anemia to 1 in 250,000 for maple syrup urine disease. The cost of the screening program is $27 per infant.

SCREENING FOR PRESYMPTOMATIC INDIVIDUALS AT RISK FOR ADULT-ONSET GENETIC DISEASE

The identification of genes that appear to confer susceptibility to serious and potentially preventable diseases of adult life, such as cardiovascular disease and cancer, raises the possibility of genetic screening programs to identify individuals at risk. An instructive example is that of the *BRCA1* and *BRCA2* genes discussed in chapter 11. Mutations in these genes account for the ma-

Table 12.9. Michigan Newborn Screening Program

Disease	Inheritance	Incidence	Screening Test	Treatment
Phenylketonuria (PKU)	AR	1/10,000	Rapid flow fluorometric assay (RFA)	Dietary restriction of phenylalanine
Congenital hypothyroidism	Usually sporadic	1/4,000	Radioimmunoassay of T4	Thyroid hormone replacement
Sickle cell anemia	AR	1/2,600 (1/400 blacks)	High-performance liquid chromatography	Close medical care, penicillin prophylaxis
Congenital adrenal hyperplasia (CAH)	AR	1/14,000	Immunofluorometric assay of 17-OH progesterone	Cortisol
Galactosemia	AR	1/50,000 to 1/100,000	RFA for galactose and galactose-1-phosphate	Soy formula, galactose restriction
Biotinidase deficiency	AR	1/50,000 to 1/100,000	Enzymatic assay (colorimetric)	Pharmacologic doses of biotin
Maple syrup urine disease (MSUD)	AR	1/200,000 to 1/250,000	Bacterial inhibition assay (detects leucine)	Dietary restriction of branched-chain amino acids

AR, autosomal recessive.

jority of breast cancer in multiplex families (containing four or more affected close relatives) with breast cancer, and an even higher proportion of those families with both breast and ovarian cancer. Although many different mutations have now been identified in these two genes, in the Ashkenazi Jewish population, two mutations in *BRCA1* and one in *BRCA2* account for most of the familial breast and ovarian cancer. The combined frequency of these three mutant alleles is almost 2.5% in this population, making this one of the most common serious genetic diseases in any population group. As discussed in chapter 11, several major problems remain to be solved before generalized genetic screening programs might be undertaken for this condition. It is reasonable to expect, however, that the lessons learned from *BRCA* screening will be applicable to comparable situations involving other gene mutations conferring high risk of serious adult-onset disease.

SCREENING FOR CARRIERS OF RECESSIVE GENETIC DISEASES

To establish a cost-effective program for screening carriers of a recessive genetic disease several criteria should be met: (*a*) the disease is clinically significant and severe enough to warrant such a screening program; (*b*) a high-risk population can be identified in which to focus screening efforts; (*c*) an inexpensive test is available with adequate sensitivity and specificity; (*d*) definitive tests are available for specific diagnosis in individuals identified as being at high risk by carrier detection tests; and (*e*) reproductive options are available to couples found to be at risk. The best example of the successful application of such a carrier detection test is screening for carriers of Tay-Sachs disease in the Ashkenazi Jewish population. Tay-Sachs disease is an autosomal recessive disorder characterized by a deficiency of the α subunit of N-acetyl-β-D-glucosaminidase (hexosaminidase A). Deficiency of this enzyme results in accumulation of G_{M2} gangliosides in neurons, causing a severe neurologic degenerative disease resulting in blindness, loss of neurologic function, and death between the ages of 2 and 4 years. There is no known therapy. Although less than 0.3% of the general population are carriers of this disease, 3% of Ashkenazi Jews are carriers of Tay-Sachs disease; thus, screening programs can be focused on this well-defined population. An inexpensive test is available for measuring heat-labile hexosaminidase A (hex

A) activity in blood; carrier status can be confirmed by a definitive measurement of hex A activity in white blood cells. (Because serum hex A activity is increased in pregnancy, leukocyte assay is necessary for screening pregnant women.) Three mutations account for 98% of Tay-Sachs disease in Ashkenazi Jews; therefore, definitive DNA diagnosis is also available. Prenatal diagnosis is available for Tay-Sachs disease, thereby offering couples at risk the option of terminating a pregnancy with an affected fetus. Widespread application of this testing in the Ashkenazi Jewish population has virtually eliminated Tay-Sachs disease in this group during the last 25 years. More than a million individuals have been tested, and the frequency of Tay-Sachs disease has been reduced by 95% in this population.

Other examples of diseases amenable to such testing are the β-thalassemias in Mediterranean populations, α-thalassemias in Asian populations, and sickle cell anemia and other hemoglobinopathies in the black population. β-thalassemia screening programs in Sardinia and parts of Italy, coupled with selective termination of affected pregnancies, have reduced the frequency of this disease by 95%.

Cystic fibrosis (CF) is the most common severe autosomal recessive disorder in whites, with an incidence of approximately 1 in 2500 live births in the United States, and a carrier frequency of approximately 1 in 25. More than 600 mutations have now been described in the *CFTR* gene, although most of these are very rare. A single mutation, ΔF508, accounts for approximately 70% of CF chromosomes in people of Northern European origin, and approximately 50% in people of Southern European origin. By testing for 70 of the most common mutations, including ΔF508, at a cost of approximately $150, it is possible to identify 90% of Northern European carriers of cystic fibrosis. Ironically, in the Ashkenazi Jewish population, in which the frequency of cystic fibrosis is lower, the analysis of only five mutations can identify 97% of CF carriers. Thus, in some centers, CF testing has been added to already existing Tay-Sachs disease-screening programs. In the black population, 61% of carriers can be detected. Prenatal diagnosis of affected fetuses is available. Unlike the situation in Tay-Sachs disease, however, CF is treatable, and improvements in therapy during the past several decades have resulted in a marked increase in life expectancy of individuals with CF, to approximately 30 to 40 years, today. Thus, carrier testing for CF becomes a much more complex psychological and ethical issue.

Implications for Health and Social Policy

The increasing use of genetic screening tests will raise important issues for health and social policy. Genetic testing, which has been the province largely of medical geneticists in academic institutions, will become routine medical practice carried out by primary care physicians and commercial laboratories. Clearly, there is a need for better and more extensive training of health professionals, and of the public as well, in genetics and its application to health care. The development of genetic screening tests for serious diseases of adult onset, as discussed above for breast cancer, raises a number of new and important issues. The potential of future genetic tests to detect susceptibility to major psychiatric illnesses, such as schizophrenia and manic-depressive illness, will raise even greater dilemmas. Public health policy oriented toward the reduction in the frequency and burden of genetic diseases may collide with the need to maintain individual autonomy of decision making. Some of these issues will be dealt with in greater detail in chapter 14.

The objective of prenatal diagnosis is to offer prospective parents, who so choose, the assurance of having unaffected children when the risk of having an affected child is unacceptably high. This is NOT equivalent to the assurance of having normal children. Prenatal diagnosis allows one to convert a probability statement about the risk of a specific disease to a certainty; however, it does not address all possible birth defects or genetic diseases.

Prenatal diagnosis represents a paradigm of the application of basic scientific techniques to clinical problems. The development of these diagnostic procedures in the 1960s resulted from advances in obstetrical techniques, in the ability to culture human cells, and in cytogenetics and (later) molecular genetics. Prenatal diagnosis uses both invasive (amniocentesis, chorionic villus sampling, and percutaneous blood sampling) and noninvasive (ultrasonography) techniques.

Prenatal Diagnosis of Genetic Disease

AMNIOCENTESIS

Amniocentesis involves removal of a small amount (usually 20 mL) of amniotic fluid (Fig. 12.17). The amniotic fluid, which bathes the developing fetus during the early part of pregnancy, is thought to represent a transudate; its composition reflects that of fetal extracellular fluid. Found within this fluid are cells sloughed from the fetal skin and from epithelial linings of the gastrointestinal, respiratory, and genitourinary tract. Later in the pregnancy, as the volume of amniotic fluid increases, the major contributor to the fluid is fetal urine. Amniocentesis must be done early enough to be useful, i.e., to allow a specific diagnostic test to be carried out such that the results may be used to decide whether to continue or terminate a pregnancy within safe and legal limits, and yet late enough to be safe, i.e., so that the removal of a small amount of amniotic fluid does not alter subsequent fetal

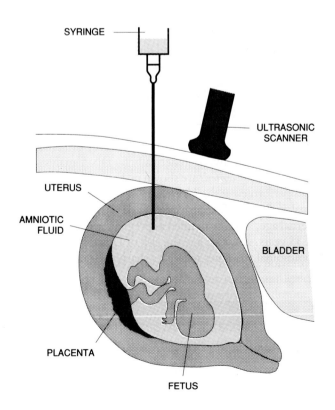

Figure 12.17.   Diagram of amniocentesis.

DNA in maternal cells is preferentially amplified and difficult to distinguish from that of the fetus. However, sickle cell anemia and β-thalassemia have recently been diagnosed successfully after isolation of individual fetal cells. Cytogenetic diagnoses, directed primarily at the detection of aneuploidy, can be carried out by FISH, which can identify abnormalities in chromosome number in interphase nuclei. Studies to assess the sensitivity and specificity of cytogenetic diagnosis in fetal cells in maternal circulation are currently being performed.

APPLICATIONS OF DNA ANALYSIS TO PRENATAL DIAGNOSIS

Many genes are expressed in a tissue-specific manner. This limits biochemical diagnostic techniques to those diseases for which the gene products are expressed in amniocytes or chorionic villus cells. Deficiency of gene products expressed only in specialized tissues such as liver (e.g., ornithine transcarbamylase) could not be diagnosed by such biochemical techniques. Because the DNA in all somatic cells is essentially the same, the ability to detect mutations at the DNA level overcomes this limitation. Several techniques can be used for DNA analysis (Table 12.11).

To detect known point mutations, splicing mutations, or small deletions or insertions, the relevant regions of the gene can be amplified by PCR and analyzed by several techniques. If a single base change causes an altered restriction site, then one can readily diagnose the condition prenatally by restriction enzyme analysis. An example of this is sickle cell anemia in which the causative mutation causes the loss of an MstII site (as discussed in chapter 6). A more generally applicable technique at present is the use of allele-specific oligonucleotides (see chapter 5). This technique is particularly useful when most cases of a disease are caused by one or a limited number of mutations, as is the case for α_1-antitrypsin deficiency, Tay-Sachs disease, and sickle cell anemia, or when the specific mutation in a family has been defined. In the case of β-thalassemia, where there are multiple mutations, the technique can still be applied in situations in which a small number of particular mutations is especially common in a defined population (e.g., the splice mutation at position 110 of IVS-I in certain Mediterranean populations or the β^{39} nonsense mutation in Sardinia). Similarly, for *BRCA1* and *BRCA2*, although more than 100 mutations have been defined, only three mutations account for the great majority of mu-

---

Table 12.11.   Diagnosis by DNA Analysis

1. Detection of known point mutations, splicing mutations, or small insertions or deletions by:
   a. Restriction endonuclease analysis to detect mutations that alter restriction sites.
   b. Allele-specific oligonucleotide hybridization.
   c. PCR amplification and direct automated sequencing.
2. Detection of unknown mutations by PCR amplification followed by:
   a. Single-strand conformation polymorphism analysis.
   b. Heteroduplex analysis.
   c. Mismatch cleavage.
   d. DNA sequencing.
3. Detection of large insertions, expansions, deletions, or other major structural rearrangements by:
   a. Southern blot analysis.
   b. PCR amplification.
4. Linkage-based analysis using intragenic DNA polymorphisms to diagnose diseases in which there are many pathogenic mutations, and the specific mutation in a family is unknown.

PCR, polymerase chain reaction.

tations in the Ashkenazi Jewish population. Finally, with the development of automated microchip DNA sequencing technology, direct sequencing may become an increasingly feasible approach to DNA diagnosis, especially when a limited number of mutations are known to cause most cases of the disease.

Unknown mutations can be detected by PCR amplification of exons followed by physical or biochemical analyses, as discussed in chapter 5. These include single-strand conformation polymorphism (SSCP) analysis, heteroduplex analysis, and mismatch cleavage methods. Putative mutations are confirmed by direct sequencing. Although these approaches are not generally used for prenatal diagnosis, they are valuable postnatally for defining previously unknown disease-causing mutations.

Large deletions, insertions, expansions, or other major structural rearrangements can be detected by Southern blot analysis or PCR. Currently, multiplex PCR analysis is most useful in the prenatal diagnosis of Duchenne muscular dystrophy, in which more than 60% of cases are the result of deletions in this very large gene. Southern blot analysis is also used for the diagnosis of α-thalassemia and for hemophilia A resulting from gene inversion. Southern blot analysis is the method of choice for the diagnosis of the massive triplet-repeat expansions in fragile X syndrome and in congenital myotonic dystrophy, whereas PCR is more useful for detecting fragile X premutations and for the triplet-repeat expansion in Huntington disease.

Linkage-based analysis using intragenic DNA polymorphisms requires family study to be useful, but this is the most generally applicable technique for prenatal diagnosis of single-gene disorders in which there are multiple pathogenic mutations and the specific mutation in a family is unknown. Examples in which this technique has been used include hemophilia, familial hypercholesterolemia, Duchenne muscular dystrophy families without a deletion in the dystrophin gene, α_1-antitrypsin deficiency, and adult polycystic kidney disease.

Finally, if multiple unique mutations can result in the formation of an incomplete, nonfunctional protein product, then protein truncation assays may be useful, as in the diagnosis of neurofibromatosis 1 and familial polyposis of the colon. The list of diseases diagnosable by DNA analysis (Table 12.12) is growing rapidly and includes the hemoglobinopathies, hemophilia A and B, α_1-antitrypsin deficiency, PKU, Duchenne muscular dystrophy, and cystic fibrosis, as well as such late-onset diseases as adult polycystic kid-

---

Table 12.12. Selected Single-Gene Diseases Amenable to Prenatal or Presymptomatic Diagnosis by DNA Analysis

Autosomal dominant
  Myotonic dystrophy
  Adult polycystic kidney disease
  Huntington disease
  Neurofibromatosis 1
  Familial breast cancer
Autosomal recessive
  Sickle cell anemia
  β-thalassemia, α-thalassemia
  Cystic fibrosis
  Phenylketonuria
  α_1-Antitrypsin deficiency
  Tay-Sachs disease
X-linked recessive
  Hemophilia A and B
  Duchenne and Becker muscular dystrophy
  Fragile X syndrome
  Ornithine transcarbamylase deficiency

ney disease and Huntington disease. In many cases a combination of the above techniques can be, and are, used to make the diagnosis.

ETHICAL QUESTIONS

A more extensive discussion of ethical issues in clinical genetics is found in chapter 14. A major ethical issue raised by prenatal diagnosis is that related to abortion. Should a couple undergoing prenatal diagnosis, which carries a small but finite risk, have made a commitment to terminate a pregnancy carrying an affected fetus? It should be noted that less than 5% of fetuses examined by prenatal diagnostic techniques are, in fact, affected with the disease being sought. Therefore, the outcome for the vast majority of women undergoing prenatal diagnosis is reassurance that they are carrying a fetus that is not affected with the disease in question. Furthermore, a woman who finds that she is carrying an affected fetus should have the opportunity to make the best decision for her circumstances, without prior commitment.

A second issue is how to handle unrequested or unexpected information. Because a karyotype and α-fetoprotein analysis are done on all amniocenteses whatever their primary indication, unexpected information may be obtained. However, the same consideration holds for many other medical diagnostic tests, and most genetic counselors feel that full disclosure with appropriate supportive counseling should be provided. How does one handle the situation of twin pregnancies and specifically, twins discordant for a serious genetic disease? For example, what if one twin has Down syndrome and the other does not? A number of such cases have been reported in which it has been possible to selectively abort the affected fetus, allowing the birth of the unaffected twin. The situation emphasizes again the limitation of prenatal diagnosis; it is possible to terminate the life of a fetus affected with a genetic disease, but not yet possible, except in rare circumstances, to treat the affected fetus. For the couple faced with the anguish of carrying a fetus with a severe or lethal genetic disease, this option nevertheless may be a more humane and satisfactory one than any of the alternatives.

EFFECT OF PRENATAL DIAGNOSIS ON GENE FREQUENCY AND DISEASE FREQUENCY

Prenatal diagnosis coupled with therapeutic abortion of affected fetuses has no effect *per se* on the gene frequency of an otherwise lethal genetic disease. Without prenatal diagnosis, an affected child would die without reproducing. The effect on gene frequency of a lethal autosomal recessive disease would depend on whether carriers would have more (or fewer) children if they could avoid having affected children, and thus, might actually pass more (or fewer) mutant alleles on to the next generation. In contrast, prenatal diagnosis and selective termination of fetuses with a genetically nonlethal, autosomal dominant disease (e.g., Huntington disease or familial breast cancer), could have a dramatic effect on gene frequency.

The effect of prenatal diagnosis on disease frequency depends on whether it is offered to all women at risk, or only to those who have already had an affected child. For example, the frequency of neural tube defects in the general population is about 1 in 1000; for a woman who has had a child with a neural tube defect, the recurrence risk is approximately 2–5%. Prenatal detection and therapeutic abortion of affected fetuses, if limited to women who have already had one affected child, will have a very small impact on the overall frequency of neural tube defects in the population. (This is not to say that it will not have a major emotional and medical impact on specific families.) If, however, prenatal diagnosis is coupled with genetic screening programs (e.g., maternal serum α-fetoprotein screening to detect women at higher risk of carrying a fetus with a neural tube defect), then one can offer this test to the majority of women at risk, and this could have a significant impact on the population frequency of this birth defect. Similarly, the availability of amniocentesis and CVS, offered to pregnant women older than 35 years of age, has not yet had any significant impact on the incidence of Down syndrome. Triple marker screening, offered to all pregnant women, and the development of techniques to isolate and analyze fetal cells in maternal blood, however, could have a much greater impact.

In summary, rapid advances in molecular genetics, and in the mapping and cloning of genes and identification of disease-causing mutations, have dramatically increased the scope of prenatal diagnosis. Combined with sensitive and supportive genetic counseling, the availability of prenatal diagnosis allows couples at risk for having a child with a serious genetic disease to choose among reproductive options and to avoid, if they so choose, the birth of an affected child.

PRINCIPLES

Treatment of Genetic Disease

Treatment of genetic diseases, paradoxically, usually involves *environmental* manipulation rather than genetic manipulation (gene therapy is discussed in chapter 13). It should be kept in mind that genetic diseases are no less treatable than most "nongenetic" diseases faced by the physician. Avoidance of genetic disease by genetic screening, counseling, prenatal diagnosis, and early intervention is closely intertwined with treatment. Medical genetics offers a notable example of the emphasis on preventive medicine rather than simply treatment of established disease. Finally, treatment of genetic diseases at the environmental level generally involves a combination of the application of the three *R*'s: restriction, replacement, and removal.

RESTRICTION OF POTENTIALLY TOXIC ENVIRONMENTAL AGENTS

Dietary therapy is an important part of the treatment of several genetic metabolic diseases. The restriction of dietary phenylalanine in PKU can prevent the development of profound mental retardation. In familial hypercholesterolemia, restriction of dietary cholesterol and saturated fats is a helpful adjunct in lowering serum cholesterol. Restriction of drugs and toxins is critically important in certain other diseases. For example, individuals with G6PD deficiency must avoid oxidant stresses such as antimalarial drugs and certain antibiotics. In α_1-antitrypsin deficiency, cigarette smoking (a serious hazard for any individual) is a particular hazard and can be shown to accelerate the destruction of lung tissue and the development of severe emphysema.

REPLACEMENT

Replacement of deficient products, or even organs, can be therapeutic or even curative. In hemophilia A, replacement of factor VIII is a successful therapy in the great majority of patients. In the case of α_1-antitrypsin deficiency, there is evidence that intravenous administration of human α_1-antitrypsin can result in levels of this inhibitor in alveolar fluid sufficient to neutralize elastase (Fig. 12.22). However, replacement of deficient or abnormal α_1-antitrypsin would not be expected to prevent the liver damage

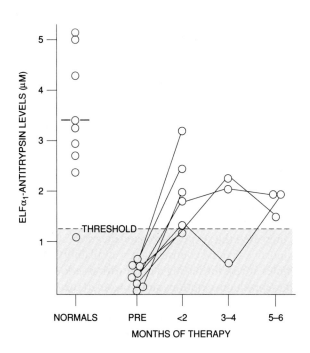

Figure 12.22. Effect of intravenous administration of purified human α_1-antitrypsin on levels of this inhibitor in alveolar fluid. Patients with α_1-antitrypsin deficiency received weekly infusions of purified inhibitor for the times indicated. The *red dashed line* represents the theoretical protective level of α_1-antitrypsin in lung epithelial lining fluid (ELF). (From Wewers MD, Cosolaro MA, Sellers SE, et al. Replacement therapy for α_1-antitrypsin deficiency associated with emphysema. N Engl J Med 1987;316:1055–1062. Reprinted by permission from The New England Journal of Medicine.)

that occurs in some patients with this disease secondary to the accumulation of the abnormal protein in that organ.

Liver transplantation has been carried out in patients with homozygous familial hypercholesterolemia with successful reversal of the metabolic defect. Bone marrow transplantation with HLA-matched marrow is curative in some patients with severe combined immunodeficiency disease secondary to adenosine deaminase deficiency, and has now been used successfully in sickle cell anemia. Kidney transplantation in cystinosis (in which the kidney is damaged by accumulation of intracellular cystine) can correct the most severe problem associated with this disease.

REMOVAL

Removal of toxic substances or organs at risk of damage has also been used successfully. Wilson's disease is an autosomal recessive disease characterized by hepatic and neurologic damage secondary to copper accumulation. Chelation of copper by penicillamine is a highly effective, though sometimes toxic, treatment to prevent the damage associated with this disease and has even been shown to reverse liver cirrhosis in a limited number of patients. Neurologic symptoms are often reversed if treatment is begun early enough (Fig. 12.23). Similarly, phlebotomy to remove iron in hemochromatosis can successfully prevent the progressive damage to liver, heart, pancreas, and other organs (see chapter 9). In familial polyposis of the colon there is a virtually 100% risk of malignant degeneration of the multiple polyps leading to cancer of the colon. Although not trivial therapy, removal of the colon can completely prevent cancer of the colon from developing and can be a lifesaving procedure.

In addition to the three *R*'s, a number of metabolic tricks can be used to treat genetic metabolic diseases. In familial hypercholesterolemia secondary to LDL-receptor deficiency, endogenous cholesterol biosynthesis can be blocked by statins, competitive inhibitors of HMG-CoA reductase, which in turn cause an increase in cellular LDL receptors and normalization of serum cholesterol (see Fig. 7.15).

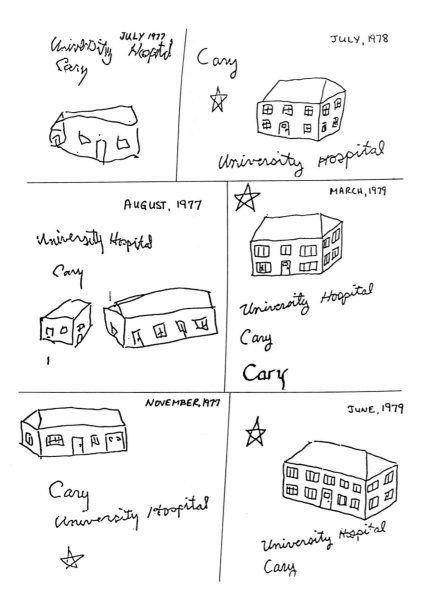

Figure 12.23. Samples of handwriting and drawing by a 21-year-old man with Wilson disease treated with penicillamine to chelate and remove copper. The first sample of writing was obtained before initiation of therapy (July 1977); the subsequent samples, during the first 2 years of his treatment. This is a convenient method for assessing the degree of tremor and dystonia (abnormal muscle tone).

In summary, rapid and dramatic advances in medical genetics, particularly in the area of molecular genetics, have indeed propelled the geneticist from the role of "bookie" to that of "fixer." Nowhere is this more striking than in the area of prenatal diagnosis. Clinical genetics has benefited from impressive progress in gene mapping and in recombinant DNA technology and from parallel advances in nongenetic medical diagnosis and therapy. The diagnosis, treatment, and prevention of genetic diseases has moved to the mainstream, and indeed forefront, of medical practice.

SUGGESTED READINGS

Genetic Counseling

Baker DB, Schuette J, Uhlmann W, eds. A guide to genetic counseling. New York: John Wiley & Sons, 1998.

Emery AEH, Pullen IM, eds. Psychological aspects of genetic counselling. New York: Academic Press, 1984.

Gelehrter TD. The family history and genetic counseling: tools for preventing and managing inherited disorders. Postgrad Med 1983; 3:119–126.

SOMATIC GENE THERAPY

GERMLINE GENE THERAPY

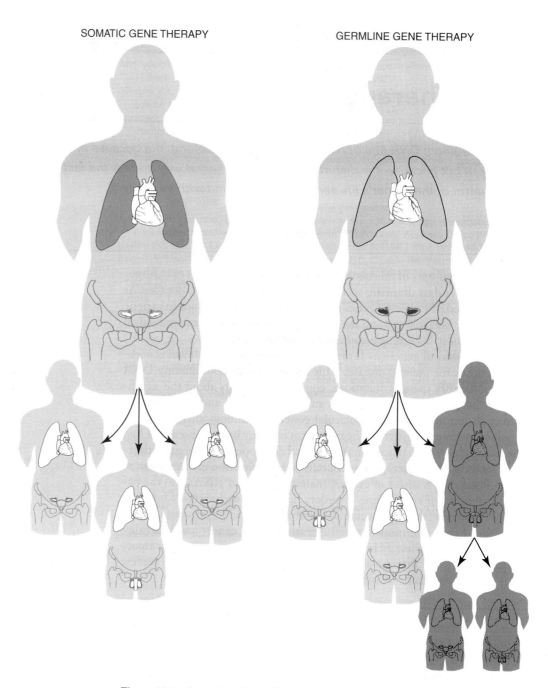

Figure 13.1.   Somatic and germline gene therapy.   In somatic cell gene therapy, the exogenous genetic material is only introduced into somatic cells of the patient, and not into any germ cells in the ovaries or testes. As a result, this treatment has no effect on subsequent generations. In contrast, germline gene therapy genetically modifies germ cells in the gonads, often along with other somatic cell types. As a result, these genetic alterations may be passed on to the patient's offspring and subsequent generations.

worry that an inadvertent DNA modification introduced into the germline could create a new, unexpected human disease or interfere with human evolution in an unanticipated way. Permanent modifications to the human genome of this type raise difficult moral, ethical, and scientific questions that will undoubtedly be debated for a number of years to come. Though not currently feasible, perhaps future scientific advances will make it possible to

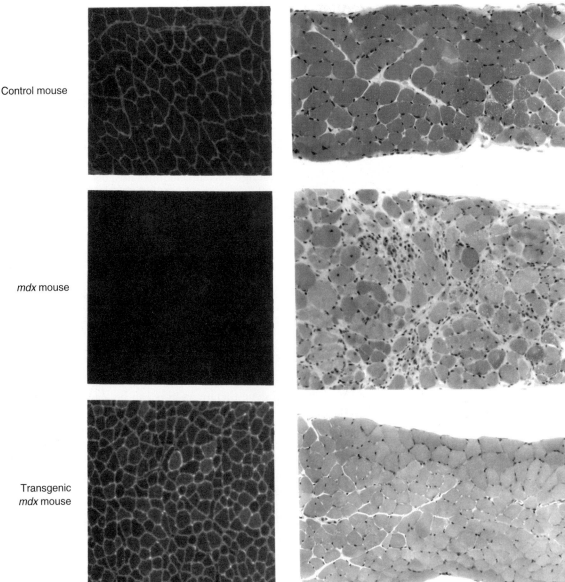

Control mouse

mdx mouse

Transgenic
mdx mouse

Figure 13.2.   Correction of the muscle defect in the *mdx* mouse with a dystrophin transgene.   The *mdx* mouse is a model for Duchenne muscular dystrophy (see chapter 9). Like DMD patients, the *mdx* mouse carries a mutation in the dystrophin gene on the X chromosome. These mice develop many of the features of human DMD, including progressive myofiber degeneration and fibrosis. In the experiment shown here, the full-length murine dystrophin cDNA, under the control of a muscle-specific promoter and enhancer (from the muscle creatine kinase gene) was used to generate a transgenic mouse line (see chapter 5). The transgenic mice were then crossbred with *mdx* mice. The *top row* are muscle sections from a control normal mouse, the *middle row* from an *mdx* mouse, and the *bottom row* from an *mdx* mouse also carrying the dystrophin transgene. For each row, the section on the *left* is an immunohistochemical stain for dystrophin protein, in skeletal muscle, similar to that shown for human muscle in chapter 9 (Fig. 9.23). Dystrophin staining is seen at the periphery of the normal muscle fibers and is absent in the *mdx* mouse, with increased expression evident in the transgenic *mdx* mouse. The micrographs on the *right* show the histologic appearance of tissue sections from the diaphragm. Muscle fibers in the *mdx* mouse show prominent muscle degeneration and fibrosis, which is completely corrected by the dystrophin transgene. (Used with permission from Cox GA, Cole NM, Matsumura K, et al. Overexpression of dystrophin in transgenic *mdx* mice eliminates dystrophic symptoms without toxicity. Nature 1993;364:725–729.)

precisely correct a disease mutation in the germline with high efficiency, in a manner that may prove acceptable and lead to the lifting of the current unofficial moratorium on germline gene therapy.

Methods for Introducing Foreign DNA into Somatic Cells

Gene therapy generally requires the expression of an exogenously introduced gene in a target host tissue. A number of approaches have been explored as a means of introducing foreign DNA into a cell. The agent used to facilitate the delivery of the therapeutic gene to its target is referred to as a **vector.** Vectors can be of either viral or nonviral origin.

The entry of foreign nucleic acid into a host cell is a regular event in the life cycle of naturally occurring RNA and DNA viruses. These infectious agents have been selected during evolution to efficiently introduce their genome into a target cell and also to evade normal host defenses. As we shall see, gene therapists have exploited the bag of tricks developed by several such viruses.

RETROVIRUSES

The first viral system to be adapted as a gene therapy vector was the retrovirus. This class of viruses was first discussed in chapter 11 because of its central role in the discovery of oncogenes. As you will recall, acute transforming retroviruses that have "captured" a normal cellular gene now direct expression of this gene in an aberrant way, leading to the development of cancer. Retroviral gene therapy vectors can be viewed as the helpful "Dr. Jekyll," in contrast to the destructive "Mr. Hyde" of the acute transforming retrovirus, similarly exploiting the viral machinery for the efficient introduction of a gene into a cell, but substituting a therapeutic gene for the tumor oncogene.

The retroviral lifecycle was discussed in chapter 11 (Fig. 11.3A). Retroviruses can efficiently adsorb to and enter a target cell, where the RNA genome is copied into DNA by reverse transcriptase. This proviral DNA can subsequently integrate stably into the chromosomal DNA, a step generally requiring that the target cell be undergoing cell division and DNA replication. The integrated provirus then directs expression of the viral genes it carries.

The general scheme for the use of retroviruses in gene therapy is depicted schematically in Figure 13.3. The original viral genes (*gag*, *pol*, and *env*) are removed and replaced with the therapeutic gene. Since this artificial vector sequence no longer contains the viral genes required to reproduce an infectious virus, a trick is used to generate the recombinant viral particle. The gene therapy vector DNA is transfected into a specially designed producer or **packaging cell line.** These cells have been engineered to carry sequences for a defective retrovirus that expresses the *gag*, *pol*, and *env* viral genes. This "helper" virus is missing a critical segment of DNA that serves as a packaging signal (Ψ) required for recognition of the viral RNA genome for assembly into a mature virus particle. Though deleted from the defective helper virus, this packaging signal is maintained in the engineered viral vector. The viral coat proteins produced by the helper virus are unable to package the helper virus RNA, but efficiently package the RNA genome of the gene therapy vector to form infectious retroviral particles that are released from the cell. The recombinant retroviruses produced in this way are now collected and used to infect target cells. These particles carry all the required viral components for adsorption and entry into the target cell, where the vector RNA genome is uncoated, copied into DNA, and stably inte-

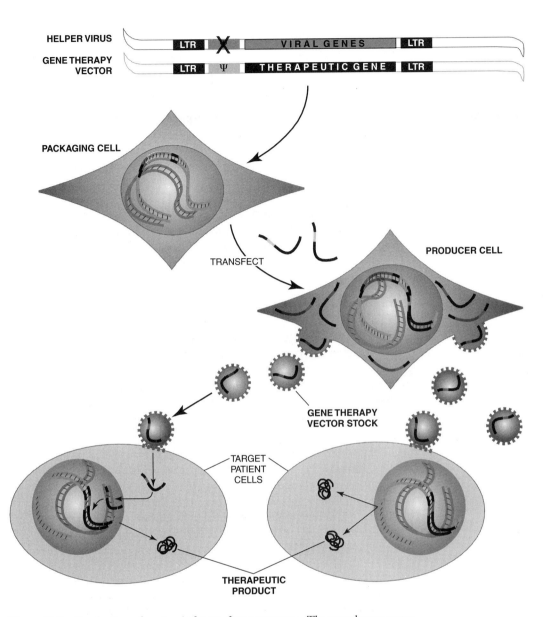

Figure 13.3.   Production of a retroviral gene therapy vector.   The gene therapy vector
DNA contains retroviral long-terminal repeat (LTR) sequences at both ends. The LTR is required for efficient integration into chromosomal DNA. The Ψ signal is a sequence required
for packaging of the viral RNA genome into an infectious virus particle. This sequence is disrupted in the helper virus but intact in the gene therapy vector. The remaining retroviral gene
sequences have been replaced in the vector with the desired therapeutic gene. The gene therapy vector is assembled using conventional recombinant DNA cloning methods, as described
in chapter 5. The packaging cell is a stable tissue culture line carrying an integrated copy of
the helper virus DNA. These cells are transfected with the gene therapy vector DNA and potential viral genome RNA molecules are produced from both the helper virus and gene therapy vector sequences. However, only the gene therapy vector RNA has an intact Ψ signal allowing it to be packaged and released in infectious virus particles. When target cells of the
patient are exposed to the gene therapy vector, the vector RNA is efficiently introduced into
the cell, reverse transcribed into DNA, and stably integrated into the chromosomal DNA, as
would occur in the normal retroviral lifecycle (see Fig. 11.3). However, because the genes for
the essential viral proteins are not present, no further infectious virus particles can be generated. Instead, the gene therapy vector DNA only directs expression of the therapeutic gene
product in the target cells.

Table 13.1. Gene Therapy Vectors		
Vector	*Advantages*	*Disadvantages*
Retrovirus	High-efficiency transduction of appropriate target cells Long-term expression-integration into chromosomal DNA	Potential for insertional mutagenesis Requirement for dividing cells Limited size of DNA insert
Adenovirus	High transduction efficiency Broad range of target cells Does not require cell division Low risk of insertional mutagenesis	Transient expression Immunogenicity Direct cytopathic effects of virus
Adeno-associated virus	Does not require cell division site-specific integration	Potential for insertional mutagenesis if integration not site-specific Limited size of DNA insert
Nonviral vectors	No infectious risk Completely synthetic No limitation on insert size	Low efficiency Limited target cell range Transient expression

grated into the genome. The inserted vector DNA can now direct expression of the desired therapeutic gene. Because the target cell does not contain helper virus sequences, the retroviral infection process ends here, with no further production of infectious particles.

Retroviral vectors offer a number of distinct advantages, as outlined in Table 13.1. Perhaps most importantly, this is the only currently available system that will reliably produce stable integration of recombinant DNA sequences into the host genome. Cells successfully transduced by a retroviral vector should carry the therapeutic gene permanently and continue to pass it on to all progeny cells after cell division. In addition, retroviral infection can be an extremely efficiently process. Under the right conditions nearly 100% of a target cell population can be transduced. However, there are also significant potential drawbacks to this approach. The size of the retroviral genome is limited and as a result, these vectors can only accommodate small- to moderate-sized genes ($\leq$8 kb). As noted above, retroviral DNA integration into the genome generally requires that the cell be undergoing cell division. This requirement significantly limits the range of cell types that can be effectively targeted, excluding terminally differentiated cells, such as neurons and cardiac and skeletal muscle cells. Recently, a new class of retroviral vectors based on the HIV virus (lentiviruses) have been developed that appear to overcome this limitation, permitting transduction of nondividing cells.

Perhaps the most important obstacle to the widespread use of retroviral vectors is the concern for potential complications resulting from the integration of the proviral DNA into the chromosome. The site of integration is essentially random, so there is always some small risk for disruption of a critical gene or aberrant expression of a nearby gene through the influence of viral regulatory sequences. Indeed, retroviruses have been demonstrated to produce cancers by both of these mechanisms (see chapter 11). However, as we will discuss later, retroviruses have already been used in a number of human gene therapy trials and the risk of retrovirally induced cancer appears to be low.

ADENOVIRUSES

The adenovirus, a natural viral pathogen of humans, has also been heavily investigated as a potential tool for gene therapy. Adenoviruses carry a double-stranded DNA genome, can infect many different types of cells, and cause only a mild illness in humans (one form of the common cold). The adenoviral genome is approximately 36 kb and thus gene therapy vectors based on this virus could potentially accommodate fairly large genes.

The strategy for producing recombinant adenoviral vectors is illustrated schematically in Figure 13.4. Similar to the approach for retroviral vectors,

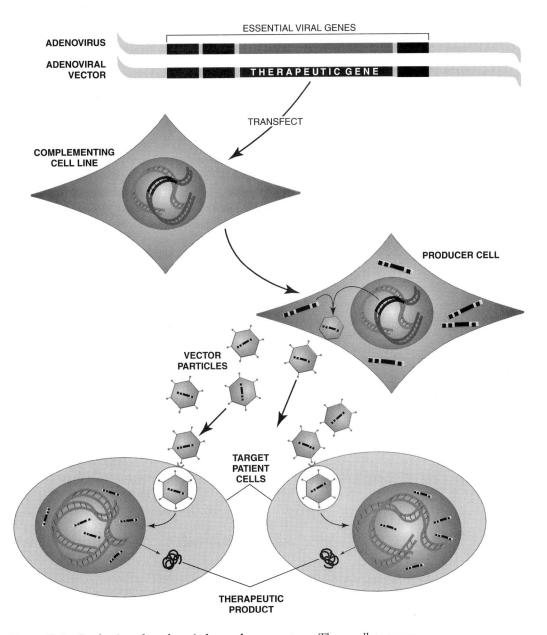

Figure 13.4. Production of an adenoviral gene therapy vector. The overall strategy resembles that described for retroviral vectors in Figure 13.3. Again, a segment of essential viral genes has been removed from the adenoviral genome to make room for a therapeutic DNA sequence and to render the recombinant adenovirus incapable of self-replication. The complementing cell line expresses the essential viral genes that are deleted in the vector DNA, allowing the production of infectious viral particles containing the recombinant viral vector genome. The vector particle can infect a wide range of host cells, efficiently introducing its DNA as an episome into the nucleus. There the therapeutic gene sequence can be expressed, producing the desired protein product. Because the host target cell should not contain the missing essential viral genes, no additional viral particle should be produced.

essential genes are removed from the wild-type adenovirus, both to make room for the therapeutic gene and to cripple the adenovirus so that it cannot propagate and spread within the host or outside of the treated individual. As with the retrovirus, special packaging cell lines have been developed that can complement the essential factors missing from the recombinant adenovirus, permitting it to be packaged as an infectious particle to produce a high-titer viral stock.

The wide host range of the adenovirus and high efficiency of infection are major advantages of this system. In addition, adenovirus infection does not require a dividing cell. The viral DNA exists as an episome and does not stably incorporate into a chromosome of the target cell. This latter feature is both an advantage and a disadvantage. Though the risk of oncogenesis by integration into a critical gene, as discussed for retroviruses, may be eliminated, the gradual loss of the episome with time will generally result in transient expression, particularly in dividing cells.

The immune reaction of the host to the adenovirus is also a major limitation for this vector. Because adenoviruses are a natural pathogen of humans, most individuals already have some degree of immunity directed against adenoviral coat proteins, or develop it rapidly after treatment. This inflammatory response is a major factor in the transient expression often observed with adenoviral vectors. The inflammatory response to the adenovirus can in itself be a significant complication, as observed in at least one patient in an early gene therapy trial for cystic fibrosis (see below). Additional modifications to the adenoviral vector that reduce its immunogenicity may offer solutions to some of these problems.

ADENO-ASSOCIATED VIRUS

Adeno-associated virus (AAV) is a small DNA-containing parvovirus that requires coinfection with adenovirus for its replication. AAV replicates as a double-stranded DNA but is packaged as a single strand. The wild-type virus generally integrates into the genome of the target cell at a specific location on human chromosome 19. This feature offers the potential advantage of stable chromosome integration without the danger of random gene inactivation, as discussed for retroviruses. Unfortunately, the capacity for site-specific integration seems to be lost in the recombinant AAV vectors examined to date.

Nearly all of the AAV genome can be removed for replacement with the therapeutic gene, though there are significant size limitations, given the 4.7-kb size of the wild-type virus. Recent experiments have produced promising levels of expression in animal model systems using AAV, but there are still a number of significant problems to overcome.

OTHER VIRAL VECTORS

The herpes viruses, large double-stranded DNA viruses that include several well-known human pathogens, have also been studied as potential gene therapy vectors. Like adenoviruses, herpes viruses exist as episomes in the target cell, and do not stably integrate into the genome. The large size of the genome can potentially accommodate very large target genes. Herpes viruses have been explored in a limited number of settings, particularly for the introduction of genes into the central nervous system. A number of other viruses including vaccinia and influenza are also being investigated as potential vehicles for gene therapy, although these studies are in a much earlier phase.

NONVIRAL VECTORS

Because of the problems inherent in all of the viral vectors we have discussed so far, a number of approaches have been developed using DNA alone, without the assistance of viral machinery for infection. Though simple injection of naked, purified DNA results in remarkably efficient uptake by muscle cells and subsequent expression of the encoded genes, this approach does not appear to work well in other tissues. Nonetheless, this could be a useful approach when targeting to muscle is the objective or the specific cell type is not critical.

A number of enhancements of the nonviral DNA strategy have been developed including coating of the DNA in a lipid layer (**liposomes**). Coating the liposome-packaged DNA with a ligand for a specific receptor on a target cell type may also provide a useful method for selective DNA delivery. These and other approaches offer promise for the efficient introduction of DNA into cells without the problems associated with viral components. Liposome-mediated gene transfer has already been used in several human gene therapy trials.

Therapeutic Strategies

There are two general approaches for the delivery of the desired gene therapy vector to the patient, as illustrated in Figure 13.5. In ex vivo gene therapy, cells are removed from the patient and exposed to the vector in a tissue culture dish. Cells that have taken up the desired DNA are then returned to the patient. This approach has the advantage of precisely controlling the type of cells that are exposed to the gene therapy vector and also facilitating exposure of the cells to a high concentration of vector and whatever other conditions might be necessary to optimize the process.

In vivo gene therapy introduces the vector directly into the patient by intravascular infusion or injection directly into a specific site or tissue. This approach is often much simpler and less technically demanding and also allows delivery of the vector to sites that might not be easily accessible for ex vivo manipulation. Disadvantages of in vivo gene therapy include difficulty in controlling the conditions of exposure to the vector and the potential for more widespread dissemination of the recombinant sequences, including inadvertent contamination of the germline.

So far in this chapter, we have discussed the techniques that can be used to introduce foreign DNA into a target cell. The next major issue is selecting which genes to transfer and into what types of target cells. The general strategies that are being explored are illustrated schematically in Figure 13.6. The introduced DNA may encode a protein that replaces a deficient factor or may exert its therapeutic effect through aberrant expression of a normal host gene or a novel foreign gene. This gene may then act locally, perhaps within the cell, or at more distant sites.

Perhaps the most obvious and direct strategy is the treatment of a recessive genetic deficiency with replacement of the missing DNA sequence. This is exemplified by experimental gene therapy trials that have used adenoviral vectors to introduce the normal cystic fibrosis transmembrane regulator (CFTR) sequence into the lungs of cystic fibrosis (CF) patients. Ideally, this approach would fully replace the missing gene in the critical cell type, leading to complete correction of the genetic disease. This is a particular challenge for genetic diseases such as CF or muscular dystrophy in which the therapeutic gene must be targeted to a very specific cell population. In addition, it may be necessary to replace the gene with high efficiency

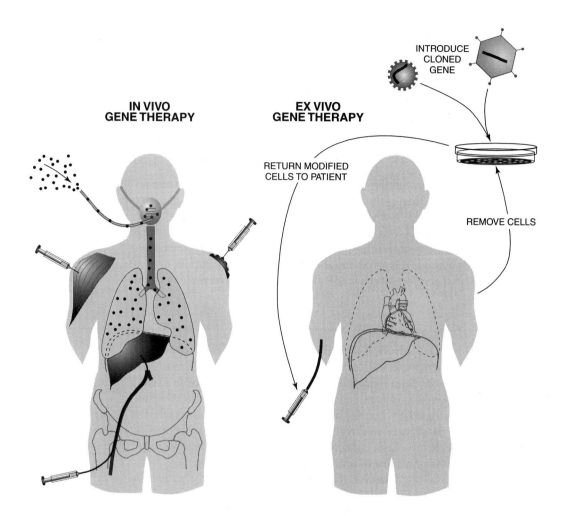

Figure 13.5.   General approaches for delivery of the gene therapy vector. In in vivo gene therapy, the therapeutic genetic material is introduced directly into the patient. Examples include injection of DNA directly into muscle or into a tumor, direct intravascular infusion to deliver vector DNA to the liver or other organ, or administration of an aerosol to deliver a vector to the lung. In ex vivo gene therapy, the target cells are first removed from the patient and exposed to the gene therapy vector in the tissue culture dish. After optional amplification or selection of the desired cell population, the genetically modified cells are returned to the patient, usually by intravascular infusion.

in all or nearly all cells of the critical type. Most dominant genetic diseases are also likely to prove very difficult to approach with gene therapy, particularly when the mechanism is a dominant negative or gain of function effect of the mutant protein.

For many genetic diseases, correction of the defect by gene therapy will also require precise transcriptional regulation of gene expression. For example, correction of β-thalassemia (see chapter 6), by introduction of normal recombinant β-globin gene sequences into bone marrow cells, would require that the expression of the introduced gene be restricted only to the maturing red blood cell lineage and that high level expression, close to that of the normal β-globin gene, be achieved. You will recall that expression of the α-globin and β-globin genes is carefully coordinated and that an excess of either α or β chains results in β- or α-thalassemia, respectively. Such pre-

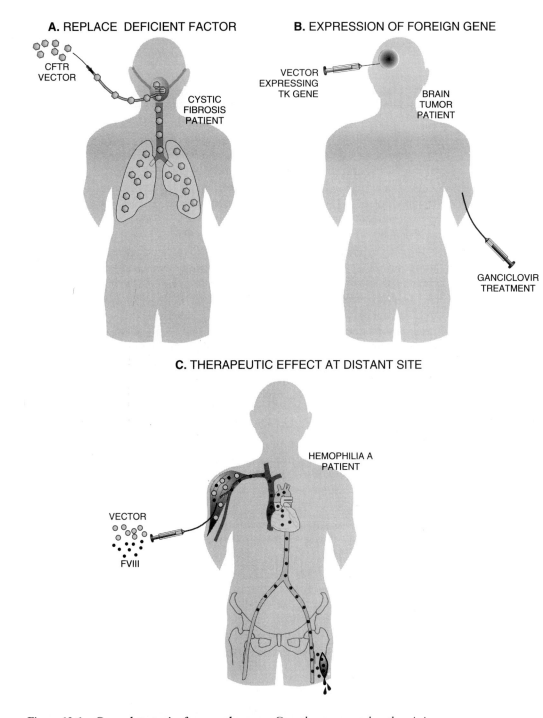

A. REPLACE DEFICIENT FACTOR

CFTR
VECTOR

CYSTIC
FIBROSIS
PATIENT

B. EXPRESSION OF FOREIGN GENE

VECTOR
EXPRESSING
TK GENE

BRAIN
TUMOR
PATIENT

GANCICLOVIR
TREATMENT

C. THERAPEUTIC EFFECT AT DISTANT SITE

HEMOPHILIA A
PATIENT

VECTOR

FVIII

Figure 13.6.   General strategies for gene therapy.   Gene therapy can replace the missing factor in a patient with genetic deficiency, such as introduction of the CFTR gene into the lungs of a cystic fibrosis patient by aerosol inhalation (**A**). Gene therapy can also aim to express the host gene in a novel way or use a foreign gene. In (**B**), the thymidine kinase gene (TK), which sensitizes cells to the action of the drug ganciclovir, is directed to a brain tumor. These cells can now be killed by the drug while sparing normal host cells. The examples in (**A**) and (**B**) both depend on the local action of the gene therapy vector at the site of administration. (**C**) illustrates a treatment in which the therapeutic gene product acts at a distant site. In this example, a gene therapy vector introduced into a muscle in the arm of a hemophilia A patient produces factor VIII, which corrects the clotting deficiency throughout the circulation, preventing serious hemorrhage from a wound at a distant site.

cise control of gene expression remains a very difficult challenge for the field of gene therapy and it will undoubtedly be a number of years before diseases for which this degree of regulation is required can be successfully approached.

Though precise control of gene expression in vivo is not yet feasible, there are a number of diseases for which expression of the therapeutic gene, within a broad range of levels and in any of a number tissues, could be potentially beneficial. Hemophilia A (see chapter 7) is an example of a human genetic disease for which precise regulation of recombinant gene expression may not be required. Because the site of action of the factor VIII blood clotting protein that is deficient in these patients is in the blood, nearly any accessible tissue is a potential target for gene therapy, as long as it is able to direct secretion of factor VIII into the circulation. In addition, elevation of the plasma factor VIII level to even 1% of normal could be of significant clinical benefit in a patient with severe hemophilia A. Also, overexpression of the protein is unlikely to be harmful, as levels two to three times normal are observed under some circumstances without obvious adverse consequences.

In addition to replacement of the normal sequence in a patient with genetic deficiency, a number of gene therapy protocols rely on aberrant expression of a normal or foreign gene. For example, overexpression of a normal sequence, such as that for a therapeutic growth factor, may be of potential value in several disease settings. Perhaps one of the most promising applications of gene therapy is in the area of DNA vaccines. Intramuscular injection of DNA directing the expression of a critical antigen for a microbial pathogen or even a cancer cell may prove to be a very effective method for immunization in some circumstances.

A number of gene therapy strategies direct the expression of a toxin to a target cell, most commonly a cancer cell. This toxin may directly kill the cancer cell or, alternatively, could be a "pro-drug," which sensitizes the cancer cell to a subsequent treatment. For example, the enzyme thymidine kinase (TK), encoded by the herpes simplex virus genome, converts the ordinarily nontoxic drug ganciclovir into a compound that is highly toxic for mammalian cells. This is the basis for the use of ganciclovir as a therapy for herpes virus infection, efficiently killing virus-infected cells. Introduction of the TK gene into a cancer cell renders that cell sensitive to subsequent administration of ganciclovir. This approach has the advantage of potentially also killing cancer cells in the vicinity of the target cell by a "bystander" effect, even though these cells might not themselves be transduced by the vector. This mechanism may enhance the effectiveness of a gene therapy vector that only gets into a subset of the tumor cells.

Some gene therapy experiments are designed to block the effects of a harmful gene expressed by the target cell, such as a tumor oncogene or a gene required for assembly of a virus (e.g., HIV). This can be accomplished by directing the synthesis of antisense DNA (DNA complementary to the mRNA for the target host gene). The antisense DNA hybridizes with the target gene and blocks its transcription, RNA processing, or translation into protein. The antisense strategy may also be accomplished by short sequences including synthetic oligonucleotides. A gene therapy vector may also direct the expression of a recombinant protein that interacts with a host protein and blocks its function. Finally, a class of RNAs called **ribozymes** may prove to be a useful gene therapy tool. These molecules are derived from naturally occurring RNAs that were identified as components of some plant viroids (virus-like particles) and as self-splicing introns in some lower organisms. Ribozymes can be engineered to inactivate a target mRNA by cleaving at a specific sequence and are also being explored as a mechanism to potentially catalyze precise correction of disease-causing point mutations.

Human Gene Therapy
Experiments

In response to the prospect of human gene therapy, the Recombinant DNA Advisory Committee (RAC) of the National Institutes of Health created a gene therapy subcommittee to review the scientific and ethical challenges raised by this new approach. Beginning with the first approved study in 1989, the RAC effectively reviewed all proposed human gene therapy experiments performed in the United States, until 1996 when much of this responsibility was transferred to the Food and Drug Administration (FDA). The first approved human gene therapy trial was begun in 1990, for the treatment of two patients with severe combined immunodeficiency (SCID) as a result of adenosine deaminase deficiency.

EX VIVO GENE THERAPY

Adenosine deaminase (ADA) deficiency is an autosomal recessive disorder caused by inactivating mutations in the ADA gene on chromosome 20. Adenosine deaminase is an important enzyme in purine metabolism and its deficiency results in the accumulation of metabolites that are particularly toxic for T lymphocytes. Severely affected patients experience a nearly complete loss of T cells, resulting in a profound immune deficiency that, if untreated, is generally fatal in early childhood. This condition was particularly attractive as a candidate for a gene therapy approach for several reasons. First, ADA deficiency can be cured by bone marrow transplantation in patients with an appropriately matched bone marrow donor. In addition, significant improvement can often be observed in patients after a simple blood transfusion. These results indicate that replacement of the enzyme within the bone marrow compartment is sufficient and that even very low levels of enzyme activity may significantly improve the clinical course. The subpopulation of bone marrow cells successfully transduced by the gene therapy vector, and thus expressing ADA, might also have a selective survival advantage over the patient's original ADA-deficient cells, leading to gradual repopulation of the bone marrow by the corrected cells. Finally, the grim prognosis for patients without a suitable bone marrow donor justified the potential risk of this new experimental treatment.

This initial trial was an example of ex vivo gene therapy. T cells collected from two ADA-deficient children were treated in the tissue culture dish with a retroviral vector directing ADA gene expression. The first two patients treated in this way have now been followed for more than 5 years. The number of T cells and several measures of immune function have all significantly improved, and integrated vector DNA and ADA gene expression remained detectable for at least several years after the end of treatment.

Although these results are encouraging, the interpretation is complicated by the lack of a suitable control group for comparison and the simultaneous administration to these patients of a modified form of the purified ADA enzyme (an effective standard therapy in many patients). Thus, the direct therapeutic contribution of the gene transfer itself is still unclear.

Familial hypercholesterolemia, discussed in detail in chapter 7, was the next genetic disease to be treated by an ex vivo gene therapy approach. The drastically shortened survival of these patients justified the experimental procedure, which began with surgical resection of part of the liver. Hepatocytes prepared from this liver section were grown in tissue culture to induce cell division, as required for stable DNA insertion into the genome after infection with the retroviral gene therapy vector. The virus was engineered to express the normal LDL receptor gene. After gene transfer, the transduced hepatocytes were reinfused into the patient through the portal vein. Though a modest reduction in LDL cholesterol was observed in the first reported patient, interpretation of this experiment is complicated by the partial nature of the LDL-receptor gene defect in that patient, which may have permitted a response to other aspects of the treatment protocol unrelated to the gene transfer.

IN VIVO GENE THERAPY

The first in vivo gene therapy experiment was directed at the treatment of metastatic malignant melanoma. Skin tumors were injected directly with plasmid DNA designed to express the HLA class I gene, B7, which was chosen to be mismatched with the patient's HLA type (see discussion of HLA in chapter 9). It was hoped that introduction of this foreign gene into tumor cells would stimulate immune recognition and rejection by the patient's own immune system. Given the low apparent risks of this nonviral approach and encouraging preliminary results, this strategy is being extended to other tumor types.

Animal models have been employed extensively for the evaluation of a variety of in vivo gene therapy approaches, with some dramatic examples of significant and prolonged levels of therapeutic gene expression and biologic effect. Significant levels of clotting factor IX have been obtained in hemophilic dogs with adenoviral vectors and a variety of protein products have been expressed with these and other vectors, including retroviruses, AAV, and nonviral vectors. However, the number of human in vivo experimental trials is still relatively small.

The first human genetic disease to be approached by in vivo gene therapy was cystic fibrosis. A number of patients have now been treated with adenoviral vectors expressing the normal CFTR gene (see chapter 9), administered as an aerosol to the lung. However, the results so far have been disappointing, with no clear evidence of a detectable therapeutic effect. In vivo gene therapy trials have now been initiated for a number of other genetic diseases and considerable new information and improvement in the technology can be expected during the next few years.

Gene Therapy for Cancer

Because of concerns about potential risks of gene therapy approaches through the creation of unanticipated genetic alterations, particularly the possibility of oncogenic effects of retroviral-mediated insertional mutagenesis, gene therapy experiments have generally been confined to patients with serious, life-threatening illnesses and short life expectancy. In addition to the introduction of the HLA B7 gene into melanoma cells described above, a number of other strategies have been employed to modulate the immune response to the tumor, including the introduction of a variety of different types of growth factors. Attempts have also been made to interfere with the function of a mutant oncogene or replace loss of a tumor suppressor gene, such as P53. Several experiments have attempted to introduce "suicide genes" into tumor cells to directly kill the cells or to sensitize them to later drug or radiation therapy. Although a few of these studies have shown encouraging evidence for induction of the desired immune response, there is not yet a clearly documented example of a clinically significant tumor response to a gene therapy approach, and thus these techniques remain confined to the experimental arena.

Figure 13.7 summarizes the types of gene therapy protocols that had been submitted for review by the RAC or the FDA, through June of 1997. The vast majority of these studies have been performed in patients with forms of cancer that are either untreatable or have failed standard treatment. A number of specific genetic diseases have also been targeted, though here also, the initial subjects have been primarily limited to patients with an otherwise poor prognosis for whom effective alternatives do not exist.

As of June 1995, 597 patients had been treated in a total of 106 RAC-approved gene therapy protocols. With the exception of one CF patient treated with an adenoviral vector who developed transient deterioration of pulmonary function, there have been no instances of serious clinical complications directly related to the gene therapy vector or therapeutic gene itself. The remarkable lack of significant complications or toxicities in these initial trials, particularly when compared with other experimental treatments for these illnesses, is reassuring. However, only limited follow-up for late complications is available, because of the nature of the patient population. The most feared complication, carcinogenesis as a result of retroviral insertion, may require many years to become clinically apparent, because the gene altered by the retrovirus may only be the "first hit" in the development of such a cancer (see chapter 11). Nonetheless, current experience suggests that somatic gene therapy is generally safe and that the risks are small.

What about the benefits? Though several of the gene therapy experiments we have discussed give suggestive and encouraging evidence for clinical benefit, none of the more than 100 approved gene therapy protocols have yet provided definitive evidence for therapeutic efficacy. Although the prospect of gene transfer for the treatment of disease has been under investigation for nearly 20 years, the field of gene therapy must still be considered to be in its infancy.

The Risks and Benefits of Gene Therapy

Although not generally considered a form of gene therapy, production of recombinant therapeutic proteins through DNA technology is having an increasing impact on medical practice. Table 13.2 lists a number of new "drugs" whose development would not have been possible before the advent of modern molecular genetics. Some of these recombinant proteins are used

Other Recombinant DNA-Based Therapies

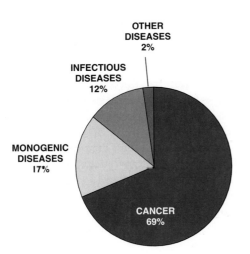

Figure 13.7. Human gene therapy protocols submitted to the RAC or FDA. A total of 161 gene therapy protocols have been submitted for review as of June 1997. One hundred ten of these have been directed at the treatment of cancer. Seventy-four of the cancer trials involved immunotherapy, with about half of these using an in vivo gene therapy approach. Twenty-two of the cancer trials used the TK gene to sensitize tumor cells to ganciclovir. Only 28 protocols have been submitted for the treatment of monogenic diseases, with more than half of these aimed at cystic fibrosis. All 19 infectious disease trials are directed at the treatment of AIDS. The "other diseases" category includes one protocol each for treatment of peripheral artery disease, rheumatoid arthritis, arterial restenosis, and cubital tunnel syndrome.

Table 13.2. Pharmaceuticals Produced by Recombinant DNA Technology

Recombinant Product	Disease Target	Advantages Over Existing Drugs
Human insulin	Diabetes	Less immunogenic than porcine or bovine insulin
Growth hormone	Growth hormone deficiency	No infectious risk Increased availability
Recombinant factor VIII	Hemophilia A	No infectious risk ? Less immunogenicity
Tissue plasminogen activator	Acute coronary thrombosis (myocardial infarction) and stroke	Increased efficacy (compared with natural bacterial product, streptokinase) Less immunogenic
Erythropoietin	Anemia	NA
Granulocyte colony-stimulating factor (G-CSF)	Neutropenia after chemotherapy	NA
Hepatitis B vaccine	Prevention of hepatitis B	No infectious risk
α Interferon	Hairy cell leukemia, chronic hepatitis	No infectious risk
β Interferon	Multiple sclerosis	NA
γ Interferon	Infections in chronic granulomatous disease patients	NA

NA = No equivalent drug was available before development of the recombinant product.

in place of natural proteins that had previously been purified from human or animal tissues by standard biochemical techniques.

Human insulin, produced by recombinant DNA methods, is now often used in place of bovine insulin, purified from bovine pancreas. Several other recombinant proteins also replace protein products that have been previously purified from human plasma and tissue sample. The recombinant protein should be free of the risk of contamination with human pathogenic viruses, which must always be a concern in protein products prepared from human tissues. Recombinant growth hormone has replaced the product previously purified from human pituitaries and potentially contaminated with "slow viruses," which could cause catastrophic neurologic degenerative diseases. The contamination of the blood supply in the early 1980s with the HIV virus resulted in the inadvertent administration of HIV-laden factor VIII to the majority of severe hemophilic patients treated during that time and the subsequent death of a large segment of the hemophilic population of AIDS. This tragedy was a major factor behind the cloning of the factor VIII gene and the production of recombinant factor VIII that is free of viral risk. Recombinant protein engineering has also have been used to generate vaccines, such as that for hepatitis B, which were previously based on viral antigens isolated from human blood.

Recombinant technology has also made novel biologic drugs available, which could not otherwise have been obtained in sufficient quantities. Examples include a number of therapeutically useful growth factors, such as erythropoietin, which stimulates red blood cell production and corrects the anemia associated with kidney failure, and granulocyte colony-stimulating factor (G-CSF), which counteracts the dangerous decrease in white blood count that frequently complicates cancer chemotherapy.

Recombinant protein therapeutics are generally produced in bacteria or yeast, or in mammalian cells in tissue culture. Transgenic approaches have also been used to generate the expression of recombinant proteins in livestock, including sheep and goats. Recombinant proteins have been directed to the milk in this way, where they can potentially be produced cheaply and efficiently in large quantities.

Future Directions

Though interest in gene therapy has expanded dramatically during the past few years, it is likely that the techniques of this developing field will eventually merge with other aspects of medical treatment. Rather than defining a new and separate field, the tools of recombinant DNA technology may simply expand the potential of existing fields of medical treatment. For example, many gene therapy approaches, including several current trials for the treatment of ADA deficiency (see above), rely on ex vivo introduction of the target gene into bone marrow cells and the return of these bone marrow cells to the patient by standard bone marrow transplantation. This could be viewed as a technical enhancement of existing bone marrow transplantation methods. Indeed, all allogeneic bone marrow transplantation (introduction of bone marrow from another individual into a patient) can be viewed as a complete form of gene therapy, replacing the entire genome of the patient's bone marrow cells with that of another individual who carries a normal copy of the disease-causing gene. Similarly, induction of expression of a potentially immunogenic gene in a tumor cell through gene therapy is closely related in concept to more traditional immunologic approaches, including the injection of immunogenic bacterial products directly into tumors.

Finally, a promising new direction for gene therapy is the creation of bioreactors that can be implanted into the patient for long-term production of therapeutic protein. Cells engineered to express the recombinant protein are grown in an implantable device, which allows nutrients to enter to support cell growth, and the recombinant therapeutic protein to diffuse out into the circulation, but protects the cells from immune destruction by the host. Such implantable devices could find widespread application for the treatment of many protein deficiency disorders and may offer significant safety advantages over other forms of gene therapy. This approach is similar in concept to the more conventional infusion of therapeutic protein or drug into the patient.

Gene therapy and other related applications of recombinant DNA technology to the treatment of human disease hold great promise for the future. Improved technology for the delivery of therapeutic DNA sequences and for efficient regulation of gene expression may open up exciting new approaches to the treatment of many genetic and acquired disorders, including common multifactorial diseases such as atherosclerosis, diabetes, hypertension, and cancer. With the continued identification of genetic factors that predispose to the latter group of diseases, it may become possible to identify highly susceptible patients before they become symptomatic, permitting preventive gene therapies to be initiated. Advances in recombinant DNA technology may eventually make it possible to precisely correct a specific genetic defect at the actual site of the authentic gene, without the risk of other untoward effects elsewhere in the genome. With continued progress in these and other areas, it is likely that the dramatic impact of molecular genetic technology on the diagnosis of human disease will soon begin to realize its promise in the realms of treatment and prevention.

SUGGESTED READINGS

Friedmann T. A brief history of gene therapy. Nat Genet 1992;2:93–98. *A historic perspective on gene therapy, beginning with the early cell transformation studies in the 1960s.*

Blaese RM, Culver KW, Miller AD, et al. T lymphocyte-directed gene therapy for ADA-SCID: initial trial results after 4 years. Science 1995;270:475–480. *Follow-up report on the first approved clinical gene therapy study.*

Wivel NA, Walters L. Germ-line gene modification and disease prevention: some medical and ethical perspectives. Science 1993;262:533–538. *A discussion of the issues surrounding germ-line gene therapy from the directors of the Recombinant DNA Advisory Committee (RAC).*

Crystal RG. Transfer of genes to humans: early lessons and obstacles to success. Science 1995;270:404–410. *A general overview of the gene therapy field.*

Rosenfeld MA, Collins FS. Gene therapy for cystic fibrosis. Chest 1996;109:241–252. *A review of current progress and the major obstacles to gene therapy for cystic fibrosis.*

Roth JA, Cristiano RJ. Gene therapy for cancer: what have we done and where are we going? J Natl Cancer Inst 1997;89:21–39. *A detailed summary of the current status of cancer gene therapy, including trials completed or in progress worldwide.*

Orkin SH, Motulsky AG. Report and recommendations of the panel to assess the NIH investment in research on gene therapy. 1996. *The report of an expert panel appointed by the Director of the NIH to review the status of gene therapy. The report can be obtained through the internet at the home page for the Office of Recombinant DNA Activities (ORDA) at **http://www.nih.gov/od/orda/index.html**. This website is also a useful resource for additional up-to-date information about gene therapy, such as the complete list of approved gene therapy protocols and their current status, including the number of patients enrolled and complications observed.*

Ethical Considerations

"It is but sorrow to be wise when wisdom profits not."

—SOPHOCLES

Medical genetics, once the province of a relatively small number of special-ists, is now moving into the mainstream of clinical medicine, thanks to dra-matic advances in the identification of the causes of genetic disease. But ge-netic medicine, whether in clinical care or research, often presents difficult choices—for the patient, the research subject, the family, the physician, the investigator, and society. Some of these dilemmas are not so different from those faced in other branches of medicine—the available options may be less than ideal, the information on which to make a decision may be fragmentary, and thus the patient and physician are forced to choose a path forward in the best way possible, without assurances that it will succeed. In the medical ge-netics arena, additional complexities may arise: genetic information is partic-ularly powerful, and its ethical implications particularly profound, because it may predict future illness in a currently healthy individual, and because there may be significant consequences for other family members (born or unborn).

Throughout this text, the reader has probably been troubled at times by the ethical aspects of some of the clinical situations presented. The purpose of this concluding chapter is to outline certain general ethical principles, in order to allow the framing of such challenging situations in clearer terms. Through the use of illustrative cases, four major principles of medical ethics will be out-lined and applied to genetics. The reader should not, however, expect simple answers to complex questions; some of the most difficult debates in medical ge-netics arise when two of these principles conflict. In many actual clinical situa-tions, however, the apparent ethical conflicts will be seen to be partly a result of inadequate communication between patients, caregivers, and families.

Before considering these principles, it is appropriate to inquire briefly about the moral perspectives on which they rest. What determines the good-ness of an act? Whether the person performing it met his or her duties and obligations? Whether the motives of that person were virtuous? Or simply the consequences of the act? The three traditional ethical theories (duty-based theory, virtue ethics, and consequentialism) represent respectively those three points of view. Other contemporary theories reach out beyond the individual to incorporate the community and the broader social context. A full consideration of the theoretical basis of medical ethics is well beyond the scope of this chapter, and the interested reader is referred to authorita-tive references at the end of this chapter.

Respect for Autonomy

The first principle to consider is that of respect for autonomy of the indi-vidual. Autonomy is synonymous with self-determination, self-rule, or self-governance. Respect for autonomy arises from the assertion that indi-viduals are capable of reasoning, deciding, willing, and acting, and thus

Figure 14.8.

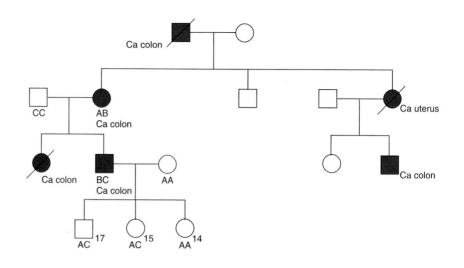

the diagnosis of their cancer, making a diagnosis of familial polyposis almost certain (see chapter 11). A linkage study is carried out using probes from the *APC* gene on chromosome 5q, and the disease gene is found to be traveling with the B allele of an intragenic marker (see Fig. 14.8). Familial polyposis is one of those conditions in which testing in childhood is offered, since interventions may need to begin before age 18. With full informed consent, assent of the children, and extensive education of the family, linkage testing is carried out on the three children with the closely linked marker. By linkage analysis, it is determined that the two older children have received the normal gene from their father. DNA testing for the youngest child, however, is incompatible with the father being her biological father. Analysis of a number of other polymorphic markers confirm the high likelihood that her biological father is someone else. In a private conversation with the mother, she admits the possibility that this daughter might well have been fathered by a different man through a long past affair that she now regrets. She pleads with the clinic staff to keep this information confidential. Accordingly, the clinic staff simply inform the parents and all three children that in this instance the father's familial polyposis mutation has not been passed to any of his three children.

Comment

Discovery of misattributed paternity is not a rare event in a medical genetics clinic that performs DNA analysis. In fact, the possibility of such an outcome should always be presented before testing as one of the possible risks of the procedure. Although some would argue that the father's right to know the biological status of his daughter forces disclosure of this unexpected information, the confidentiality of the relationship with the mother and her desire to keep this information private is generally considered to carry greater weight.

CASE 9—WHEN DUTY TO WARN COLLIDES WITH CONFIDENTIALITY

A couple comes to the clinic because their firstborn child, now 1 week old, has been diagnosed with Down syndrome (Fig. 14.9). Physical exam reveals typical stigmata, and a karyotype reveals 46,XX,−14,+t(14;21). The parents are informed that this type of Down syndrome could potentially have a high recurrence risk (see Chapter 8), and they request chromosome studies. The

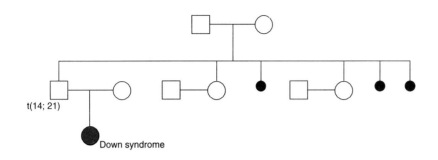

Figure 14.9.

father is found to carry a t(14;21) Robertsonian translocation. Given that his mother has a history of three first-trimester miscarriages, the possibility that this translocation was inherited has to be considered. In this case his two sisters could also be carriers, and would therefore be at increased risk of having a child with Down syndrome. When the possibility of testing his parents is raised, the father adamantly refuses to discuss it. The relationships in the family are already strained, and he feels a considerable burden of shame and guilt for carrying a chromosome rearrangement that has led to the birth of a child with Down syndrome. The father is determined that the rest of his family not learn of this information. The counselor is thus caught between the duty to warn his two sisters, who are about to begin childbearing, that they may be at elevated risk for Down syndrome, and the need to respect the confidentiality of the provider-patient relationship.

Comment

The first responsibility of the genetic counselor in this circumstance is to explain thoroughly the consequences of nondisclosure to relatives. The purpose is to help the father think through those outcomes, recognizing that these could potentially be much worse than the immediate consequences he fears. In almost all instances, with some time and opportunity for reasoned discussion, family members will recognize the need for disclosure when there is a genuine risk to relatives. In those rare circumstances in which such a resolution cannot be achieved, there is currently no solid guidance to assist the health care provider in deciding which of these rather sacred principles is preeminent, and the severity of the risk to others has to be a major determinant in the decision made.

Justice and Equity

The principles of equity and justice refer to how an individual is treated in the context of the rest of society. Are benefits distributed fairly? Are burdens shared? Is access to medical care, social goods, and potentially beneficial research studies limited to those with financial resources or perceived social worth?

CASE 10—THREATENED LOSS OF JOB OPPORTUNITY FROM GENETIC PREDISPOSITION

An asymptomatic woman, age 25, with a family history of colon and endometrial cancer, is evaluated at a genetics clinic. The family history strongly suggests hereditary nonpolyposis colon cancer (HNPCC) (see Chapter 11). As part of a research protocol, her family is evaluated and a mutation is found in the *MSH2* gene. The patient wishes to know her status, and after extensive education about possible outcomes, the test is carried out

Glossary

Acrocentric chromosome—a chromosome in which the centromere lies near the end of the chromosome.

Additivity principle—if two events are mutually exclusive, the probability of obtaining one or the other is the sum of their separate probabilities.

Allele—alternative forms of a gene at a given locus.

Allele-specific oligonucleotide (ASO)—synthetic oligonucleotide designed to hybridize to a specific sequence and, under the right conditions, to fail to hybridize to a related sequence. Even a single nucleotide variation can readily be detected by hybridization with ASOs designed to match each of the allelic sequences. ASOs are also used as PCR primers in several methods similarly designed to distinguish between closely related alleles.

Allelic heterogeneity—similar or identical phenotypes caused by different mutant alleles at the same genetic locus.

α_1-Antitrypsin—a serine protease inhibitor that inhibits the activity of elastase. Absence of this inhibitor as in α_1-antitrypsin deficiency results in chronic severe pulmonary disease and liver disease.

Alu repetitive sequence—moderately repetitive sequence located within intergenic or intronic DNA, containing a recognition site for the restriction enzyme *Alu*I. These sequences are about 300 bp long, and occur about 500,000 times in the human genome.

Amniocentesis—a prenatal diagnostic procedure, generally performed during the second trimester of pregnancy, in which amniotic fluid is withdrawn from the amniotic sac surrounding the fetus.

Amplification—the production of multiple copies of a DNA sequence.

Aneuploid—any chromosome number that is not an exact multiple of the haploid number. Usually aneuploid refers to an extra copy of a single chromosome (trisomy) or the absence of a single chromosome (monosomy), resulting from nondisjunction during meiosis or mitosis.

Anticipation—the occurrence of a genetic disease at an earlier age of onset or with increasing severity in successive generations.

Antisense strand (of DNA)—the noncoding strand of double-stranded DNA. It is complementary to the mRNA and serves as the template for mRNA synthesis.

Apoptosis—programed cell death.

Ascertainment—the selection of individuals for inclusion in a genetic study.

Association—in a population the occurrence together of two or more different phenotypes more often than expected by chance (not the same as linkage).

Assortative mating—nonrandom mating in which a member of a particular subpopulation is more likely to mate with other members of that subpopulation (positive) or less likely (negative).

Autoimmune disorder—a disorder characterized by the presence of antibodies directed against the individual's own antigens.

Autosomal disease—a disease encoded by a gene on one of the 22 pairs of autosomes.

Autosome—any chromosome other than the sex chromosomes or the mitochondrial chromosome.

Auxotrophic mutants—mutant cells dependent on an exogenous nutrient because they lack the ability to catalyze a specific metabolic step.

B cells—small lymphocytes that respond to antigenic stimulation by producing humoral antibodies.

Bacterial artificial chromosome (BAC)—a recombinant plasmid designed for the cloning of large fragments of DNA between 50–200 kb. BACs are propagated in a host bacterial cell.

Bacteriophage—bacterial virus. In molecular biology, these are used as vectors in cloning.

Barr bodies—sex chromatin as seen in female somatic cells (derived from the inactivated X chromosome).

Base pair (bp)—in double-stranded DNA there is complementary purine-pyrimidine hydrogen bonding (adenine must always pair with thymine, and guanine with cytosine). The hydrogen-bonded residue pair is designated as 1 bp. This unit is used for measuring the length of pieces of DNA.

Bayes' theorem—a theorem using conditional probability to incorporate all pertinent information relevant to estimating the likelihood that an individual at risk is affected with, or a carrier of, a genetic disorder. See text for explanation.

Candidate gene—a gene, mapped to a region known to be linked to a specific disease, whose protein product has characteristics suggesting that it may be the actual disease-associated gene. In practice, when the physical location of the disease gene has been narrowed to a small region containing a limited number of genes, any gene that also maps to this small interval may be referred to as a candidate gene.

Cap—a modified nucleotide, 7-methylguanosine, added at the 5' end of the growing mRNA chain, which appears to

341

be necessary for normal processing, stability, and translation of mRNA.

Cap site—site of initiation of transcription.

Carrier—an individual heterozygous for a mutant allele that generally causes disease only in the homozygous state.

CCAAT box—a region found 75–80 bp upstream from the transcription initiation site of many, but not all, genes that seems to be important for quantitatively efficient transcription.

CentiMorgan (cM)—a unit of genetic distance. Two loci are 1 cM apart if there is a 1% chance of recombination between them in a given meiotic event.

Centromere—central constriction of the chromosome, a heterochromatic region by which the chromatids are held together and to which the kinetochore is attached.

Chain terminator mutations—nonsense or frameshift mutations that result in premature cessation of translation of the mRNA.

Chimera—an individual formed by cells derived from more than one zygote. In the preparation of knockout mice, ES cells carrying the desired gene alteration are mixed with normal donor embryonic cells. The mice produced from these embryos are derived from a mixture of ES cells and the normal donor cells and are thus referred to as chimeras.

Chorionic villus sampling—a procedure used for prenatal diagnosis at 8–10 weeks gestation. Fetal tissue for analysis is aspirated under ultrasonic guidance from the villous area of the chorion (chorion frondosum).

Chromatids—the two parallel identical strands, connected at the centromere, of the doubled chromosome after chromosomal replication but before anaphase.

Chromatin—the nucleic acids and proteins of which chromosomes are made.

Chromosomal disorder—disorders that are the results of addition or deletion of entire chromosomes or parts of chromosomes (e.g., Down syndrome, trisomy 21).

Chromosome aberration—an abnormality of chromosome number or structure.

Clone—a group of genetically identical cells derived by mitosis from a single ancestral cell.

Codon—a triplet of three bases in a DNA or RNA molecule, specifying a single amino acid.

Coefficient of relationship (r)—the probability that two persons have inherited a particular allele from a common ancestor. Also, the proportion of all genes that are identical by descent from a common ancestor.

Complementary—the interaction of purine-pyrimidine base pairs of a nucleic acid by hydrogen bonding (thus adenine with thymine, guanine with cytosine) to provide the geometry for nucleic acid secondary structure.

Complementary DNA (cDNA)—DNA synthesized from an mRNA template, using reverse transcriptase.

Complementation analysis—a genetic test for whether two mutations producing a similar phenotype are allelic.

Compound heterozygote—an individual with two different mutant alleles at a given locus.

Concordant—a twin pair in which both members exhibit the same phenotype or trait.

Conditional probability—the probability of the joint occurrence of two nonindependent events is the product of the probability of one event times the probability of the second event given that the first event has occurred.

Consanguinity (consanguineous)—genetically related by descent from a common ancestor (literally of the same blood).

Consensus sequence—a nucleotide sequence, such as CCAAT, TATA, or the splice donor, which plays an important functional role in gene expression. Such sequences may not be identical from gene to gene, but tend to share certain features, which are denoted as consensus sequences.

Consultand—the individual seeking, or referred for, genetic counseling.

Contact inhibition—the condition in which normal cells will stop growth when they touch each other.

Contiguous gene syndrome—a usually sporadic syndrome, with a consistent but complex phenotype, associated with a small deletion involving two or more contiguous loci. *See also* microdeletion syndrome.

Crossing over—reciprocal breaking and rejoining of homologous chromosomes in meiotic prophase I that results in exchange of chromosomal segments.

Cytotrophoblast—rapidly dividing cells obtained from fetal chorionic villi by chorionic villus sampling; used for karyotyping and DNA analysis.

Deformation—an abnormal form, shape, or position of a part of the body caused by mechanical forces that may be either extrinsic or intrinsic to the fetus.

Degeneracy of the code—several codons code for the same amino acid.

Denaturing gradient gel electrophoresis (DGGE)—a method used to detect differences between closely related DNA sequences. Double-stranded DNA samples are fractionated in an increasing gradient of a denaturant. Melting of the double strand, resulting in altered mobility, occurs at varying places along the gel, depending on the DNA sequence content.

Diploid—the number of chromosomes in most somatic cells, which is double the number found in the gametes (the haploid number). In humans the diploid chromosome number is 46.

Discordant—a twin pair in which one member exhibits a certain trait and the other does not.

Disruption—a morphologic defect resulting from the extrinsic breakdown of, or interference with, an originally normal developmental process.

Dizygotic—the product of fertilization of two separate eggs by two separate sperm; nonidentical twin pair.

DNA, deoxyribonucleic acid—the ultimate molecule of life. The polymer of which eukaryotic genes are composed.

DNA ligase—enzyme that catalyzes religation of two fragments of DNA.

DNA methylation—covalent attachment of methyl groups to DNA. Most commonly in eukaryotes this involves methylation of cytosine residues and is associated with reduced levels of transcription of a gene.

DNA polymerase—enzyme responsible for replication of DNA, which is accomplished by using each complementary strand of the DNA double helix as a template for the synthesis of a new strand.

DNA rearrangements—somatic recombination of DNA segments. In cells of the immune system, the variable (V), diversity (D), and joining (J) regions rearrange to generate functional antibody genes.

Domain—a region of the amino acid sequence of a protein that can be equated with a particular function, or a corresponding segment of a gene.

Dominant (trait)—those conditions that are expressed in heterozygotes (i.e., individuals with one copy of the mutant gene and one copy of the normal allele).

Dosage compensation—mechanism to account for the observation that the amount of a product encoded by a gene on the X chromosome is the same in males and females.

Double heterozygote—an individual with one mutant allele at each of two different loci.

Duffy blood group locus—the first autosomal gene placed on a chromosome (chromosome 1) by Donahue in 1968.

Dysmorphology—the area of clinical genetics concerned with the diagnosis and management of congenital anatomic abnormalities.

Dysplasia—the abnormal organization of cells into tissues, and its morphologic consequences.

Dystrophin—the protein encoded by the X-linked gene, which, when mutated, causes Duchenne or Becker muscular dystrophy. Dystrophin is presumed to be involved in anchoring the contractile apparatus of striated and cardiac muscle to the cell membrane.

Ecogenetic disorder—a disorder resulting from the interaction of a common environmental factor with a specific genetic predisposition to disease (e.g., cigarette smoking causing emphysema in α_1-antitrypsin deficiency).

Electroporation—application of a short high-voltage electric pulse to cells in the presence of DNA to permit DNA to enter the cells.

Empirical recurrence risks—recurrence risks for siblings or offspring, calculated by actual observed frequency of the trait in families rather than on knowledge of the exact inheritance pattern of the trait.

Endonuclease—an enzyme that cuts DNA at an internal site.

Restriction endonucleases cut DNA at specific nucleotide sequences.

Enhancers—DNA sequences that act in *cis* to increase transcription of a nearby gene. Enhancers can act in either orientation, may be either 5' or 3' to the gene, and may act at considerable distance from the gene.

Euchromatin—the chromatin that is light staining with trypsin G banding and is thought to contain genes that are, or have the potential to be, actively transcribed.

Euploid—any exact multiple of the number of chromosomes in a normal haploid gamete. In a normal somatic cell, the number of chromosomes is 2N, or diploid.

Exon—the transcribed regions of the gene that are present in mature mRNA and usually contain coding information.

Expressivity—the nature and severity of the phenotype of a mutant allele are a reflection of its expressivity. Variable expressivity is a frequent characteristic of autosomal dominant traits.

False-positive rate—proportion of all positive tests occurring in individuals who are not affected.

False-negative rate—proportion of all negative results in individuals with the trait or disease.

Familial—any trait that is more common in relatives of an affected individual than in the general population; could be related to genetic or environmental causes.

Familial hypercholesterolemia—an autosomal dominant disease in which there is a deficiency of low density lipoprotein (LDL) receptors, resulting in elevated serum cholesterol and LDL-cholesterol.

Favism—acute hemolytic anemia in certain G6PD-deficient individuals, resulting from ingestion of fava beans.

α-Fetoprotein—a protein produced by the fetus and found in amniotic fluid. The amounts increase during normal pregnancy up to the 34th week, but abnormally high levels are found under certain normal (i.e., multiple births) or pathologic (i.e., neural tube defects, fetal death) conditions.

Fitness (f)—a measure of fertility and therefore of the contribution to the gene pool of the succeeding generation. For a given genotype, the number of offspring surviving to reproductive age relative to the number for the wild-type genotype.

Fluorescence in situ hybridization (FISH)—identification of chromosomes and chromosomal loci using nucleic acid probes that can be detected by fluorescence tagging. This technique may be used to study chromosomes in interphase cells, as well as in cells arrested in metaphase.

Founder effect—the high frequency of a mutant gene in a rapidly expanding population founded by a small ancestral group in which one or more of the founders was, by chance, a carrier of the mutant gene.

Frameshift mutation—a mutation involving a deletion or insertion that is not an exact multiple of 3 bp, which changes the reading frame of the gene. All coding regions 3′ to the frameshift mutation will thus be read as gibberish, usually soon encountering a stop codon.

Gene flow—gradual diffusion of genes from one population to another, as a result of migration and intermarriage.

Gene therapy—the treatment of human disease by introduction of recombinant nucleic acid sequences into the cells of a patient.

Genetic code—the base triplets that specify the 20 different amino acids.

Genetic counseling—a communication process, the intent of which is to provide individuals and families having a genetic disease or at risk of such a disease with information about their condition and to provide information that would allow couples at risk to make informed reproductive decisions. (For details, see text.)

Genetic drift—random fluctuations in gene frequencies, most evident in small populations.

Genetic heterogeneity—different mutations can cause a similar phenotype; *allelic heterogeneity* refers to different mutations at the same locus, whereas *locus heterogeneity* refers to mutations at a different loci.

Genetic lethal—a genetic disease that prevents fertility. It need not cause illness or death, but must prevent reproduction.

Genetic locus—a specific position or location on a chromosome.

Genetic map—the relative position of genes and markers along a chromosome, as determined by genetic linkage information. This map can be contrasted with the physical map in which the actual location of the genes along the chromosome have been determined by direct physical techniques, such as restriction mapping and physical cloning.

Genetic screening—testing on a population basis to identify a subset of individuals at high risk of having a specific disorder, or of transmitting a specific genetic disorder.

Genome—the complete DNA sequence of an organism containing its complete genetic information.

Genomic imprinting—differential expression of genetic information depending on whether it was inherited from the father or the mother. Imprinting is thought to reflect differential activation or inactivation during gametogenesis in the male and female parents.

Genotype—the genetic constitution of an individual or, more specifically, the alleles at specific genetic loci.

Germline gene therapy—the introduction, intentionally or unintentionally, of genetic alterations into cells of the germline (i.e., oocytes and sperm, or their precursors). Germline gene therapy has the potential of altering genes in subsequent generations. This is to be contrasted with somatic gene therapy.

Germline mosaicism—two or more genetically distinct germ cell lines derived from a single zygote, but differ-

ing because of somatic mutation or nondisjunction. Also called gonadal mosaicism.

Giemsa banding—characteristic light and dark bands, unique for each human chromosome, obtained by staining with Giemsa stain after gentle trypsin treatment.

Glucose-6-phosphate dehydrogenase (G6PD)—enzyme catalyzing the first step in the hexose monophosphate shunt pathway.

Guthrie test—bacterial inhibition test used to screen for the presence of phenylketonuria.

Haploid—the chromosome number of a normal gamete, with only one member of each chromosome pair. In humans, the haploid number is 23.

Haploidentical—the sharing of one haplotype for a specific locus among two individuals who differ at the second allele. In HLA typing, for example, a parent and child are always haploidentical because the child has inherited one HLA allele from that parent and the second allele from the other parent.

Haplotype—genotype of a group of alleles from two or more closely linked loci on one chromosome, usually inherited as a unit, e.g., the HLA complex.

Hardy-Weinberg equilibrium—the law that relates gene frequency to genotype frequency in a population at equilibrium and permits determination of allele frequency and heterozygote carrier frequency in a population for which the frequency of a trait is known.

Hemoglobin Bart's—the tetramer of 4 γ-globin subunits. This is the major form of hemoglobin that accumulates in hydrops fetalis (complete absence of α-globin gene expression).

Hemoglobin H—the tetramer of 4 β-subunits. This insoluble form of hemoglobin accumulates in hemoglobin H disease.

Hemoglobinopathies—disorders caused by either quantitative or qualitative abnormalities of hemoglobin. These include the thalassemias (quantitative disorders), as well as a variety of qualitative hemoglobin disorders as a result of mutations that affect hemoglobin function, such as sickle cell anemia.

Heterochromatin—chromatin that stains darkly with trypsin and Giemsa and is composed of repetitive DNA.

Heteromorphism—a normal variant of a chromosome.

Heteroplasmy—two or more genetically distinct populations of mitochondria in a somatic cell tissue.

Heteropyknotic—dense and dark staining, suggestive of inactive chromatin.

Heterozygote (heterozygous)—an individual who has two different alleles at a given locus on a pair of homologous chromosomes.

Histones—proteins associated with DNA in the chromosomes, rich in basic amino acids (lysine or arginine) and virtually unchanged throughout eukaryote evolution.

Homogeneously staining region (HSR)—a cytogenetically

detectable expanded region in a chromosome resulting from many fold amplification of a discrete segment of DNA, termed an amplicon. Similarly amplified sequences existing outside of the chromosome are referred to as double minutes.

Homozygote (homozygous)—an individual possessing a pair of identical alleles at a given locus on a pair of homologous chromosomes.

Housekeeping genes—genes that encode enzymes required for basic functions that are present in virtually all cells.

Human Genome Project—the plan to map and sequence the entire 3 billion bp of the human genome.

Hybridization (or reannealing)—in molecular genetics, complementary pairing of an RNA and a DNA strand or of two different DNA strands. In somatic cell genetics, fusion of two somatic cells to form a hybrid cell containing genetic information from both parental cells.

In situ hybridization—one of the most direct means for mapping a gene; the molecular hybridization of a cloned DNA sequence to metaphase chromosomes spread on a microscope slide.

Inborn error of metabolism—a genetically determined biochemical disorder in which a specific enzyme defect produces a metabolic block that may have pathologic consequences. The concept put forward by Archibald Garrod in 1908 that, in effect, established the field of biochemical genetics.

Independence principle—the probability of a joint occurrence of two or more independent events is the product of their separate probabilities.

Index case—proband.

Insertion—a structural chromosomal abnormality in which part of the material from one chromosome is inserted into a nonhomologous chromosome.

Intergenic DNA—relatively long stretches of DNA in between the transcribed genes, without known function.

Intervening sequence (IVS)—an intron.

Intron—a segment of a gene that is initially transcribed into RNA but is then removed from the primary transcript by splicing together the exon sequences on either side of it. Intronic sequences are not found in mature mRNA.

Inversion—a structural abnormality of a chromosome in which a segment of a chromosome is reversed end to end; may be pericentric when inverted segment includes the centromere, or paracentric when it does not.

Isochromosome—an abnormal chromosome in which one arm is duplicated (so that two arms of equal length are formed with the same loci in reverse sequence) and the other arm is deleted.

Karyotype—the chromosome constitution of an individual (number of chromosomes, sex chromosome constitution, and any abnormalities in number or morphology). Also commonly used term for a photomicrograph of the chromosomes of an individual arranged in the standard classification and for the process of preparing such a photomicrograph (karyotyping).

Kilobase (kb)—one thousand base pairs in a DNA sequence.

Kinetochore—a structure at the centromere to which the spindle fibers are attached.

Knockout—this term is used to refer to the inactivation of a specific target gene by homologous recombination methods. Mice produced by this procedure are referred to as knockout mice. Knockouts for a large number of genes have been generated, serving as useful models for the corresponding human genetic deficiencies.

Library—a large collection of recombinant DNA clones, in which genomic or cDNA fragments have been inserted into a particular vector.

Linkage—coinheritance of two or more nonallelic genes because their loci are in close proximity on the same chromosome, such that after meiosis they remain associated more often than the 50% expected for unlinked genes.

Linkage disequilibrium—the preferential association of a particular allele, for example, a mutant allele for a disease with a specific allele at a nearby locus more frequently than expected by chance.

Linkage map—a chromosome map showing the relative positions of genetic markers of a given species, as determined by linkage analysis; not the same as a physical map or a gene map that uses linkage analysis, cytogenetic examination, and physical techniques to generate the map.

Lipofection—a procedure using lipids to efficiently introduce DNA into a target cell.

Liposome—a synthetic lipid particle designed to transport DNA for efficient introduction into a target cell.

Locus control region (LCR)—a segment of DNA that regulates the expression of a cluster of genes, often in a tissue-specific manner. The LCR can be located at distances up to 10–100 kb away from the genes it regulates.

Locus heterogeneity—similar phenotypes caused by mutations at different genetic loci.

Lod score—a statistical method that tests whether a set of linkage data indicates two loci are linked or unlinked. The lod score is the base 10 logarithm of the odds favoring linkage. By convention, a lod score of +3 (1000:1 odds) is taken as proof of linkage; a score of −2 (100:1 odds against) indicates no linkage.

Loss of heterozygosity (LOH)—loss of one allele in a tumor cell from a chromosomal region for which the individual's normal cells are heterozygous. LOH is detected using polymorphic DNA markers that can distinguish between the two alleles.

Lyonization—one of the two X chromosomes in female somatic cells is randomly inactivated early in embryonic development. As a result, the female is a mosaic of cells each functionally hemizygous for one or other X chromosome.

Major histocompatibility complex (MHC)—the complex of human leukocyte antigen (HLA) genes on the short arm of chromosome 6. Because it is so polymorphic, this complex is an ideal marker for linkage studies.

Malformation—a morphologic defect of an organ, or part of an organ, resulting from an intrinsically abnormal developmental process.

Marker locus—a locus whose alleles are readily detectable. It may or may not be part of an expressed gene.

Maxam-Gilbert method—method for determining the exact nucleotide sequence by a chemical degradation process.

Meiosis—special type of cell division occurring in the germ cells of sexually reproducing organisms during which gametes containing the haploid chromosome number are produced from diploid cells. Two meiotic divisions occur, meiosis I and meiosis II; reduction in number takes place during meiosis I.

Messenger RNA (mRNA)—the template on which polypeptides are synthesized; the crucial connecting link between information contained in a gene and its end result as the specific amino acid sequence of a protein.

Metacentric chromosome—chromosome in which the centromere is in the middle of the chromosome.

Microdeletion syndrome—a syndrome resulting from a chromosomal deletion too small to be observed microscopically. *See also* contiguous gene syndrome.

Missense mutation—a single DNA base substitution resulting in a codon specifying a different amino acid.

Mitochondrial DNA—the DNA in the circular chromosome of the mitochondria, cytoplasmic organelles that possess their own unique DNA. Mitochondrial DNA is present in many copies per cell, is maternally inherited, and evolves 5 to 10 times as rapidly as genomic DNA.

Mitosis—process of nuclear division, occurring in five stages (prophase, prometaphase, metaphase, anaphase, and telophase) in which one cell divides to give rise to two that are genetically identical to the parent.

Molecular hybridization—the ability of a single-stranded DNA or RNA to anneal to its complementary single strand by Watson-Crick base pairing.

Monosomy—a condition in which one chromosome of a pair is missing, as in 45,X Turner syndrome.

Monozygotic—arising from a single zygote or fertilized egg; genetically identical twin pair.

Mosaicism—condition in which an individual has two or more genetically distinct cell lines derived from a single zygote, but differing because of mutation or nondisjunction.

Multifactorial inheritance—those traits resulting from interplay of multiple environmental factors with multiple genes.

Mutagen—a chemical or physical agent that increases the mutation rate by causing changes in DNA.

Mutation—any permanent heritable change in the sequence of genomic DNA.

Mutation rate (μ)—the frequency of mutation expressed as the number of mutations per locus per gamete per generation.

Nondisjunction—the failure of two homologous chromosomes to disjoin during meiosis I, or two chromatids of a chromosome to separate in meiosis II or mitosis, so that both pass to the same daughter cell and the other daughter cell receives neither.

Nonpenetrance—lack of clinical expression of the mutant phenotype in an individual with the appropriate genotype.

Nonsense mutation—a single DNA base substitution resulting in a stop (termination) codon.

Northern blot—blotting technique, analogous to Southern blotting, for detecting RNA fragments by hybridization. The blot reveals the size and abundance of the RNA complementary to the probe used.

Nucleosome—the basic structural units of chromatin. They consist of 146 bp of DNA wrapped around a core of eight histone molecules.

Nude mice—immunologically deficient mice used to permit growth of tumor cells from mouse and other species, such as human.

Obligate heterozygote—an individual who is clinically unaffected but, on the basis of pedigree analysis, must carry the mutant allele. (See text for discussion.)

Oligogenic diseases—diseases or traits that result from the effects of relatively few genes, some of which have rather large effects.

Oligonucleotide—a short segment of DNA or RNA anywhere from a few to a hundred nucleotides in length. DNA oligonucleotides are routinely produced on automated devices designed for their synthesis.

Oncogene—an altered version of a proto-oncogene (resulting from mutation, overexpression, or amplification) that contributes to neoplastic transformation.

p—designation for the short arm of a chromosome, from the French *petit*.

Packaging cell line—a cell line engineered for the production of recombinant retroviruses by introduction of essential viral genes missing in the recombinant gene therapy vector.

Palindrome—a DNA sequence that contains the same 5′ to 3′ sequence on both strands, e.g., 5′ GAATTC 3′ 3′ CTTAAG 5′.

Pedigree—from "pied de grue" or crane's foot; a diagram of a family history indicating the family members, their relationship to the proband, and their status with respect to a particular hereditary condition.

Penetrance—an all-or-none phenomenon that refers to the observable expression, or lack of it, of the mutant gene; for a dominant disease, defined quantitatively by determining the proportion of obligate gene carriers (heterozygotes), for a mutant gene, who express the phenotype.

Peptide fingerprint—chromatographic pattern of peptides obtained after partial hydrolysis of a protein or polypeptide. The technique may also be applied to DNA and RNA.

Pharmacogenetics—study of the genetic basis for differences in response to drugs.

Phase—the determination of whether the alternative alleles for two linked loci are on the same or different chromosomes.

Phenocopy—a phenotype produced by environmental factors that mimics a genetically determined trait.

Phenotype—the observed result of the interaction of the genotype with environmental factors, the observable expression of a particular gene or genes.

Philadelphia chromosome (Ph¹)—structurally abnormal chromosome 22, a reciprocal translocation between the distal portion of this chromosome and of chromosome 9, occurring in a proportion of bone marrow cells in patients with chronic myelogenous leukemia.

Physical map—the actual location of genes and markers along a chromosome as determined by direct physical techniques, such as restriction mapping and physical cloning. This map can be contrasted with the genetic map, in which the relative positions are determined by genetic linkage information.

Phytohemagglutinin—lectin from the red bean used to agglutinate red blood cells and stimulate lymphocytes to divide; used in preparation of peripheral blood karyotypes.

Plasmid—independently replicating, extrachromosomal circular DNA molecules often bearing antibiotic resistance genes and propagated in bacteria; used in recombinant DNA technology as vectors to carry cloned DNA segments.

Platelet-derived growth factor (PDGF)—a protein, produced by platelets and other cells, that strongly stimulates cell growth and division and is involved in normal wound healing. The gene for PDGF is identical to the proto-oncogene *sis*.

Pleiotropy—the diverse effects of a single gene or gene pair on several organ systems and functions.

Point mutation—substitution of one nucleotide for another.

Polyadenylation—the addition of about 200 adenosine residues at the 3′ end of messenger RNAs, apparently involved in their transport out of the nucleus and stability.

Polygenic diseases—diseases (or traits) that result from the interaction of multiple genes, each of which has a relatively minor effect.

Polymerase chain reaction (PCR)—a technique for amplifying a short stretch of DNA. The method depends on the use of two flanking oligonucleotide DNA primers and repeated cycles of primer extension using DNA polymerase.

Polymorphism—in a population the occurrence of two or more genetically determined alternative phenotypes at such a frequency that the rarest could not be maintained by recurrent mutation alone. In practice, a genetic locus is considered polymorphic if the rare allele has a frequency of at least 0.01, such that heterozygotes carrying this allele occur at a frequency greater than 2%.

Polysome (polyribosome)—structures composed of multiple ribosomes attached to mRNA in the process of translation.

Population genetics—the study of distribution of genes in populations and of the factors that maintain or change the frequency of genes and genotypes from generation to generation.

Positional cloning—the application of human gene mapping to clone the gene responsible for a disease, when no information about the biochemical basis of the disease is available.

Positive predictive value (PPV)—the probability that an individual with an abnormal test result has, or will develop, the disease for which he has been tested.

Premutation—an intermediate-size expansion of a triplet repeat region (such as the CGG repeat in fragile X syndrome) that does not itself cause the disease, but is unstable when transmitted and is likely to increase in size during meiosis (in the mother in the case of the fragile X syndrome).

Primary transcript—the direct RNA transcript of a gene, containing introns as well as exons.

Proband (propositus; proposita)—index case; the affected person through which a pedigree is discovered and explored.

Probe—in molecular genetics, a labeled DNA or RNA sequence used to detect the presence of a complementary sequence by molecular hybridization; a reagent capable of recognizing the desired clone in a complex mixture of many DNA or RNA sequences.

Promoter—the sequence elements located 5′ to the gene. These elements fix the site of initiation of transcription and control mRNA quantity and sometimes tissue specificity.

Protein suicide mechanism—in dominant disorders, one mutant subunit leads to the loss of function of an entire multimeric protein, e.g., collagen.

Proto-oncogene—the normal cellular homologue of an oncogene. These genes are generally involved in control of cell growth and have been preserved throughout evolution.

Pseudogenes—DNA sequences that have the structures of expressed genes, and were presumably once functional, but have acquired one or more mutations during evolution that render them incapable of producing a protein product.

q—designation for the long arm of a chromosome.

Quasidominance—the pattern of inheritance produced by the mating of a homozygous affected individual with an individual heterozygous for the same recessive trait, so that homozygous affected members appear in two or more successive generations.

Reading frame—one of the possible ways of reading a nucleotide sequence as a series of triplets. An open reading frame contains no termination codons and thus is potentially translatable into protein.

Recessive (trait)—those conditions that are clinically manifest only in individuals homozygous for the mutant gene (i.e., carrying a double dose of the abnormal gene).

Reciprocal translocation—exchange of material between two nonhomologous chromosomes.

Recombinant chromosome—chromosome in an offspring that has a genotype not found in either parent, as a result of crossing over in meiosis.

Recombinant DNA technology—techniques of genetic analysis in which the DNA from one gene or part of a gene from one organism is inserted into the genome of another organism.

Recombination—the formation of new combinations of linked genes by crossing over (breakage and rejoining) between their loci.

Recombination fraction (θ)—in linkage analysis, the fraction of meiotic events that show a recombination between two loci.

Recurrence risk—the probability that a genetic disorder that has occurred in a family will recur in another member in the same or in future generations.

Restriction enzymes—endonucleases purified from bacteria that can cut double-stranded DNA at a specific nucleotide sequence. Each enzyme is designated by the organism from which it was obtained, e.g., *Eco* RI from *Escherichia coli* RY13, which cleaves at the sequence GAATTC.

Restriction fragment length polymorphism (RFLP)—a variation in DNA sequence that alters the length of a restriction fragment. These may be simple point mutations, which create or destroy a restriction site, or variable length regions (so-called VNTRs, for variable number of tandem repeats). RFLPs provide convenient markers for linkage analysis.

Restriction map—a map of a DNA sequence, usually in base pairs, indicating the location of restriction sites.

Reticulocyte—precursor of mature erythrocyte.

Retrovirus—RNA viruses that are reverse transcribed into a DNA copy on entering a host cell and subsequently are stably inserted into chromosomal DNA.

Reverse transcriptase—an enzyme that catalyzes the synthesis of DNA on an RNA template.

Ribosome—cytoplasmic organelle composed of ribosomal RNA and protein, on which polypeptide synthesis from messenger RNA occurs.

Ribozyme—an RNA molecule capable of catalyzing specific reactions, including DNA cleavage.

Ring chromosome—a structurally abnormal chromosome in which the end of each arm has been deleted and the broken arms have rejoined in ring formation.

RNA polymerases—DNA-template-dependent transcription enzymes that synthesize RNA from ribonucleoside triphosphate precursors.

RNA, ribonucleic acid—the ribonucleotide polymer, containing ribose instead of deoxyribose, into which DNA is transcribed.

Robertsonian translocation—a translocation between two acrocentric chromosomes by fusion at the centromere with loss of the short arm and satellites.

Sanger method—enzymatic method for determining the exact nucleotide sequence of a cloned fragment of DNA.

Segregation—in genetics, the separation of allelic genes at meiosis. Because allelic genes occupy the same locus on homologous chromosomes, they pass to different gametes; that is, they segregate.

Selection—the action of environmental factors on a particular phenotype, and hence its genotype, based on differences in biologic fitness.

Semiconservative replication—as applied to DNA, each daughter DNA strand contains one parental strand and one newly synthesized strand.

Sensitivity—as applied to a diagnostic test, the frequency with which the test yields a positive result when the disease is present.

Sequence (dysmorphic)—a pattern of multiple anomalies derived from a single prior anomaly or mechanical factor, as in the Potter sequence.

Sex chromosomes—X and Y chromosomes.

Sibship—group comprising all the siblings (brothers and sisters) in a family.

Silent gene—a mutant gene that has no detectable phenotypic effect.

Simple sequence repeat (SSR)—a segment of DNA consisting of a multiply repeated short sequence element. Repeats of a 2-bp unit are referred to as dinucleotides, those with 3 bp as trinucleotides, etc. Longer repeats are particularly likely to have multiple polymorphic alleles with variable lengths. Polymorphic SSRs are a major source of genetic markers for the Human Genome Project.

Single-gene disorders—disorders caused by single mutant genes with a large effect on the patient's phenotype (e.g., sickle cell anemia).

Single-strand conformer polymorphism (SSCP)—a method for detecting single nucleotide differences between sequences based on alterations in gel mobility as a result of changes in the conformation of single-stranded DNA.

Sister chromatids—two identical strands of DNA generated during the S phase (DNA synthesis) of the cell cycle and held together at the centromere until mitosis or meiosis II anaphase.

Somatic cell—any cell of an organism not involved in the germline.

Somatic cell hybrid—a hybrid cell made by fusing different cells (usually from different species) together. For human gene mapping, human and rodent cell hybrids are commonly used.

Somatic gene therapy—insertion of new DNA material into a particular tissue of an affected individual in such a way that the inserted DNA does not enter the germline.

Southern blot—a technique, devised by Edward Southern, for transferring DNA fragments separated by agarose gel electrophoresis to a nitrocellulose filter, on which specific DNA fragments can then be detected by their hybridization to radioactive probes.

Specificity—as applied to a diagnostic test, the frequency with which the test is negative when the disease is absent.

Splicing—removal of introns in the generation of mature mRNA.

Submetacentric chromosome—a chromosome in which the centromere is somewhat distant from the center of the chromosome.

Synapsis—in meiosis, the pairing of homologous chromosomes in meiotic prophase I.

Syndrome—a pattern of multiple anomalies thought to be pathogenically related.

Synteny (syntenic genes)—the property of occurring on the same chromosome. Groups of genes that occur together on the same chromosome in one species and are conserved in a similar grouping in another species are said to show "conservation of synteny."

TATA box—a conserved sequence 25–30 bp upstream from the start site of transcription in many, but not all, genes that is apparently involved in the initiation of transcription.

T cells—small lymphocytes committed by the influence of the thymus gland to be responsible for cell-mediated response to antigens.

Telomere—specialized protein-DNA structures containing long stretches of TTAGGG hexameric repeats at the ends of chromosomes.

Teratogen—a chemical or physical agent that produces or raises the incidence of congenital malformations.

Termination (or stop) codon—one of the three codons, UAG, UAA, or UGA, that causes termination of protein synthesis (also called a nonsense codon).

Thalassemias—disorders of hemoglobin in which the mutation has caused a quantitative abnormality, e.g., deficiency of α-globin, α-thalassemia; deficiency of β-globin, β-thalassemia.

Transcription—the synthesis of a single-stranded RNA molecule from a double-stranded DNA template in the cell nucleus, catalyzed by RNA polymerase.

Transfection—transfer of a specifically altered gene or segment of a gene into prokaryotic or eukaryotic cells.

Transfer RNA (tRNA)—in cooperation with the ribosomes, transfer RNAs bring amino acids into position along the messenger RNA template and are used to carry out the translation from mRNA sequence to protein sequence.

Transforming retrovirus—a retrovirus carrying an additional DNA sequence (often an oncogene) that confers the ability to transform infected cells to a malignant phenotype.

Transgenic—an experimentally produced plant or animal in which foreign DNA has been artificially introduced and stably incorporated into the germline. For mice, the term "transgenic" encompasses mice generated by standard pronuclear microinjection as well as knockout mice produced by embryonic stem cell techniques.

Translation—the process of synthesizing a polypeptide directed by the sequence of a specific mRNA.

Translocation—exchange of chromosomal material between two or more nonhomologous chromosomes; may be balanced or unbalanced.

Trisomy—the state of having an additional copy of a chromosome or three copies instead of the normal two.

Tumor suppressor gene—a normal cellular gene that, when homozygously deleted, can contribute to tumor development. Tumor suppressor genes generally operate in a recessive manner, requiring loss of both copies for tumorigenesis, in contrast to oncogenes, which can exert their effects in a dominant fashion.

Unequal crossing over—crossing over between similar DNA sequences on chromosomes that are misaligned, resulting in a deletion or duplication of nucleotides. Such unequal crossing over accounts for several variants of hemoglobin, e.g., α-thalassemia and Lepore hemoglobins. (See text for explanation.)

Uniparental disomy—the presence of two copies of a specific chromosome inherited from one parent, and no copies of that chromosome inherited from the other parent.

Variable expressivity—refers to the variable severity of a genetic trait. Individuals with the same mutant gene with pleiotropic effects frequently show variable expressivity as a result of either environmental effects or effects of other genes modifying the expression of the mutant gene.

Variable number tandem repeat (VNTR)—a class of DNA polymorphisms resulting from multiply repeated segments of DNA. VNTRs are sometimes referred to as minisatellites. VNTRs are similar in concept to SSRs, though with a longer, more complex repeated unit. Polymorphic VNTR markers are very useful for gene mapping, but have largely been replaced by SSRs.

Vector—the carrier of recombinant DNA or RNA material. In cloning, the vector is generally autonomously replicating DNA, such as a plasmid, phage, or YAC, into which a cloned DNA segment can be inserted. In gene therapy, the vector is used to efficiently introduce the recombinant DNA into a target cell.

Western blot—blotting technique, analogous to Southern blotting, for detecting proteins, usually by immunologic methods.

X-autosome translocation—reciprocal translocation between the X chromosome and one of the auto-somes.

X-chromosome inactivation—*see* lyonization.

X-linked disease—a disease encoded by a mutant gene on the X chromosome.

Yeast artificial chromosome (YAC)—a cloning vector, propagated in yeast, which can carry large inserts of DNA up to one megabase in length. YACs contain the control elements required for autonomous replication in yeast.

Zinc finger proteins—transcription-activator proteins containing fingerlike structures containing a zinc atom.

Zygote—the diploid cell resulting from the union of the haploid male and female gametes.

Study Questions and Answers

Chapter 1: Questions

*1. Discuss the relative contributions of heredity and environment in the following clinical cases:
   a. Mental retardation in a boy with phenylketonuria
   b. Squamous cell carcinoma of the cheek in an English farmer on a penal colony in Australia
   c. Intellectual regression in a child with Tay-Sachs disease
   d. Myocardial infarction in a 52-year-old male cigarette smoker
   e. Faintness and syncope in a middle-aged hypertensive patient 1 day after starting therapeutic doses of a new blood pressure medication

2. How can mutations in the same gene result in a number of different clinical disorders or in no disease at all?

Chapter 1: Answers

*1. All disease should be viewed as the result of an interaction (albeit sometimes complex) between heredity and environment.
   a. Phenylketonuria, a hereditary defect in the gene encoding phenylalanine hydroxylase, predisposes to severe mental retardation due to markedly elevated blood phenylalanine levels in infancy. This serious consequence can be avoided by dietary control of phenylalanine intake. Thus, two individuals with the same genetic make-up (i.e., deficiency of a particular enzyme) can have vastly different clinical outcomes depending on environmental factors.
   b. The incidence of skin cancer in sun-exposed areas due to excessive exposure to ultraviolet light from the sun is much higher among Caucasians than among black individuals, demonstrating how genetic differences (in this case, those relating to skin color) can lead to differing disease susceptibilities to a common environmental agent.
   c. In Tay-Sachs disease, clearly the overwhelming contribution to clinical disease is the genetic deficiency in hexosaminidase A with very little environmental contribution.
   d. Cigarette smoking is a known risk factor but hereditary components in blood lipids and family history of heart disease are also important contributing factors.
   e. Hereditary differences in drug metabolism are becoming increasingly recognized and should always be considered when a patient suffers an adverse reaction to medication. One such genetic difference is known in the cytochrome P-450 metabolizing system in the liver, which leads to marked differences in the rate at which certain drugs, including commonly used antihypertensive medications, are metabolized.

2. As is described in much more detail in Chapter 2 and Chapter 5, a gene contains a great deal of coding information. Not all mutations in a gene will completely destroy the function of that gene, and therefore, different mutations are capable of resulting in different effects. The human hemoglobin genes (Chapter 6) are a good example and have already been alluded to in this opening chapter. A mutation in the human β-globin gene is the cause of sickle cell anemia. However, different mutations in the human β-globin gene can lead to a hemoglobin with an unusual oxygen affinity, which gives rise to a different clinical problem. Many simple mutations in the human β-globin gene lead to no disease at all, because the protein product is still fully functional. A "knock-out" mutation of the gene, however, results in a different disorder called β-thalassemia, which is more thoroughly described in Chapter 6.

Chapter 2: Questions

1. Draw a schematic diagram of a methionine codon (ATG) in double-stranded DNA. Label the following structures:
    a. 5' ends
    b. 3' ends
    c. Phosphodiester backbones
    d. 2' carbons
    e. The "bases"
    f. The chemical bonds responsible for Chargaff's base-pairing rules

2. During normal spermatogenesis in man, spermatogonia serve both as self-renewing stem cells as well as a source of cells that can mature into primary spermatocytes. Primary spermatocytes enter meiosis, giving rise after meiosis I to secondary spermatocytes, which in turn give rise to spermatids following meiosis II. Spermatids mature into spermatozoa without further cell divisions. For each type of cell and cell cycle stage in the following table, provide the total number of DNA base pairs per cell, the number of chromosomes per cell, and the number of chromatids per cell. Designate the "ploidy" (haploid, diploid) for each.

	DNA (bp)	Chromosomes	Chromatids	Ploidy
Spermatogonia at G1				
Spermatogonia at G2				
Primary spermatocyte				
Secondary spermatocyte after meiosis I				
Spermatid after meiosis II				

3. During DNA replication (or RNA transcription), the appropriate nucleotide triphosphate is used to add a base to a preexisting DNA (or RNA) strand. To which end, 5' or 3', is the new nucleotide added? What determines which nucleotide, A, G, C, or T (U for RNA), is added? What would happen if a synthetic *3'-deoxy* nucleotide were added to a growing nucleic acid strand?

4. It is a truism that each of us is the beneficiary of genetic information inherited from both parents, four grandparents, eight great grandparents, etc. What is the chance that a child might carry information from only

two of his/her four grandparents? For example, what is the chance that a child would have no genetic information from his/her grandmothers and has information only from his/her grandfathers? (Assume that no crossing over occurs.) What would the sex of this child be?

5. The following sequence of amino acids represents part of a protein. What kind of mutation is most likely represented by each of the following amino acid sequences?

Normal   Glu-Cys-Met-Phe-Trp-Asp
Mutant A   Glu-Cys-Ile-Phe-Trp-Asp
Mutant B   Glu-Val-Cys-Ser-Gly-Thr
Mutant C   Glu-Cys-Met-Phe
Mutant D   Glu-Met-Tyr-Val-Leu-Gly

Chapter 2: Answers

1.

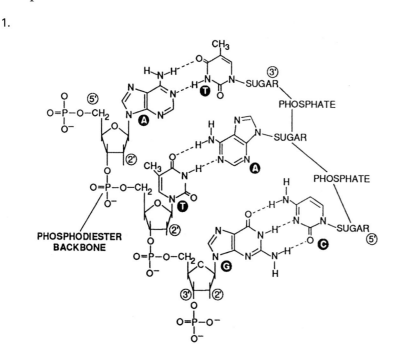

2.

	DNA (bp)	Chromosomes	Chromatids	Ploidy
Mitosis				
Spermatogonia at G1	6×10^9	46	46	Diploid
Spermatogonia at G2	12×10^9	46	92	Diploid
Meiosis				
Primary spermatocyte	12×10^9	46	92	Diploid
Secondary spermatocyte				
after meiosis I	6×10^9	23	46	Haploid
Spermatid after meiosis II	3×10^9	23	23	Haploid

3. Nucleotides are always added to the 3′ end. In DNA replication, the parental DNA strand is used as a template to direct the synthesis of the

new DNA strand using the base pairing rules (Fig. 2.4). In RNA transcription, the nonsense strand of the double helical DNA is used as a template to synthesize the growing RNA strand, again using base pairing rules (Fig. 2.6). For both DNA and RNA, a 3′ deoxynucleotide will block further extension of that strand, as the absence of a hydroxyl group in the 3′ position will prevent the next nucleotide from attaching.

4. One member of each of the 23 pairs of chromosomes in the child's father was inherited from the child's paternal grandfather; with independent assortment, there is $(1/2)^{23}$ that these 23 paternal grandfather's chromosomes all segregate into the same gamete and are passed on to the child. Likewise for the mother's father's chromosomes. Thus, there is $(1/2)^{46}$ or 1.4×10^{-14} chance that the child would inherit only his maternal and paternal grandfathers' chromosomes. The child would be a male because he would have received his paternal grandfather's Y chromosome.

5.

Mutant A.	Missense [ATG (Met) → ATT, ATC, or ATA (all give Ile)]
Mutant B.	Frameshift (deletion of first T in cysteine codon (TGT)—note that resulting amino acid sequence reveals exactly which codon was used for normal sequence)
Mutant C.	Nonsense [TGG (Trp) → TGA or TAG (STOP)]
Mutant D.	Frameshift [insert A after the first, second, or third nucleotide of the first codon (Glu, GAA, or GAG)]

Chapter 3: Questions

1. Both X-linked dominant and autosomal dominant traits are inherited vertically in families. What are four characteristics you might look for that would help you distinguish between X-linked dominant and autosomal dominant inheritance in a set of families all showing the same vertically inherited trait?

2. Choose the term from the following list that best describes the situations labeled a through f below:

   i.   Allelic heterogeneity
   ii. Pleiotropy
   iii. Variable expressivity
   iv. Anticipation
   v.   Consanguinity
   vi. Locus heterogeneity

   a. A 65-year-old man shows no signs of myotonic dystrophy save cataracts, but his 25-year-old daughter has significant muscle weakness and wasting, and has recently had a baby girl with severe muscle weakness and developmental delay.
   b. Variegate porphyria, an autosomal dominant inborn error of porphyrin biosynthesis, can cause blistering skin photosensitivity, abdominal pain, peripheral neuropathy, and psychotic episodes.
   c. A man with severe scoliosis and hundreds of subcutaneous neurofibromata has a sister with a disfiguring plexiform neurofibroma, and a 30-year-old son with a few Lisch nodules and axillary freckles.

    d. A rare form of autosomal recessive growth hormone deficiency occurs only in certain small isolated villages in the Swiss Alps.

    e. A nonsense mutation and a deletion in the ornithine transcarbamylase (OTC) gene both cause lethal neonatal hyperammonemia due to absence of OTC, an important hepatic enzyme in the urea cycle.

    f. Retinitis pigmentosa, a form of retinal degeneration, occurs in autosomal and X-linked forms.

3. True/False:

    a. For a disease to be considered a genetic lethal, it must cause the patient to die before he/she reaches puberty.

    b. When an individual inherits a disease-causing mutant gene from a parent, the gene is present in utero and therefore is present at birth; therefore, all hereditary disease is congenital.

    c. Whenever an autosomal dominant disease occurs in a child born to two unaffected parents, the disease is the result of a new mutation.

    d. It is unlikely that a patient has a genetic disorder if he/she is the only one in the family with the disease.

4. A woman has cystic fibrosis. She is the only person in the family with this disease. What is the carrier risk for her mother, her father, her daughter, her daughter's son, her brother, her brother's child?

5. A woman is a carrier of hemophilia, an X-linked disorder. What is her chance of having a son? Call this probability P1. What is her chance of having an affected child? Call this probability P2. What is her chance of having a child who is both male *and* affected? Is it P1 times P2? Why or why not?

*6. A hematologist has collected data on 25 unrelated children with sickle cell anemia and their siblings. Of a total of 165 children in these 25 families, a total of 60 have sickle cell anemia. Because sickle cell anemia is an autosomal recessive disorder, the hematologist expected 25%, or 41 of the 165 children, to have the disease, and is puzzled that there seem to be too many affected children in the families. Can you help her out?

Chapter 3: Answers

1.

    a. In X-linked dominant (XLD), there is no male-to-male transmission, whereas a male affected with an autosomal dominant (AD) would pass the trait to, on average, half his sons.

    b. In XLD, all daughters of an affected male would inherit the trait while, in AD, only 50% on average would.

    c. When many families with the disorder are studied, twice as many affected females will be present as affected males, because females have two X chromosomes and therefore have twice the chance of having a disease allele on one of their two X chromosomes. In AD disorders, the ratio of affected females to males in a large set of families is 1:1.

    d. Females with XLD tend to have a milder form of the disease than do males with XLD who only have one X chromosome.

2.
  a. Anticipation
  b. Pleiotropy
  c. Variable expressivity
  d. Consanguinity
  e. Allelic heterogeneity
  f. Locus heterogeneity

3.
  a. False. A genetic lethal is defined by the fact that it prohibits reproduction, which may or may not reflect a shortened life span.
  b. False. Congenital refers to whether or not the *phenotype* is apparent at birth.
  c. False. One of the parents may have carried the gene but may have been nonpenetrant, or a different biological father may have been involved.
  d. False. This situation is more the rule than the exception for autosomal recessive disorders (Fig. 3.15) and may also occur for other forms of inheritance.

4.
  Mother: 100%
  Father: 100%
  Daughter: 100% (assuming her husband is not a carrier)
  Daughter's son: 50%
  Her (unaffected) brother: 67% (Being the unaffected child of two carrier parents, he has 1/3 chance of being homozygous normal and 2/3 chance of being a carrier.)
  Her brother's child: 33%

5. Her chance of having a son is 50%. Her chance of having an affected child is 25%. Her chance of having an affected son is 25% which is **not** the product because these two events are not independent.

*6. She has been led astray by ascertainment bias. Because all the families were originally identified as having at least one patient with sickle cell anemia, this is not a random sample of all families in which the parents are carriers, since those families with two carrier parents and no affected children are missed. There are a number of ways to correct for this ascertainment bias. One simple way is simply to subtract out all the patients that were used to ascertain the families in the first place. Thus, the corrected estimate would be 60 − 25 = 35 affected out of a total of 165 − 25 = 140, which agrees with the expected 25%.

Chapter 4: Questions

1. Two large tribes of equal size live on separate neighboring islands but are unaware of each other's existence. In tribe 1, the incidence of one form of autosomal recessive albinism is 1 in 10,000 whereas in tribe 2 the same disease is 100 times more common. Volcanic activity suddenly produces a land bridge and the two tribes quickly find each other and begin to mix and mate freely. (Assume no selective disadvantage to this form of albinism). Answer the following questions:

a. What were the allele frequencies for the normal and albinism alleles in each tribe prior to the appearance of the land bridge?

b. What were the allele frequencies for the normal and albinism alleles in the two tribes taken as a whole immediately after the tribes mixed? What was the frequency of the disease at that time?

c. What were the allele frequencies and disease frequency in the mixed tribe after one generation?

2. In a population study, 5000 individuals were typed for the MN locus, an autosomal codominant trait. There were 2400 MM individuals, 2400 MN individuals, and 200 NN individuals. What are the allele frequencies for M and N alleles? Is this population in Hardy-Weinberg equilibrium?

3. A Finnish woman is the mother of a child with Meckel syndrome (a rare autosomal recessive disorder occurring in 1/9000 births in her part of Finland). She is widowed and is now going to remarry. What is the risk of the disease in a pregnancy in her new marriage if her new husband is

a. an unrelated Finnish man from her geographic area?

b. her former husband's brother?

c. her own first cousin?

*4. Gyrate atrophy of the retina is an autosomal recessive retinal disease with onset in late childhood and adolescence. Suppose the disease occurs with a frequency of 1 in 324 individuals in a particular population. Nine couples with normal vision from this population split off and form a new genetic isolate by moving to a remote area to begin homesteading. What is the probability that the new isolate will not have the gene for gyrate atrophy in its gene pool? What is the chance that the gene will be about as common in the isolate as in the original population? More common?

5. Every occurrence of a genetic lethal autosomal dominant disorder is a new mutation. Why?

6. In the table below are shown concordance rates for three different disorders in monozygotic twins, dizygotic twins, and siblings. Comment on the probable roles played by heredity and environment for each disorder. If heredity plays a major role in any of these disorders, can you form any hypotheses concerning the number of loci involved?

| Disorder | Concordance | | |
	Monozygotic	Dizygotic	Siblings
	%	%	%
A	100	25	25
B	50	6	6
C	10	10	0.1

*7. A particular clinical syndrome can be inherited either as an autosomal recessive trait or as a completely nonhereditary phenocopy with no known environmental cause. If the phenocopy form of the syndrome accounts for 80% of all cases of the disease, what would you expect the recurrence risk to be for a couple with one child with the disorder?

8. The risk of developing ankylosing spondylitis, a chronic inflammatory arthritis, is 90 times higher in individuals who carry the B27 allele at the HLA-B locus than it is in the general population. Does this mean that the gene for ankylosing spondylitis is closely linked to the HLA-B locus?

9. Apply the correct descriptive term to each of the following observations concerning studies of HLA in a hereditary disease:

   Linkage
   Association
   Linkage disequilibrium

   a. A particular allele at the HLA B locus is found in 75% of individuals with a hereditary disease and 4% of normal controls.
   b. In families with multiple siblings with the disease, affected individuals often inherit the same alleles from their parents while unaffected individuals often have the other parental alleles in common.
   c. In a disease known to be linked to HLA, two particular alleles at the HLA A and B loci are found 15 times more frequently in individuals affected with the disease than in matched controls.

Chapter 4: Answers

1.
   a. In tribe 1, the albinism allele has a frequency of $\sqrt{(1/10,000)} = 0.01$. In tribe 2, the allele has a frequency of $\sqrt{(1/100)} = 0.1$ (assuming the tribes are in Hardy-Weinberg equilibrium prior to the appearance of the land bridge).
   b. The allele frequency is the simple average since the two tribes are of equal size. Allele frequency $= 1/2(0.01 + 0.1) = 0.055$
      The frequency of the disease is also the average $= 1/2(1/10,000 + 1/100) = 0.00505$
   c. Normal allele frequency $= 1 - 0.055 = 0.945$
      Albinism allele frequency $= 0.055$
      Disease frequency $= (0.055)^2 = 0.003$ (assuming random mating within and between the newly mixed tribes)

2. The 5,000 individuals represent 10,000 alleles as shown in the table:

		M Alleles	N Alleles
MM individuals		4,800	0
MN individuals		2,400	2,400
NN individuals		0	400
	Total	7,200	2,800

Thus, the frequency of the M allele is 7,200/10,000 = 0.72 and of the N allele 2,800/10,000 = 0.28. If the population were at Hardy-Weinberg equilibrium, one would predict $(0.72)^2 \times 5,000 = 2,592$ MM individuals, $2(0.72)(0.28)(5,000) = 2,016$ MN individuals and $(0.28)^2(5,000) = 392$ NN individuals, which is quite different than the observation.

3. By definition, the Finnish woman is a carrier for Meckel syndrome and in the general population of her part of Finland, $q = \sqrt{1/9,000} \cong 0.0105$.

a. The unrelated new husband would have a risk of carrying the Meckel syndrome gene of 2pq, or 2(0.9895)(0.0105) = 0.0209. Even if both parents are carriers, the risk that a subsequent child will be affected is 1/4, so the total risk is 0.0209 × 1/4 = 0.0052, or 0.52%.

b. Her former husband must also be a carrier for Meckel syndrome, which he must have inherited from one of his parents. His brother, therefore, has a 1/2 risk of carrying the same gene. In this situation, the risk of an affected child is 1/2 × 1 × 1/4 = 1/8.

c. These questions are best answered by drawing a hypothetical pedigree and calculating the risk that an individual carries the gene through a loop of the family until reaching the person of interest. This leads to a calculation that the woman's first cousin has a 1/8 chance of carrying the same gene, so the risk of an affected child is 1/8 × 1 × 1/4 = 1/32.

*4. Allele frequency for gyrate atrophy in this population = $\sqrt{(1/324)}$ = 1/18. Use the binomial distribution for these calculations. Among the nine couples with normal vision, there are 18 people, or 36 alleles. Think of sampling 36 alleles from a population in which 1/18 of the alleles are mutant alleles for gyrate atrophy and 17/18 are normal. For each allele, there is a 17/18 chance that it will be normal. For all 36 alleles, the probability that a random sample contains only normal alleles is given by $(17/18)^{36}$ = 13%. Probability that only one of the 36 alleles is the mutant allele is given by 36 × $(17/18)^{35}(1/18)$ = 27%. (The 36 in front is due to the fact that any one of the 36 alleles could be the mutant one.) The probability that two of the 36 alleles are mutant alleles is given by $[36!/(2!34!)](17/18)^{34}(1/18)^2$ = 28%, where the term in front (=630) gives the number of different ways that 2 of 36 could be the mutant alleles (alleles 1 and 2, 1 and 3, 1 and 4,..., 2 and 3, 2 and 4, ...).

(This is not quite the right result because we are not correcting for the small chance that both mutant alleles are in the same individual, which we said is not the case because all 18 homesteaders had normal vision. The more correct term would be 630 − 18 = 612 because we will not allow both mutant alleles to be in the same individual, which can happen in any one of 18 ways). Thus, the chance the new isolate will not have the gene at all = 13%. The chance that it will be as frequent = the chance that 2/36 are mutant =28%. The chance the mutant allele will be more frequent = 1 − (13% + 27% + 28%) = 32%. This demonstrates how allele frequencies, even for deleterious genes, can be higher than expected through random events operating on small populations (genetic drift) of which this is one particular example, known as the founder effect.

5. Because an autosomal dominant genetic lethal disorder, by definition, cannot be inherited (otherwise it would not be a genetic lethal), every time it occurs, it must have arisen through new mutation.
(Although the preceding statement is generally true, there is one important exception: An individual can inherit a genetic lethal autosomal dominant disorder from a parent who is a gonadal mosaic for the disease-producing mutation. In this way, the parent can reproduce and pass the mutation on to more than one child and yet have the disease be a genetic lethal.)

6. In disorder A, the very high rate or concordance in monozygotic twins suggests an overwhelming, nearly exclusive, contribution of heredity to the etiology of the disorder. The fact that dizygotic twins and siblings have the same concordance, at about one-fourth that of monozygotic twins, suggests the disorder is inherited as an autosomal recessive trait at one locus.

In disorder B, the high rate of concordance in monozygotic twins when compared to dizygotic twins suggests a significant hereditary component, although the lack of complete concordance in the monozygotic twins suggests a significant environmental contribution. The ratio of concordance in monozygotic versus dizygotic twins of ~8 suggests that alleles at two unlinked loci contribute to the disease.

In disorder C, the low concordance in monozygotic twins suggests a strong environmental component. The fact that all twins seem to have the same concordance, but siblings significantly less than dizygotic twins, suggests that hereditary components may be very minimal and that intrauterine environment may be a much more important contributory factor.

*7. The couple's risk of recurrence would be 25% if the disorder was always autosomal recessive. If the chance of that inheritance pattern is only 20%, however, one might then quote a recurrence risk of $0.2 \times 0.25 = 0.05$. In reality, however, additional information about the family might be useful in coming up with the most accurate prediction. For instance, if this couple has previously had 10 normal children, the chance of the autosomal recessive pattern of inheritance is considerably decreased, and the chance of the phenocopy goes up.

8. No. The correlated occurrence of the B27 allele with ankylosing spondylitis is an *association*. Establishing that the gene responsibile for ankylosing spondylitis is *linked* to the HLA-B locus would require demonstrating the co-segregation, in families, of alleles at the B27 locus with the disease. In linkage studies, the specific allele co-segregating with the disease only serves as a marker of the locus; the specific allele will be different in different families. In contrast, association studies depend on the simultaneous occurrence of a specific allele at a given locus in all or a large proportion of individuals affected with the disease.

9.
   a. Association
   b. Linkage
   c. Linkage disequilibrium

Chapter 5: Questions

1. A gene for an enzyme is made up of three exons. Shown below is the sequence of the DNA of the sense strand for the first two exons (*capital letters*) as well as some of the sequence (*lower case letters*) around these exons.

. . . accggcagtagATATCAGACCATGCTAATCGCTCCCCGACAGgtaagttgca . . .

atgaacgcaatatccttcctctcgacagGGGTAGTTT . . .

a. How many bases are in the first exon? How many amino acids in the enzyme are encoded by this exon? Write them down. (Hint: Where does translation of this exon start?)

b. Where will the 7-methylguanosine cap be placed in the mRNA made from this gene?

c. What is the effect on expression of this gene if base number 14 in the first exon were changed from C to T?

d. Where is the stop codon?

e. What is the effect on expression of changing base number 26 in the first exon from C to T?

f. Write a "D" and arrow pointing to the splice donor site(s) and an "A" and arrow pointing to the splice acceptor site(s).

*2. You have identified an enzymatic activity in cell extracts that catalyzes the conversion of metabolite A to product B. Outline three different strategies you could use to isolate a cDNA representing the mRNA that encodes all or part of the protein for this enzyme.

3. Shown below is a Southern blot of human DNA cut with three different restriction enzymes. Each *lane* is labeled B, E, or H representing DNA digested with *Bam* HI, *Eco* RI, and *Hind*III, respectively, alone or with two of the enzymes in a double digestion. The probe is a 2.3-kb *Hind*III fragment of human genomic DNA. Draw the two possible maps of the restriction endonuclease sites in and around the probe sequence.

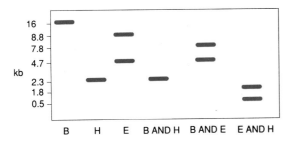

*4.

a. Describe at least three methods you might use to efficiently screen a large gene (100 kb, 15 exons, 6 kb total coding sequence) for point mutations.

b. What types of defects would you miss?

c. How would your approach differ for a small gene (1 kb, 2 exons, 500 bp coding sequence)?

d. If the same single point mutation were identified in a large subset of patients, how would you screen multiple DNA samples for the presence or absence of this particular mutation?

5. You have just identified a C→T substitution in exon 26 of the factor VIII gene in a patient with hemophilia A.
   a. Is this the defect responsible for hemophilia A in this patient? How else could you explain this nucleotide change?
   b. If this substitution alters an amino acid (a CGC codon→TGC, resulting in an Arg→Cys substitution), would this change your answer to a?
   c. How could you prove that this is an authentic hemophilia A mutation?

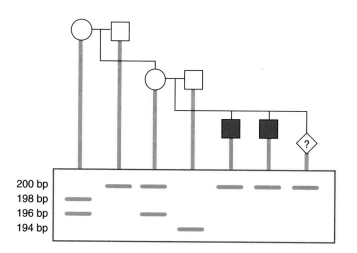

6. The filled squares in the above pedigree represent individuals with severe hemophilia A. Open symbols are unaffected. DNA from each individual has been amplified by PCR for a segment within an intron of the FVIII gene and the PCR products separated on the gel shown below the pedigree.
   a. What is the origin for the different sized DNA fragments seen in the gel?
   b. Can you conclude anything about the origin of the mutation in this family?
   c. What is the sex of the fetus (the diamond)?
   d. Is the fetus affected with hemophilia A?

Chapter 5: Answers

1.
   a. 31 bases in the first exon. Seven amino acids are encoded: ATG methionine, CTA leucine, ATC isoleucine, GCT alanine, CCC proline, CGA arginine, and CAG glutamine.
   b. On the 5′ end of the first base in the primary RNA transcript. One can infer from the information given above that the RNA polymerase initiated transcription at the first capital letter A. This is where the cap would be placed.
   c. TTA still encodes leucine, so this is a silent base change, with no effect on gene expression.
   d. TAG (bases 4–6 in exon 2)

e. This changes arginine to a premature stop codon, resulting in truncation of the protein when it is translated. This would be very deleterious to gene expression.

f.
$$D$$
$$\downarrow$$
. . . accggcagtagATATCAGACCATGCTAATCGCTCCCCGACAGgtaagttgca . . .

atgaacgcaatatccttcctctcgacagGGGTAGTTT . . .
$$\nwarrow$$
$$A$$

*2.

a. Purify the enzyme, obtain amino acid sequence, infer which nucleic
acid sequences would encode these amino acids, and use a set of
chemically synthesized pieces of DNA corresponding to these sequences to probe a cDNA library.

b. Purify the enzyme, use it as an antigen to raise a specific antibody
for the protein, and screen a cDNA library cloned in such a way that
cDNA sequences in the library are expressed in the bacteria carrying the cloning vector. Use the antibody to screen the library for
production of antigen recognized by the antibody.

c. Make a cDNA library in a system that allows expression of the
cloned cDNAs in cultured cells. Introduce clones from the library
into cultured cells that lack the enzymatic activity and test them for
expression of the enzymatic activity.

3.

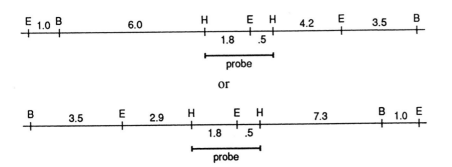

*4.

a. It is generally not practical to screen the entire sequence of a large
gene like this. Thus, one should concentrate on the coding regions
and the immediately adjacent splice signals. Multiple small segments of the gene containing each of the exons and exon/intron
junctions could be amplified by PCR and screened by one of a number of methods, including denaturing gradient gel electrophoresis
(DGGE), single-strand conformational polymorphism (SSCP) analysis, or mismatch cleavage methods (see Figure 5.26). As an alternative approach, if cells expressing the gene of interest can be readily obtained, for example if the gene is expressed in blood cells,
then the mature mRNA sequence could be amplified by PCR and
analyzed by any of the above screening methods, or even by direct
DNA sequence analysis.

b. Chemical mismatch cleavage methods can detect nearly 100% of mutations. DGGE is considerably less efficient, though using a heteroduplex procedure nearly all mutations may be detected in some systems. SSCP is probably the easiest of these methods, but will miss 20% or more of mutations. Since only the exons and exon/intron junctions of this large gene are being screened, mutations within the introns, potentially affecting splicing or other aspects of RNA processing, would be missed. Also mutations in the promoter or other transcriptional regulatory signals would also not be detected.

c. For a very small gene (similar in size to β-globin) direct sequence analysis of genomic DNA would be the most straightforward approach and should pick up nearly all mutations.

d. If the single base change results in the loss or gain of a restriction enzyme recognition site, then screening can be easily accomplished by PCR followed by restriction enzyme digestion and gel analysis. If no restriction site is changed, then allele specific oligonucleotide hybridization (ASO) can be performed to distinguish mutant and normal alleles. Note that ASO can be applied to any mutation, including those that change restriction sites. A number of other rapid and efficient screening methods are also available. Like ASO, most of these approaches rely on sensitive hybridization conditions that can distinguish even a single base difference.

5.

a. Though this certainly could be the defect responsible for hemophilia A, the single nucleotide change could also represent a silent DNA sequence variation that does not alter the amino acid sequence.

b. The fact that this single nucleotide change alters an amino acid certainly strengthens the evidence that it might be the defect in this patient. It is also worth noting that this is a nonconservative amino acid substitution. Also, note that this is a C->T transition at a CpG dinucleotide, a hot spot for mutation in the human genome. However, this could still represent a neutral amino acid variation that does not affect FVIII function.

c. The most straightforward (and perhaps most definitive) way to prove that this nucleotide change represents the disease-causing mutation in this patient is to express the mutant protein by transfection of tissue culture cells and to assay the recombinant factor VIII for function. If the single nucleotide change results in loss of function, this would prove the identity of this mutation as the defect in the patient. Genetic evidence could also provide support. For example, identification of the same mutation in two or more unrelated hemophilia patients, along with failure to observe it in a large panel of normal subjects, would strongly suggest that this is an authentic mutation.

6.

a. Four different-sized bands are seen, separated by units of 2 bp in length. This is a simple sequence repeat (SSR) polymorphism, within the intron, with a dinucleotide repeat unit.

b. The two affected boys each inherited a 200 bp allele from the mother who is heterozygous 200/196. The mother in turn must have inherited her 200 bp allele from her father and the 196 bp allele from her mother. Since the grandfather did not have hemophilia A, the hemophila A mutation associated with the 200 bp allele in the 2 hemophiliac boys must represent a new mutation. (As discussed in Chapter 7, approximately 1/3 of hemophilia cases represent new mutations). This mutation most likely arose in the grandpaternal meiosis, a common scenario for the recurrent FVIII gene inversion that accounts for ~1/2 of severe hemophilia A patients.

c. The fetus is a male, since it has only inherited one X chromosome (200 bp allele). A female fetus should also have inherited the father's X (194 bp allele).

d. The fetus is affected with hemophilia A, since it has inherited the 200 bp maternal FVIII allele, the same allele present in the two affected sons. (There is a very small chance that this DNA diagnosis could be incorrect as a result of germinal mosaicism in the mother or an intragenic recombination between the polymorphic SSR marker and the FVIII gene mutation. These possibilities are discussed in Chapters 7 and 9.)

Chapter 6: Questions

1. Which of the following strategies would *not* be beneficial to a patient with β-thalassemia major?
   a. Transfusion and iron chelation therapy
   b. Increasing α-globin production
   c. Increasing β-globin production
   d. Increasing fetal hemoglobin production
   e. Decreasing α-globin production

2. A polymerase chain reaction (PCR, Chapter 5) test has been developed to detect sickle cell anemia. The sickle mutation alters codon 6 of the β-globin gene from GAG to GTG, eliminating an *Mst*II site that is normally present there. The primers used for the PCR are shown below:

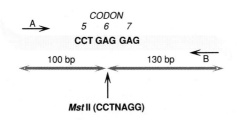

   a. What are the expected sizes of PCR products for AA (homozygous normal), AS (heterozygous "sickle trait"), and SS (homozygous affected) individuals after *Mst*II digestion?
   b. What would be the expected result for an individual homozygous for hemoglobin C (codon 6 AAG) and for an individual homozy-

gous for codon 6 frameshift β-thalassemia (one base deletion of codon 6)?

*3. You are investigating a patient with thalassemia major. On taking a family history, you are surprised to find that, although the mother is from Greece where thalassemia is common, the father and all of his known ancestors are from Russia.
   a. What are some possible explanations?
   b. You perform paternity testing on the father and find that it is very likely (>99%) that he is, in fact, the biological father of the child. However, his blood shows absolutely no evidence that he has thal trait (thal minor). How could this be explained?
   c. What is the chance that this couple's next child will have thal major? Thal minor?
   d. Intrigued by this situation, you decide to clone the β-globin genes from this patient. You obtain two clones. By sequencing, one has a nonsense mutation at codon 39, a common defect in Mediterranean populations. This mutation creates a restriction site for the enzyme MaeI, which recognizes the sequence CTAG:

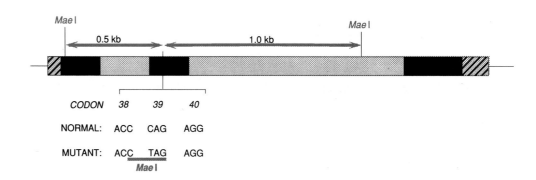

Using Southern blotting, how can you determine whether this is the mutant gene inherited from the mother? Be specific about how you set up the test. Assume you have available DNA on the mother, the father, the affected child, and any cloned DNA fragments you want from the β-globin gene. How would you do the test using PCR?
   e. The other clone does not have this same mutation. Suspecting it may harbor a heretofore undescribed mutation, and with visions of fame in your head, you sequence the clone. The entire β-globin gene is normal except for one nucleotide change at the end of the second intron:

> intron 2   exon 3
> Normal—cctcttatcttcctcccacag|CTCCTGGG
> Mutant —cctcttatcttcctcccac[t]g|CTCCTGGG

How would this cause thalassemia?
Would you expect this to be a β^0-thal or β^+-thal allele?

4. You are counseling a Greek couple because both parties have been found to be carriers of β-thalassemia in a population survey. They have

one son who tests normal (not a carrier). They wish to know whether a current pregnancy is affected. You obtain fetal DNA by amniocentesis. Using a probe 10-kb 5′ to the β gene, which detects a *Hin*cll RFLP, you obtain the following blot:

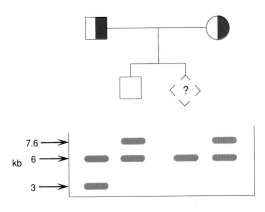

Is the fetus affected?

5. A fetus affected with severe α-thalassemia develops profound anemia and associated complications in utero (hydrops fetalis). In contrast, the anemia of severe β-thalassemia does not generally become clinically apparent until at least several months after birth. Why are the ages of onset for these two related disorders so different?

Chapter 6: Answers

1. B. Increasing α-globin production would further worsen the α/β imbalance.

2. Using primers A and B, the following would be expected:

Genotype	Mst II Digested PCR Products
AA	100, 130
AS	100, 130, 230
SS	230
CC	100, 130
Δcodon 6/Δcodon 6	230

*3.
a. Possible explanations include a low frequency Russian β-thal allele, incorrect paternity, or new mutation.
b. This suggests the paternal β-globin gene acquired a new mutation in being passed to the child.
c. It is *unlikely* that the next child will have thal major, unless the father is a germline mosaic for the β-thal mutation (see Chapter 3). Because the mother likely has thal minor, the next child's chance of also having thal minor is 50%.
d. To test by Southern blot, you would want to digest DNA from the child and both parents with *Mae*l, electrophorese, and transfer to a filter. The blot should then be probed with a β-globin sequence such as exon 2. Individuals heterozygous for the codon 39 mutation

will have 0.5, 1.0, and 1.5 kb bands, whereas individuals lacking the codon 39 mutation will have only the 1.5 kb band.

The same test can be done with PCR by designing primers on either side of codon 39, amplifying, digesting with *MaeI*, and analyzing the size of the digested products on a gel.

e. The mutation abolishes the normal splice acceptor at the end of intron 2. Because the AG in this position (now changed to TG) is absolutely required for normal splicing, this would probably be a β^0-thal allele.

4. The key to this sort of problem is to identify the allele marking the β-thal chromosome in each parent. The normal son must have inherited the *normal* chromosome from *each* parent; therefore, the 3 kb allele of the father and the 6 kb allele of the mother are on their respective β-thal chromosomes. The fetus has inherited a normal allele from the father and a β-thal from the mother; therefore, the fetus will *not* be affected (but will be a carrier).

5. The contrasting times for the onset of symptomatology in α-thalassemia and β-thalassemia are readily explained by the developmental pattern of hemoglobin gene expression (see Figure 6.2). The switch from expression of the embryonic ζ gene to the adult α globin gene occurs very early in embryonic development. The absence of the α globin genes in severe α thalassemia results in failure to assemble hemoglobin F $(_{22})$. In contrast, the switch from expression of the fetal γ to β globin gene begins just before birth and is not complete until several months of age. The absence of the β globin genes does not produce clinical problems until this later period, as fetal hemoglobin begins to disappear.

Chapter 7: Questions

1. Why would a mutation affecting stability of an enzyme expressed in both red and white blood cells be more likely to cause a detectable phenotype in red blood cells than in white blood cells?

2. Suppose an enzyme were a tetramer consisting of four identical peptides encoded on an autosome. What would you predict to be the impact of the following mutations on the function of this enzyme in an individual *heterozygous* for each mutation?

   a. Nonsense mutation in the first exon, resulting in premature termination of translation
   b. Missense mutation in the first exon, resulting in a subunit that can participate in tetramer formation but, if present in the tetramer, destroys the active site.

   If less than 10% of normal activity of this enzyme is sufficient to cause disease, what would you expect to be the inheritance pattern or patterns of disease caused by the two mutations described above?

3. G6PD A⁻ has two base changes when compared to the wild-type gene: A → G at nucleotide 376 and G → A at nucleotide 202. The enzyme has

an altered mobility and decreased stability. How might you determine experimentally which alteration or combination of alterations is responsible for the altered mobility and decreased stability?

4. Using the data in Table 7.1, calculate the allele frequencies for Pi^Z and Pi^S. What fraction of the population will be Pi^{MS}?

5. What two therapeutic interventions have been shown to be effective in lowering blood cholesterol in heterozygotes for LDL-receptor defects?

6. Approximately 1/3 of point mutations in the Factor VIII gene causing hemophilia A, approximatley 1/3 of point mutations in the Factor IX gene causing hemophilia B, and the majority of missense mutations causing G6PD deficiency involve a C→T change where the C residue is in a CpG dinucleotide. What fraction of dinucleotides would theoretically be expected to be CpGs? Why might these dinucleotides be mutational "hot spots" in the human genome?

Chapter 7: Answers

1. Red blood cells lack nuclei and depend on the transcription and translation occurring during cell differentiation for their proteins. An unstable protein cannot be replaced. In a white blood cell, additional protein can be made; therefore, the overall activity may be maintained at a level that allows normal function. Furthermore, red blood cells have a long life (120 days), whereas many white cells survive only a few days.

2.
   a. He would make only half the normal amount of the subunit; what subunit he did make would form normal functioning tetramers and you would expect him to have approximately half normal levels of the enzyme. Depending on the clinical situation, this level of enzyme could easily be sufficient to prevent any clinical disorder from occurring.
   b. Half of the subunits have this mutation. The only way to have a functioning enzyme is if all four of the subunits in the enzyme are normal. The probability of this happening is $(1/2)^4 = 0.06$. Thus, he would have only 6% of the normal levels of enzyme activity. This low level is likely not to be sufficient to allow normal function.
       The nonsense mutation is likely to cause a trait that is inherited as an autosomal recessive while the missense mutation described above will probably result in a trait inherited as an autosomal dominant.

3. A very simple step would be to look at the amino acid changes induced by these two nucleotide alterations, because a change that results in a charge difference is more likely to result in altered mobility than one that does not. Stability, however, is more difficult to predict. The most convincing way to answer the question would be to clone the wild-type and A⁻cDNAs (see Chapter 5). One could then construct hybrid molecules that have one or the other, but not both, of the mutations found in the A⁻ form. Expression of those hybrid forms in eukaryotic cells, which could be accomplished by putting the cDNA into an "expression vector" and transfecting it into any one of the large variety of possible

tissue culture cell lines, would allow analysis of the protein product, both for stability and mobility.

4. From Hardy-Weinberg considerations, the frequency of Pi^Z is $\sqrt{1/2500}$ = 0.02; the frequency of the Pi^S allele is $\sqrt{1/1000}$ = 0.032. The frequency of the M allele is everything else, namely 1−0.02−0.032 = 0.95. Individuals with Pi^{MS} genotype will occur at a frequency of 2(0.95)(0.032) = 0.06.

5. The most effective therapy for hypercholesterolemia is the inhibition of endogenous cholesterol biosynthesis by drugs known as statins, which are competitive inhibitors of HMG-CoA reductase. Bile acid sequestration is also moderately effective in lowering cholesterol levels.

6. By random chance only 1/16 of dinucleotides should be CpG. In fact, CpG dinucleotides occur far less frequently in coding regions of genes, perhaps because such mutational "hot spots" are selected against. Clusters of CpG dinucleotides ("CpG islands") are found in the 5'-upstream regions of many genes, however. CpG dinucleotides are thought to represent mutational "hot spots" because the cytosine is often methylated, and 5-methylcytosine can undergo spontaneous deamination to thymidine resulting in a C → T transition.

Chapter 8: Questions

1. What is the difference between metacentric, submetacentric, and acrocentric chromosomes? What special structures and sequences are present in acrocentric chromosomes?

2. Which of the following individuals have aneuploid karyotypes?
   a. A female with a balanced translocation involving 11q and 22q
   b. A female with trisomy 21 Down syndrome
   c. A female with a balanced Robertsonian translocation involving chromosomes 13 and 21
   What kinds of gametes can each of the individuals in a, b, and c above produce? List the chromosomal makeup of the fertilized eggs when each of these types of gametes is fertilized by a normal sperm.

3. Why hasn't every human chromosome been found involved in chromosomal trisomy in newborns? Why might the types and frequencies of various chromosomal abnormalities seen in chorionic villus samples obtained at 9–10 weeks gestation be different from those seen in live newborns?

4. A family with a child with Down syndrome due to trisomy 21 is studied for RFLPs on chromosome 21. One such RFLP has alleles of 7, 6, 5, or 4 kb. Shown on the left is a diagram of a Southern blot for the child, her father, and her mother. Can you tell in which parent the nondisjunction event occurred? Can you tell in which stage of meiosis it occurred?

5. What kind of gonad and what internal and external genitalia would you expect in the following individuals?

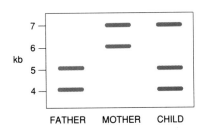

FATHER   MOTHER   CHILD

a. A 46,XY individual with a complete deletion of the SRY gene
b. A 46,XY individual homozygous for deficiency of an enzyme required for androgen biosynthesis
c. A 46,XY individual hemizygous for deficiency of the androgen receptor

6. Hemophilia A due to mutation of the X-linked gene for clotting Factor VIII is often thought of as a disease that affects males exclusively. However, there can be females with serious bleeding abnormalities due to hemophilia A. Describe four mechanisms by which females can have this disease.

7. If an individual is a mosaic for a chromosome aneuploidy, what likely inference can you make about when the event causing the mosaicism occurred?

8. Routine chromosome analysis on a child with multiple birth defects reveals an unbalanced chromosome translocation. To determine the exact chromosomes involved in this translocation fluorescence in situ hybridation (FISH) is performed. Which of the following classes of FISH probes would be most useful for this analysis: locus-specific probes, centromeric probes, or whole chromosome probes?

9. Why is it important to obtain a karyotype in a child in whom a clinical diagnosis of Down syndrome is completely obvious?

10. Why is it important to obtain a karyotype in a child in whom a clinical diagnosis of Turner syndrome is completely obvious? Will a buccal smear for Barr body count suffice?

*11. Compare the pathogenic mechanisms involved in the following diseases, all caused by triple repeat expansions: fragile X syndrome, Huntington disease, and myotonic dystrophy.

12. Choose the term from the following list that best describes the situations labeled a–c below.
    i.   Premutation
    ii. Genomic imprinting
    iii Uniparental disomy

a. A 7-year-old boy with Prader-Willi syndrome, characterized by moderate mental retardation, short stature, small hands and feet, and marked hyperphagia, is found upon molecular cytogenetic analysis to have two copies of the maternally-derived chromosome 15, and no copy of the paternal chromosome.
b. A 6-year-old girl with Angelman syndrome, characterized by severe mental retardation, seizures, jerky movements, and an enlarged jaw, is found on cytogenetic analysis to have a small interstitial deletion of her maternally-derived chromosome 15.
c. DNA analysis of the *FMR1* gene in a 32-year-old, clinically normal woman reveals one allele with 21 CGG repeats in the first exon and one allele with 92 repeats. She is counseled that she has a significant risk of having a child affected with the fragile X syndrome.

Chapter 8: Answers

1. The difference is the position of the centromere. In metacentrics, the centromere approximately bisects the chromosome. In submetacentric chromosomes, the two arms are different in size. In acrocentric chromosomes, the centromere is very near one end. The very small p arms of acrocentric chromosomes contain stalks and satellites, the location of rRNA genes.

2. b and c are aneuploid.
   a. There are six possibilities:
      Gametes with 23 normal chromosomes; Gametes with a balanced chromosome arrangement (both the derivative 11 and derivative 22); Gametes with a normal 22 and the derivative 11, resulting on fertilization with a normal sperm in partial trisomy for 22 and partial monosomy for 11; Gametes with a normal 11 plus derivative 22, resulting on fertilization in partial trisomy 11 and partial monosomy 22; Gametes with normal 11 plus derivative 11, resulting on fertilization in partial trisomy 11, partial monosomy 22; Gametes with normal 22 plus derivative 22, resulting on fertilization in partial trisomy 22, partial monosomy 11.
   b. Gametes either with 23 chromosomes (normal) or 24 with two chromosome 21. On fertilization with a normal sperm, this will yield a normal or a trisomy 21 individual, respectively.
   c. There are six possibilities:
      Normal gametes; Gametes with the Robertsonian translocation and no normal 13 or 21, resulting on fertilization in an individual with a balanced Robertsonian translocation; Gametes with 13;21 translocation and normal 21 resulting, on fertilization with a normal sperm, in trisomy 21; Gametes with 13;21 translocation and a normal 13, resulting on fertilization in trisomy 13; Gametes with a chromosome 13 and no 21, resulting in monosomy 21; Gametes with a chromosome 21 and no 13, resulting in monosomy 13.

3. Some chromosome abnormalities are not compatible with intrauterine development. Certain chromosome abnormalities may be seen in CVS samples at 9–10 weeks because it is so early that spontaneous loss of the pregnancy due to the chromosome abnormality may not have occurred yet. Also possible is that mosaicism for certain abnormalities may produce trophoblastic cells carrying an abnormal lineage in which the abnormality does not disrupt placental function while the fetus itself is actually chromosomally normal.

4. Assume the RFLP locus is very tightly linked to the centromere of chromosome 21. Because the child inherited both alleles from her father and only one from her mother, nondisjunction occurred in the father. Furthermore, because both alleles are present from the father, the nondisjunction event occurred in meiosis I.

5.
   a. This would result in sex reversal, a female with a Y chromosome.
   b. This would result in a form of pseudohermaphroditism in which gonadal sex is male (due to normal *SRY*) but internal and external

genitalia would not develop into normal male structures due to lack of androgen. Female internal genitalia would also not be present because the regression of female internal genital structures will occur, caused by factors other than steroid hormones (Müllerian inhibitory substance) produced by the male gonad. External genitalia are usually ambiguous.

c. This would result in testicular feminization, in which gonadal sex is male (due to normal *SRY*) but internal and external genitalia would not develop into normal male structures due to lack of androgen response. Female internal genitalia would also not be present because the regression of female internal genital structures will occur, caused by factors other than steroid hormones produced by the male gonad. Female external genitalia are normal.

6.

a. Homozygosity for hemophilia A mutations;

b. Turner syndrome with a mutation on the one X chromosome;

c. Balanced X;autosome translocation with the break through the hemophilia gene on the X chromosome and complete inactivation of the normal X;

d. Inactivation, by chance, of the normal X in the majority of cells making factor VIII, resulting in low levels of the clotting factor.

Finally, the possibility of a different disease, mimicking the clinical picture of hemophilia A but inherited as an autosomal trait, must be kept in mind. Type 2N von Willebrand disease, due to a mutation in the factor VIII binding domain of the von Willebrand factor, can cause a very similar clinical phenotype, including low plasma factor VIII levels.

7. The event is likely to have occurred post-conception.

8. Whole chromosome probes used to paint entire chromosomes are necessary to determine which chromosome segments have been exchanged. Centromeric probes give information only about the centromere of a given chromosome, and locus-specific probes would be useful only if one already suspected that chromosome segments containing those loci were involved in the translocation.

9. It is important for genetic counseling purposes to know if the cause of the Down syndrome is trisomy 21 or a translocation. If a translocation is responsible, the parents and other family members may be carriers and therefore at much greater risk for recurrence than if the parents have normal karyotypes and the child has trisomy 21. In addition, mosaicism for trisomy 21 may be found, which may affect the prognosis and counseling.

10. Barr body count will *not* suffice. It is important to determine if there is mosaicism for a Y chromosome bearing line, as in mixed gonadal dysgenesis, because individuals with a Turner phenotype and a cell line bearing a Y chromosome are at greatly increased risk for cancer in their dysgenetic gonads. Some prognostic information may also be obtained by an accurate karyotype.

*11. In the fragile X syndrome, triple repeat expansion in exon 1 results in hypermethylation and silencing of transcription of the *FMR1* gene and thus loss of function. In contrast, in Huntington disease, the triple repeat expansion involves the coding region and results in expression of a polyglutamine tract. Presumably this altered protein interacts with other cell components resulting in cellular abnormalities and disease. Therefore, this is an example of a gain of function mutation. The triple repeat expansion in myotonic dystrophy involves the 3′-untranslated region of the *DMPK* gene. Although this mutation may alter mRNA stability and thus affect the level of expression of this gene, the exact pathogenesis is as yet unknown.

12.
   a. Uniparental disomy
   b. Genomic imprinting
   c. Premutation

Chapter 9: Questions

1. Inspect the somatic cell hybrid panel below. Where does gene H appear to map?

Segregation of Gene H and Human Chromsomes in Human-Hamster Hybrids

Cell Hybrid	Gene H	1	2	3	4	5	6	7	8	9	10	11	12	13	14	15	16	17	18	19	20	21	22	Y	X
1	+	+	−	+	+	+	+	−	+	+	−	+	−	−	−	−	−	−	−	+	+	+	−	−	+
2	−	−	+	−	−	−	−	+	−	+	−	+	−	+	+	+	−	−	−	−	−	−	−	−	+
3	+	−	−	+	+	−	−	−	−	−	−	−	−	−	−	−	+	−	−	+	−	+	−	−	+
4	+	+	−	+	+	−	+	−	+	−	+	+	+	+	+	−	−	−	−	+	+	+	+	+	+
5	+	−	+	+	+	−	−	+	+	−	+	+	+	−	+	+	+	−	−	−	+	−	−	−	+
6	+	−	−	+	−	−	+	+	−	−	+	+	−	+	−	−	−	−	−	+	−	+	−	+
7	+	+	+	+	−	−	−	+	−	+	+	+	−	+	−	−	+	−	+	−	−	+	+	−	+
8	−	−	−	−	−	−	−	−	−	−	+	−	+	−	−	−	−	+	−	−	−	+	−	+
9	+	−	−	+	+	+	+	−	−	−	−	+	+	−	+	+	+	+	+	−	−	+	+	−	+
10	+	−	+	+	+	+	+	−	−	−	−	+	−	−	−	−	+	−	+	+	−	+	−	+	+

2. Observe the following lod score table for two markers. Graph these lod scores. What is the maximum likelihood estimate for θ? What is the lod score at that θ? Are these two markers tightly linked, loosely linked, unlinked? What can you conclude from the data?

θ	LOD
0	−∞
0.05	−10.32
0.10	−1.48
0.15	2.74
0.20	4.45
0.25	4.88
0.30	4.37
0.35	3.73
0.40	2.56
0.50	0

3. Hereditary elliptocytosis is an autosomal dominant disorder in which red blood cells have an abnormal elliptical shape and have a shortened life span, resulting in anemia due to increased destruction of red blood cells in the spleen.

In one large family, you observe the following lod scores in a linkage study between the Rh blood group on chromosome 1 and elliptocytosis:

a. What can you conclude about the relative location of elliptocytosis and the Rh locus?

θ	LOD
0	$-\infty$
0.05	4.74
0.10	5.44
0.15	5.35
0.20	4.89
0.25	4.22
0.30	3.39
0.35	2.49
0.40	1.54
0.50	0

In a second family, the following lod score results are found:

θ	LOD
0	$-\infty$
0.05	-2.9
0.10	-1.44
0.15	-0.73
0.20	-0.34
0.25	-0.12
0.30	-0.01
0.35	0.03
0.40	0.02
0.50	0

b. What can you conclude concerning the elliptocytosis and the Rh blood group loci in this family?

c. Give two explanations for the different results seen with these two families.

*4. Assume that the Hungtington disease (HD) gene had not been mapped in 1983 and subsequently cloned in 1993. Briefly describe how you would go about cloning the HD gene, using the methods and reagents available today.

5. Lict at least 3 different ways that the gene responsible for a human disease can be assigned to a specific chromosome without the use of linkage analysis to known genetic markers.

6. A and B are two families with sickle cell anemia. The affected probands (A II-1 and B II-1) are shown in red.

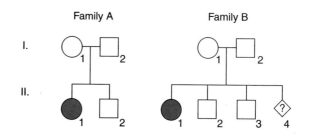

Family A   Family B

Genotype analyses by PCR for 3 RFLPs within the β-globin locus are shown below. PCR products spanning each polymorphic site were digested with the corresponding restriction enzyme and run on the gel.

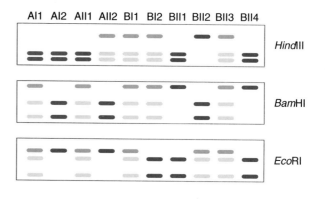

AI1 AI2 AII1 AII2 BI1 BI2 BII1 BII2 BII3 BII4

*Hind*III

*Bam*HI

*Eco*RI

a. Determine the two β-globin gene haplotypes for all the individuals in each pedigree. Denote absence of a restriction site in a given allele as "−" and presence of the site as "+".

b. What is/are the haplotype(s) for the sickle chromosome(s)? What does this tell you about the origin of the sickle mutation chromosomes in these families?

c. Is fetus B II-4 affected with sickle cell anemia? How certain are you? How could you confirm your conclusion?

d. Which individuals are sickle carriers? Are you certain of these assignments? How could they be confirmed?

Chapter 9: Answers

1. Gene H appears to map to chromosome 3, as this is the only chromosome where there is complete concordance.

2. The maximum likelihood estimate is at θ = 0.25, with a lod score of 4.88. The two markers are clearly linked with a lod score greater than 3, but there is significant recombination (25%) between them.

3.

a. The disease locus is linked to Rh in the first family. The maximum likelihood estimate is at θ = 0.10, with a lod score of 5.44.

b. The disease locus appears unlinked to Rh in this second family.

c. One possible explanation is that there are two loci for this disease, one of which is linked to Rh and one of which is not (locus heterogeneity). Another possibility is that the data are simply too limited. For example, at 10% recombination, log of odds against linkage is -1.44, or 27:1 against. At a larger value of θ, however, odds against linkage are not that high. The two data sets could represent samples of families with disease due to mutations at the same locus, but linkage is actually not as tight as the example in the first family suggests. Note that the Rh blood group and elliptocytosis are not determined by the same gene. The lod scores of $-\infty$ at $\theta=0$ indicate that there are recombinants in both families between the Rh blood group gene and the locus responsible for elliptocytosis.

*4. A search for the HD gene with today's methods would begin with a "genome scan" using a panel of markers spaced every 10–20 cM. DNA from large HD pedigrees, such as that shown in Figure 9.26, would be genotyped for these markers by PCR and the data analyzed by specialized computer programs to map the HD gene. Once the gene has been mapped, additional markers in the identified chromosomal segment would be used to type all available HD families to narrow down the candidate interval to the smallest possible region. Given the available HD pedigrees and the large number of current markers, it should be possible to reduce the interval to ≤ 1 cM. All genes known to lie within this candidate interval would then be analyzed. If necessary, physical cloning methods would be used to obtain YACs and BACs spanning the candidate region and additional genes lying within these clones would be identified using a variety of techniques. These various candidate genes would be analyzed by DNA sequencing, comparing patient and control DNAs. The identification of the HD triplet repeat expansion in all patient samples and in none of the controls would provide strong evidence that the authentic HD gene had been found.

5.

(i) X-linked inheritance. The observation that a human disease exhibits an X-linked pattern of inheritance places the responsible gene on the X chromosome.

(ii) Human disease genes are occasionally mapped through the identification of a patient with a cytogenetically identifiable deletion on a specific chromosome. Rare patients affected by two or more genetic conditions may be explained by a deletion removing several closely positioned genes (a contiguous gene syndrome, such as in patient BB described in Chapter 9).

(iii) A specific chromosome translocation disrupting the disease gene and leading to the phenotype in a rare patient may point to the gene location.

(iv) Finally, for the many human disease genes identified by functional cloning, the cloned sequences can be used to place the gene on a human chromosome by analysis of somatic cell hybrids or *in situ* hybridization techniques, such as FISH.

6.

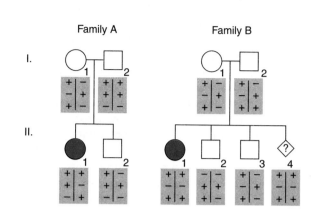

a. For each of the restriction enzymes, absence of the polymorphic restriction site ("−") results in a single large band in the restriction digest shown on the gel and presence of the site ("+") results in the
digestion of this large band to two smaller bands. Heterozygous individuals show all three bands. The bands in the homozygous individuals are darker since they contain twice as much DNA, representing both alleles. Thus, the genotypes for all the individuals can
be directly deduced from the gels. For all enzymes, those individuals with a single, dark, large band are −/−, those individuals with
only the two dark smaller bands are +/+, and the individuals with
all three bands are +/−. The next problem is to assign phase; that
is, which HindIII allele type goes with which BamHI allele type, etc.
For example, AI-2 is homozygous for all three restriction enzymes.
Thus, both chromosomes must have the haplotype ++− (HindIII,
BamHI, EcoRI). For individual AII-1, both haplotypes are + for
HindIII, but there is both a + and a − for BamHI and a + and a −
EcoRI. Figuring out the phase is determining which BamHI + or −
goes with which EcoRI. This can be deduced by looking at the parents. AII-1 must have inherited a ++− allele from his mother (AI-2).
Therefore, the other allele must be +−+ from the father. Similarly,
knowing that the father has one +−+ allele, his other allele can be
deduced to be −+−. Looking at AII-2, both haplotypes are + for
BamHI and − for EcoRI and since the HindIII is heterozygous, the
two haplotypes must be −+− and ++−. In this way, the phases can
be established for this family. Similarly, BII-1 is homozygous for the
+−+ haplotype. Since each of the two parents must have contributed a +−+ allele, you can deduce that BI-1's other allele is
−+− and BI-2's other allele is −++. BII-2 can be immediately seen
to be −++ and −+−, and BII-4, identical to BII-1, is homozygous
+−+. BII-3 is a little tricky since he is heterozygous for all three enzymes. However, looking at his parents, the + HindIII must be associated with a − BamHI and a + EcoRI and thus his two haplotypes
are +−+ and −+−. This is exactly how haplotypes are assigned at
any locus for the purpose of genetic testing or prenatal diagnosis.

b. Simply looking at the two affected individuals, AII-1 and BII-1, two
sickle chromosome haplotypes are evident. BII-1 is homozygous for
the +−+ haplotype and AII-1 has the same +−+ haplotype on one

chromosome and a $++-$ on the other chromosome. This is an example of linkage disequilibrium. The $+-+$ haplotype appears to be a common one, associated with sickle cell mutation alleles in three of the four parents. The $++-$ haplotype could possibly represent a recombination between the mutation and the *Bam*HI and *Eco*RI polymorphisms. Alternatively, it could represent a second independent occurrence of the sickle mutation, with the first event occurring on a $+-+$ haplotype background and the second on a $++-$ haplotype background. In fact, it appears that the sickle mutation has indeed occurred on four different haplotype backgrounds probably indicating four independent evolutionary origins.

c. Fetus BII-4 has inherited the same two sickle haplotype chromosomes from each parent as has the affected child BII-1. Thus, it is highly likely that the fetus has inherited sickle cell anemia. However, to be absolutely certain, one simply needs to directly look for the presence of the mutation using PCR, followed by ASO analysis or restriction digestion.

d. All four parents are obligate carriers (AI-1, AI-2, BI-1, BI-2). In addition, BII-3 has inherited the maternal sickle chromosome and thus should also be a carrier. BII-2 has inherited both normal parental alleles and is not a carrier. AII-2 inherited a $++$-allele from the mother, but since both her sickle chromosome as well as her normal chromosome have the same haplotype, one cannot distinguish which has been inherited by this child. Thus, there is a 50/50 chance of this individual being a carrier. Again, the actual mutation could be assessed as described above.

Chapter 10: Questions

1. One of the major arguments for the Human Genome Project has been the expected economy of scale in tackling the three billion base pair human genome in an organized fashion. For example, the average small molecular biology laboratory can sequence DNA at a cost of about $5.00 per finished base pair.

    a. At this efficiency, what would it cost to sequence the human genome in a "cottage industry" effort by parcelling the work out to small laboratories?

    b. In 1997, the most efficient genome centers can sequence at about $0.50/bp. What now would be the cost of sequencing the human genome? If this is spread over 9 years, what is the cost per year, and what percent does this represent of the total annual budget of the U.S. National Institutes of Health ($12 billion)?

    c. Technology development continues to drive down sequencing cost. How much is saved by each reduction of $0.01/bp?

2. Positional cloning of the cystic fibrosis gene (Chapter 19) required almost ten years of work. With the completion of the Human Genome Project such efforts will proceed much more rapidly. In the table below, fill out the actual steps an investigator had to carry out in the 1980's (pre-HGP) and what will be needed after the complete sequence is obtained (post-HGP).

Step	Pre-HGP	Post-HGP
Family collection		
Linkage analysis		
Physical mapping of region		
Identification of candidate genes		
Search for mutations		

3. You want to develop an STS from the region denoted "STS2" in Fig. 10.4.
   a. What primers would you make (be specific about 5' and 3' ends)
   b. How would you test those primers to see if they amplify a unique site in the human genome?

4. You are trying to construct a physical map of a region containing an important disease gene. You have made 5 STSs (S1-S5) but you don't know their order. Using those STSs you screen a YAC library and find 4 YACs that contain one or more of the STSs, as shown in the table below:

YAC	S1	S2	S3	S4	S5
A	+	−	+	+	−
B	−	+	−	−	+
C	−	−	+	+	−
D	+	+	−	−	−

   a. Construct a physical map (in the format of Fig. 10.5) from this data.
   b. What can you say about the overlap of YACs B and D? C and D? B and C?
   c. Can you orient this "contig" on the chromosome (i.e., can you determine which end is centromeric and which is telomeric) from this data?
   d. Could you orient the contig if S4 and S5 were also microsatellite markers, and S4 had been shown to be 4 cM distal to S5 on chromosome 11q?

5. At the outset of the Human Genome Project some argued that a uniform source of DNA should be used by all laboratories. Ideally, such a resource should be free of polymorphism, which means it should essentially be haploid. What about the following sources:
   a. Sperm
   b. Hydatidiform mole (an abnormal pregnancy where no fetus forms, only a grape-like mass of placental tissue usually found to have arisen from loss of the female pronucleus at conception, so the karyotype is 23,Y; occasionally metastasizes).

*6. The sequences of more than 400,000 human ESTs have been partially determined and deposited in a public database. Analysis of these sequences suggest that they arise from about 42,000 independent transcripts, almost half of the expected total. Since these sequences include part or most of the coding region of those genes, why do we need a Human Genome Project to sequence all the genomic DNA? Why bother with the junk?

Chapter 10: Answers

1. a. $15 billion
    b. $1.5 billion; $167 million; 1.4% (note this is an overestimate since the U.S. Department of Energy and other countries will also be participating in sequencing)
    c. $30 million

2.

Step	Pre-HGP	Post-HGP
Family collection	Ascertainment and careful phenotyping of pedigrees.	No change.
Linkage analysis	RFLPs—slow, poorly informative, holes in the map, 2 years of work.	Complete genetic map and automated genotyping readily available.
Physical mapping of region	Must handcraft a physical map (usually of YACs), with no prior milemarkers. Takes 1–2 years.	Already done and publicly available.
Identification of candidate genes	Must scan YACs or other clones of region for evidence of exons. Methods imperfect, intron/exon structure of genes difficult to obtain. Takes 1–2 years.	Already done—computer analysis of sequence of interval reveals nearly all genes, intron/exon structure, interesting homologies.
Search for mutations	Required manual sequencing of candidate genes in normals and affecteds. Often 1–2 years of work if mutations are subtle.	Mutation detection technology greatly facilitated by automation.

3. a. Primer 1   5'GGATTCCGACTAGGTCGGTCTT 3'
        Primer 2   5'ATAGCCAATACCTAGCTAATCC 3'
    b. To see whether the primer works, amplify human genomic DNA (using Taq polymerase, see Chapter 5). Run a gel of the products—you should get a single band of the size predicted from the sequence of this region. To be sure that this sequence is not also on other chromosomes (i.e., repetitive), also amplify a somatic cell hybrid (Chapter 9) containing only the chromosome of interest, and another hybrid containing several other human chromosomes but not the one where STS2 should map. The former should give a band of the expected size, the latter should give no product. (In reality, occasional STSs that pass this test still turn out not to be unique, because they derive from repetitive sequences present on only a single chromosome).

4. a.

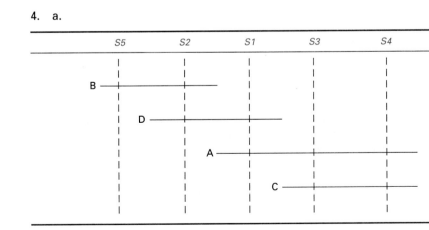

    b. B and D definitely overlap
        C and D may or may not overlap
        B and C cannot overlap

    c. From the data above, the contig cannot be oriented

    d. With this additional information, the order of the map above is centromere to the left, telomere to the right.

5. a. While a single sperm is haploid, the millions of sperm in a specimen sufficient to prepare DNA for the genome project contain all possible alleles—thus the DNA prep from a ejaculate is no less polymorphic than a lymphocyte DNA prep from the same male.

   b. A 23,Y hydatidiform male is truly haploid. However, there are reasons to believe that somatic mutations are present to allow the survival of tissue with such an abnormal karyotype, so this may be a risky source of material intended to represent the normal human genome.

*6. There are several reasons why the complete genomic sequence is needed, even though the EST sequences are of great utility (especially if mapped):

   a. cDNAs of low abundance or expressed only in inaccessible tissues or brief windows of development will be poorly represented.

   b. EST sequences will not reveal gene structure (intron/exon boundaries) or regulatory sequences (promoters, enhancers). This information is often critical in assessing the role a gene plays in disease.

   c. For large transcripts, the 5′ end is usually not obtained by the EST strategy (since the cDNAs are primed at the 3′ end, and it is difficult to obtain cDNAs longer than 3–4 kb).

   d. EST sequences will reveal little about chromosome structure and evolution, and nothing about potential functions of non-transcribed sequence (centromeres, telomeres, origins of replication, etc.).

Chapter 11: Questions

1. Name four mechanisms implicated in the activation of a proto-oncogene.

2. Explain why a patient with sporadic retinoblastoma usually has a single focus of tumor growing in one eye, while hereditary retinoblastoma often occurs in both eyes or at multiple sites in one eye.

3. A cancer develops in a patient who has inherited a germline mutation in a tumor suppressor gene. Analysis of normal and tumor DNA from the patient demonstrates loss of heterozygosity (LOH) for a polymorphism within the tumor suppressor gene.

   a. List 3 mechanisms that could account for this LOH.

   b. Analysis of a second, independent cancer from the same patient fails to identify LOH. How could this observation be explained?

4. Why do genetic disorders of DNA repair seem to predispose to malignancy?

*5.

   a. A 25 year old woman consults you because of her strong family history of cancer. Her mother underwent a mastectomy for breast cancer at age 35 and died of ovarian cancer at age 50. One of the patient's two maternal aunts also died of breast cancer at age 37. List some of the potential advantages and disadvantages of DNA testing for BRCA gene mutations in this patient.

b. If the patient were of Ashkenazi Jewish origin, would that change your answer?

Chapter 11: Answers

1. Four mechanisms implicated in the activation of a proto-oncogene are:
   a. Point mutation that interferes with normal control of the oncogene product;
   b. Amplification leading to overexpression of the oncogene product;
   c. Chromosome translocation that places a heterologous promoter upstream of the oncogene, resulting in overexpression;
   d. Chromosome translocation that produces a hybrid protein, part of which is the oncogene product that lacks a portion of the protein needed for normal regulation.

2. In sporadic retinoblastoma, both alleles in the same cell must undergo mutation to produce disease. Because it is unlikely that more than one cell will undergo such a rare event, the disease is unlikely to occur at more than one focus. In contrast, the hereditary form arises from a single mutation that affects the only remaining normal allele in a cell that already has one defective allele. With the probability of this second event sufficiently high, neoplastic transformation can occur in many cells and produce multifocal, bilateral disease.

3. a. The various mechanisms for inactivation of the normal allele in a patient carrying a germline mutation in a tumor suppressor gene are shown in Figure 11.15. The 3 mechanisms which result in LOH are (i) loss of the normal chromosome, (ii) chromosome loss and reduplication, and (iii) mitotic crossover between the normal chromosome and that carrying the mutated gene.
   b. The normal allele could also be inactivated by an independent mutation event. Combined with the germline mutation on the other allele, the result is complete loss of the tumor suppressor gene function and the development of a tumor, though LOH is not seen.

4. One reasonable explanation is that the increased mutation rate seen in these disorders results in mutation of cellular oncogenes, which become activated and cause neoplastic transformation.

*5. a. The family history of both breast and ovarian cancer in the patient's mother and the onset of these cancers at a young age in both the mother and the mother's sister is strongly suggestive of a BRCA1 or BRCA2 gene mutation. The advantages of DNA testing include more accurate assessment of the patient's risk for developing breast or ovarian cancer. Identification of a germline mutation in the patient would give her a 60–90% lifetime risk of developing breast cancer and a 20–60% risk for ovarian cancer. If the presence of a mutation could be excluded, this would reduce her risk to those of the general population (11% for breast cancer and 1.4% for ovarian cancer). Although no specific intervention is of proven benefit in preventing breast or ovarian cancer in high risk patients, options would include more frequent surveillance examinations and pro-phylactic surgery. The patient might also wish to have this infor-mation for reasons of life planning.

Disadvantages include the potential negative emotional impact of the test results, the high cost of testing, and the potential for ad-verse effects on the availability or cost of health insurance and em-ployability. It is important to note that neither of the affected rela-tives is available for testing. Thus, failure to identify a mutation in the patient would only modestly decrease her risk. A negative test result could mean either that the patient has not inherited the mu-tation or that the mutation in this family is not detected by the cur-rent analysis. In contrast, if a mutation could first be identified in an affected relative, then absence of this mutation in the patient would reduce her risk to that of the general population. It is for this reason that it is much preferred to begin analysis on an individual in the family who is known to be affected. It is sometimes possible to per-form DNA diagnostic testing on pathology specimens that might be available from deceased relatives, although such studies are still primarily restricted to the research laboratory.

b.   As noted in Chapter 11, one specific BRCA1 and two BRCA2 muta-tions appear to account for the vast majority of BRCA mutations in the Ashkenazi Jewish population. Thus, negative screening analy-sis in this population can be of considerably greater value, even in the absence of an affected individual for initial testing.

Chapter 12: Questions

1.   Interview with Thomas Smith, Jr.: *Doctor, my wife Alice and I are plan-ning on starting a family and we would like to know whether there is any risk to our children for having the nerve problem that seems to be in my family.*

My older brother, Don, started having muscle weakness and loss of sensation in his legs and feet when he was a teenager. These got pro-gressively worse until he had to go on disability ten years ago when he was 25 years old. When his problems first began, my mother told us that these problems seemed very similar to ones that my father's brother Fred Smith (age 68) and sister Sally (age 63) have, although our father, Tom, and his half brother and sister, the twins Eddie and Jane (age 73), never were bothered with these problems.

My cousins Frank and Bill seem healthy. They are in their twenties. Their father, my uncle Fred Smith, is one of my relatives with the leg muscle weakness and numbness. Cousin Frank, the older one, is mar-ried but doesn't have any children although I think his wife had a mis-carriage last year. My aunt Sally has one daughter, Linda, who also seems to have the leg weakness problem and is worried about her two children, Dick and Bob.

My father, Thomas Smith, Sr., died in an auto accident when he was 40 years old. He was the youngest in the family. His parents are dead. His father, William, was a healthy man who died of some heart problem in his 80's. His first wife died in childbirth with Eddie and Jane. His sec-

ond wife, Mary, was my grandmother. I never knew her but everyone said she always complained of 'pins and needles' in her feet and she got so weak at the end that she was in a wheelchair.

Alice's family is very healthy. Her father and mother are still alive, as are her three sisters and two brothers.

Draw the pedigree of the family portrayed above. What kind of inheritance pattern do you think the described trait is following? What else do you learn about the disease from taking this family history?

2. Why is a careful physical examination and family history an essential part of the management of a child with birth defects?

3. Choose the most appropriate diagnostic procedures and tests from the following list that are applicable to the prenatal diagnosis of the conditions labeled a through g. Numbered items may be used more than once and more than one numbered item may be used for each lettered conditon.
    1. Amniocentesis
    2. Chorionic villus sampling
    3. Ultrasonography
    4. Cytogenic analysis
    5. Southern blot
    6. PCR
    7. Allele-specifc oligonucleotide hybridization
    8. Linkage-based analysis using intragenic DNA polymorphisms

    a. Congenital myotonic dystrophy
    b. Fragile X syndrome
    c. Myelomeningocele
    d. Hemophilia A
    e. Huntington disease
    f. β-thalassemia
    g. Trisomy 13

4. Jane is a 26-year-old woman whose brother died of cystic fibrosis. Her husband Dick, also of Northern European extraction, is unrelated. Assume that the frequency of cystic fibrosis in the Northern European population is 1/2500. What is the probability that Jane is a carrier of cystic fibrosis? What is the probability that Dick is a carrier of cystic fibrosis? What is the risk that, in any pregnancy, a child will be affected with cystic fibrosis?

    Jane and Dick decide to undergo carrier testing, which, by testing for 70 of the more common mutations, can identify 90% of Northern European Caucasian carriers of cystic fibrosis. Assume that the test has no false positives. Jane's test is negative for any of the 70 CF mutations; what is her risk of being a carrier? Dick's test is positive. Now what is the risk to any child that Dick and Jane might have?

    Jane and Dick separate and divorce. Dick marries Jane's first cousin Laura. What is the risk that Laura is a carrier of cystic fibrosis and what is the couple's risk that any child born to Dick and Laura will be affected with cystic fibrosis?

5. The population of Ann Arbor (approximately 100,000) is offered a free screening test to detect carriers of a serious autosomal recessive

disease. The disease has an incidence of approximately 1/10,000 in the general population. The test is offered in a large shopping mall.

A 24-year-old man consults you. He is extremely upset and distraught. He has taken the screening test and been told that he has a positive result. He is convinced he is a carrier, despite having no family history of the disease. When you try to reassure him, he says "Don't bother. I was told this test has 98% sensitivity and 90% specificity. With that level of sensitivity the result must be correct!" What is the probability that this man is *not* a carrier of the disease for which he has been tested?

A 20-year-old woman, who has a brother affected with the disease, has had this same screening test and consults you. She is one of a group of 300 individuals who are unaffected siblings of affected individuals who have had carrier testing. She has a negative test result and wonders whether that indicates that she is really not a carrier. What is the probability that she *is* actually a carrier?

Chapter 12: Answers

1. The nerve problem described in this family appears to be inherited as an autosomal dominant disorder, which shows considerable variation in severity and age of onset (variable expressivity). The fact that Tom, Sr., who died in an automobile accident at age 40, did not manifest any signs of this disease suggests that the age of onset would have been later in him than in his affected son, Don. Although the age of onset appears to be getting earlier in subsequent generations, one cannot draw conclusions about whether or not this represents anticipation based on a single family. The arrow with the letter P refers to the proband, Don, the individual whose disease first brought the family to medical attention, and the arrow marked C is the consultand, the individual who came for genetic consultation even though he himself is not apparently affected at this time. The *red* symbols indicate individuals affected with this disorder.

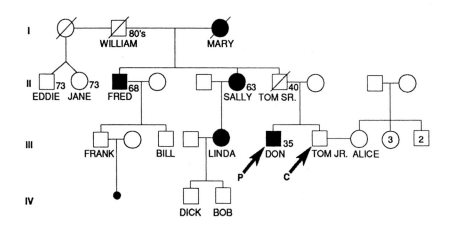

2. Obviously, a careful physical examination is essential for assessing the nature and severity of the birth defects, for attempting to give a prog-

nosis, and for planning appropriate surgical and/or other therapy. Equally important, however, the examination is an essential part of making an accurate diagnosis. It is important to document whether there is an isolated congenital anomaly or multiple anomalies, and whether multiple anomalies might be causally or pathogenetically related, as in a sequence or syndrome. An accurate diagnosis is important for providing genetic counseling, for informing parents if there is a risk of recurrence of this problem in subsequent pregnancies, and for offering counseling and intervention to other relatives who might also be at risk. The combination of the physical examination and a careful family history can also help determine which diagnostic studies, such as cytogenetic or molecular analysis, are important for diagnosis and assessing risk in patients and in other family members.

3.
   a. 1, 2, and 5.
   b. 1, 2, and 5. 6 (PCR) is useful for characterizing premutation state.
   c. 1 and 3.
   d. 1, 2, 5, and 8.
   e. 1, 2, and 6.
   f. 1, 2, and 7.
   g. 1, 2, and 4.

4. The unaffected sibling of a patient with an autosomal recessive disease such as cystic fibrosis has a 2/3 chance of being a carrier of the disease. Dick, who has no family history of CF, has a risk based on the population frequency of cystic fibrosis. Given a disease frequency of CF of 1/2500, the gene frequency (lumping all CF mutations together) is $\sqrt{1/2500} = 0.02$ or 1/50. Assuming Hardy-Weinberg equilibrium, the carrier frequency is $2pq = 2(0.02)(0.98) = 0.04$ or 1/25. The risk that both Jane and Dick are carriers is therefore (2/3) (1/25), and the risk of having an affected child in any pregnancy is 1/4 (2/3) (1/25) = 1/150 or approximately .0067 or 0.7%.

Taking into account the additional information about the DNA testing on Jane and Dick requires applying Bayes' theorem. This conditional probability calculation can be set up as shown below.

	Jane is a carrier	Jane is not a carrier
Prior risk	2/3	1/3
Conditional probability (negative test)	1/10	1
Joint probability	2/30	1/3 or 10/30
Posterior probability	$\dfrac{2/30}{2/30 + 10/30} = 1/6$	$\dfrac{10/30}{2/30 + 10/30} = 5/6$

Therefore, given her negative test result, Jane's risk of being a carrier is now 1/6 or 0.17. Dick, who had a positive test, is now known to be a carrier. Therefore the risk to any child is 1/4 (1/6) (1) = 1/24 or approximately 4%. Note that even though Jane's carrier test was negative, because of her high *a priori* risk (2/3), and because the sensitivity of the test is considerably less than 100%, she still has a 17% risk of being a carrier.

Both of Jane's parents must be heterozygous carriers of cystic fibrosis. Therefore Jane's first cousin has a 1/4 chance of also being a carrier. Because Dick is known from DNA testing to be a carrier, the risk for any children that Dick and Laura have is 1/4 (1/4) (1) = 1/16, or approximately 6%. Obviously Laura's risk could be modified by DNA testing as well.

5. This question can be answered using either a Bayesian conditional probability analysis, or a 2 × 2 grid as shown in Tables 12.6, 12.7, and 12.8.

    The man's prior risk of being a carrier, given the absence of any family history, is the population-based risk. Again, assuming Hardy-Weinberg equilibrium, if the frequency of the disease is 1/10,000, the frequency of the mutant allele (taking all mutant alleles as if they were one) is 1/100 and the frequency of heterozygous carriers 2 (1/100) (99/100) $\doteq$ 198/10,000 or approximately 1/50 or 2%. The woman who has an affected sibling has a 2/3 prior risk of being a carrier. Recall that 98% sensitivity means that there is a 98% probability that a true carrier will have a positive test and a 2% probability that a true carrier will have a negative test; a 90% specificity indicates that there is a 90% probability that a non-carrier will have a negative test but a 10% probability that a non-carrier will have a positive test.

Bayesian analysis:

	Man is a carrier	Man is not a carrier
Prior risk	0.02	0.98
Conditional probability (positive test)	0.98	0.10
Joint probability	0.020	0.098
Posterior probability	$\frac{0.020}{0.020 + 0.098} = \frac{0.020}{0.118} = 0.17$	$\frac{0.098}{0.098 + 0.020} = 0.83$

2 × 2 grid, screening for heterozygous carriers in the general population (100,000 people screened):

	Carrier	Non-carrier	Total
Positive test	1,960	9,800	11,760
Negative test	40	88,200	88,240
Total	2,000	98,000	100,000

9,800/11,760 = 83%

Despite the very high sensitivity of the screening test, because the frequency of carriers in the general population is quite low, the majority of individuals with positive tests will represent false positives rather than true carriers. Thus, this man's risk of actually *not* being a carrier is 83%. In contrast, when the prior risk of being a carrier is high, as it is for the unaffected sibling of an affected individual, then the vast majority of positive tests indicate true carriers (196/206 or 95% in the case shown below). Because the sensitivity of the test is not 100%, however, there is still a low risk (4%) that carriers will be missed.

Bayesian analysis:

	Woman is a carrier	Woman is not a carrier
Prior probability	2/3	1/3
Conditional probability (negative test)	1/50	9/10 or 45/50
Joint probability	2/150	45/150
Posterior probability	$\dfrac{2/150}{2/150 + 45/150} = 2/47 = 4\%$	$\dfrac{45/150}{2/150 + 45/150} = 45/47 = 96\%$

2×2 grid, screening for heterozygous carriers among siblings of affecteds (300 sibs screened):

	Carrier	Non-carrier	Total
Positive test	196	10	206
Negative test	4	90	94
Total	200	100	300

$$4/94 = 4\%$$

Finally, the distress suffered by the man with a positive carrier test indicates that carrier testing for genetic disease must not be carried out without concomitant counseling and education. Screening tests require careful interpretation to provide accurate and meaningful estimates of actual risk. Even more important, however, is the need for sensitive and supportive counseling. Tests for genetic susceptibility to disease, or for risk of transmitting a genetic disease, carry significant emotional content. It is not appropriate to offer such testing without requisite counseling services. These considerations are particularly important given the increasing availability of molecular diagnostic tests to assess genetic risks.

Chapter 13: Questions

*1. Briefly contrast the potential for gene therapy to treat hemophilia A and muscular dystrophy. Which do you think is more feasible over the next ten years? Why?

*2. Several patients with cystic fibrosis have been administered an inhaled aerosol to the lungs containing a replication defective adenovirus directing the expression of human CFTR. What problems might limit the effectiveness of this approach? What alternative approaches would you consider?

3.
Retrovirus
Adenovirus
Adeno-associated virus
Nonviral vector

Match each of the above gene therapy vectors with one of the following properties:
a.   No infectious risk
b.   Broad range of target cells and no requirement for cell division
c.   Potential for insertional mutagenesis
d.   Potential for site-specific chromosomal integration

4.

Inadvertent germline gene therapy
Somatic cell gene therapy
Intentional germline gene therapy

Match each of the above with one of the following descriptions:
a.   A patient is treated with an adenoviral vector directing expression of CFTR, administered through an aerosol. The patient's children, born 1 and 3 years after treatment, are all carriers of CF.
b.   A patient with ADA deficiency receives an autologous transplant of his own bone marrow cells, after *ex vivo* treatment with an ADA-expressing retrovirus. PCR analysis of DNA prepared from a sperm sample one year later detects retroviral DNA sequences.
c.   A zygote produced by *in vitro* fertilization undergoes correction of a point mutation by a targeted homologous recombination approach.

Chapter 13: Answers

*1. These two diseases are current targets for a variety of gene therapy approaches. Both genes are quite large, posing additional technical problems, but the muscular dystrophy locus is particularly difficult (dystrophin is approximately 450 kD (14kb mRNA) while Factor VIII is approximately 220 kD with a 9 kb mRNA). In order to treat muscular dystrophy, high levels of expression must be achieved specifically in muscle and there is a need for very high efficiency transduction of muscle cells.

In contrast, for hemophilia A, one must just get the protein into plasma and it could potentially come from any of a variety of different cell types including fibroblast, liver, muscle, or endothelial cells. Also precise regulation of expression is not at all critical and a wide range of levels would be tolerable. Even very low levels of expression (1 ng/ml) should be clinically useful. Taken together, hemophilia A, though also difficult, is probably an easier problem than muscular dystrophy and perhaps is more likely to succeed in the next few years.

*2. Obviously many investigators and patients participating in these trials believe that there is a significant probability of success, though there are a number of potential problems. The potential problems which might limit its effectiveness include the generally limited duration of adenovirus infection, since the DNA does not insert stably into the genome and instead exists as an episome within the cell. It is thus rapidly lost from dividing cells. In addition, infected cells may eventually be removed by the immune system. The exuberant immune response, in addition to potentially eliminating expressing cells, may also cause direct toxicity. In addition, immune response may preclude future treatment of the same patient with the same vector. There is a limitation to the size of what can be inserted into currently available adenovirus vectors, though CFTR has been effectively expressed in this way. Finally, the pathology of CF is not restricted only to the lungs and problems in other tissues would probably not be effectively addressed by this treatment. However, the lung is the major limiting organ for most patients. Alternative approaches include use of retroviral vectors either in vivo or ex vivo, and direct DNA infusion by aerosol into the lungs, potentially coupled to another agent to facilitate entry into cells (such as a liposome).

3.
   a. Non-viral vector
   b. Adenovirus
   c. Retrovirus
   d. Adeno-associated virus

4.
   a. Somatic cell gene therapy. The adenoviral vector is introduced only into the lung by the aerosol. Even if a rare particle were to be carried to the gonad, stable integration should not occur with an adenovirus. Thus germline transmission of vector sequences is very unlikely. Since cystic fibrosis is an autosomal recessive disease, the patient is homozygous (or compound heterozygous) for a mutation in the CFTR gene. Thus, all of his children are obligate heterozygotes.
   b. Inadvertent germline gene therapy. This experiment was designed as somatic cell gene therapy. However, the PCR results suggest that vector sequences inadvertently reached the gonad and were integrated into germ cells producing sperm.
   c. Intentional germline gene therapy. As discussed in Chapter 13, introduction of genetic alterations into the germline of humans is currently considered unacceptable by most scientists and physicians. However, the procedure described here is routinely performed in transgenic mouse experiments.

Chapter 14: Questions

*1. Referring to Case 1 (Fig. 14.1), how would the non-directive approach to the younger sister change if a highly effective and low-risk preventive strategy was developed for *BRCA1* mutation carriers?

*2. In Case 4 (Fig. 14.4), suppose the couple came in flatly requesting termination, feeling that they could not handle a fifth child. After talking with you, however, they realize that it would be possible to know the sex of the fetus by amniocentesis. If prenatal testing is not available, they will choose to terminate. If they are allowed to learn the fetal sex, they will allow a male pregnancy to go to term, but will terminate a female. Does this change your willingness to offer prenatal testing?

*3. Which of the following do you think a physician or genetic counselor should disclose before providing counseling?

A strong pro-life or pro-choice personal view;

Financial holdings in a company offering a test the patient is considering;

A research interest in the condition;

Personal familiarity with aspects of the pedigree, based on having previously counseled other family members.

*4. A pathologist interested in *BRCA1* has access to a large number of breast cancer samples which have been archived in the Hospital Surgical Pathology Laboratory. Using PCR it is possible to amplify DNA from such paraffin blocks and identify mutations. He studies 25 breast cancers and finds one in which a *BRCA1* mutation is present. Analyzing adjacent normal tissue in the block, he finds the same *BRCA1* mutation, indicating that it was present in the germline. Concerned that this woman may be at risk for additional cancers of breast or ovary, he requests her medical record, and then calls her on the phone to report his findings. Expecting to be thanked for his efforts, he is surprised when she questions how this could have been done without her consent. What ethical breach occurred here?

Chapter 14: Answers

*1. The non-directive stance of the provider is particularly important when there are several options of unproven benefit (as is currently the case for *BRCA1* mutation carriers). In that situation, respect for patient autonomy mitigates against a paternalistic "doctor knows best" approach. But if an intervention can be shown to be clearly beneficial, then the principle of beneficence may require the provider to be more directive. For example, a pediatrician confronted with a case of acute childhood meningitis should be VERY directive in advising IV antibiotics.

2. This subtle change in the prospective parents' presentation could have an effect on the provider's decision-making. More providers would probably acquiesce to the request for amnio if they were convinced the pregnancy would be definitely terminated without it.

*3. An open disclosure of a conflict of interest, when a provider may not be able to be completely objective, is worth considering. But it could also be distressing to the patient to learn of such conflicts if they are not really material to the case. In some instances (i.e., a research interest) the potential conflict of interest might actually turn out to provide a benefit. The non-directive stance which genetic counselors aim to adopt should theoretically prevent the outcome from being altered by provider bias—though this standard is not always achieved. Consulting with an objective colleague may be the wisest course for a provider who is aware that a potential conflict of interest may influence his/her judgement in a case. If the situation is such that the provider cannot really function in an unbiased way, the conflict of interest should be declared and another provider identified.

*4. The pathologist has carried out a research study on an identifiable sample without informed consent, thereby violating the patient's autonomy (her right to know has been overridden) and her privacy. Most observers agree that such unconsented research studies can only be allowed if personal identifiers are irreversibly stripped from the sample BEFORE the research is undertaken, so that it is not possible to identify the individual from whom the specimen was derived. If the individual is identifiable, however, even though the sample may be coded, informed consent is virtually always required.

Index

Page numbers in *italics* denote figures; those followed by "t" denote tables.

AAV. *See* Adeno-associated virus
ABL proto-oncogene, 255, *256*
ABMG. *See* American Board of Medical Genetics
Abortion
  requested for mild conditions, 332
  for sex selection, 332–333
  spontaneous
    amniocentesis and, 299, 335
    chorionic villus sampling and, 300
    due to chromosome abnormalities, 3, 153, 169–170, 170t, 301
    frequency of, 169
    as indication for chromosome analysis, 193
    percutaneous umbilical blood sampling and, 301
Achondroplasia, 26–27, *27*, 281
  diagnosis of, 283, *283*
  homozygous, 33
  mutation and, 48
  prenatal diagnosis to select for child affected by, 333–334
Acid phosphatase phenotypes, 52, *52*
Acute promyelocytic leukemia, 256
Acyl-CoA:cholesterol acyltransferase, 128
ADA deficiency. *See* Adenosine deaminase deficiency
Additivity principle, 284, 341
Adenine, 11, *12*
Adeno-associated virus (AAV), 316t, 318
Adenosine deaminase (ADA) deficiency, 308
  bone marrow transplantation for, 308, 323
  gene therapy for, 323
  immune deficiency due to, 323
  inheritance pattern of, 323
  prognosis for, 323
Adenoviruses, 88, 316t, 316–318, *317*
Advanced maternal age
  definition of, 298
  Down syndrome and, 3, 171, *172*, 282, 298
  as indication for amniocentesis, 298–299
  as indication for chorionic villus sampling, 300
  as indication for genetic counseling, 282
Age of expression of genetic diseases, *4*
Albinism, 117
Alkaptonuria, 117–120
  clinical features of, 117–118
  enzyme defect in, 118, *119*
  familial distribution of, 119
  historical studies of, 117–118
  homogentisic acid excretion in, 118
  inheritance pattern of, 119–120
  pigmentation in, 118, *118*
Alleles
  definition of, 23, 341

identical-by-descent sharing in siblings, 58, *59*
  population frequencies of, 33–34, 43–46, 44t, 45t (*See also* Hardy-Weinberg equilibrium)
  sickle cell, 50–51
Allele-specific oligonucleotides (ASOs), 84, *85*
  definition of, 341
  to diagnose α_1-antitrypsin deficiency, 126, *127*
  to diagnose hemophilia A, 84, *85*
Allelic heterogeneity, 28–29
  definition of, 28, 341
  of Ehlers-Danlos syndrome, 149
  of familial hypercholesterolemia, 29, 130, 132–135, *133*
  of glucose-6-phosphate dehydrogenase deficiency, 29, 123
  of osteogenesis imperfecta, 29
  of β-thalassemia, 29, 108
Alu repetitive sequence, 63, 131, 154, 252
  definition of, 341
  role in unequal crossing over, 131, *132*
Alzheimer disease
  Down syndrome and, 171, 173
  epsilon 4 allele of apolipoprotein E gene and, 58
  gene mapping in, 227
American Board of Genetic Counselors, 273, 290
American Board of Medical Genetics (ABMG), 273
American College of Medical Genetics, 240, 273
American Society of Human Genetics, 240
Americans with Disabilities Act, 240
Amino acids
  genetic code for, 14–15
  mutations and, 21–22
Amish, Ellis-van Creveld syndrome in, 47, *47*
Amniocentesis, 3, 292, 297–299
  appropriateness if pregnancy termination is not a consideration, 335
  cost-effectiveness of, 299
  definition of, 297, 341
  error rate for, 299
  genetic counseling for, 298
  indications for, 298t, 298–299
  procedure for, *297*, 298
  risks and complications of, 299, 335
  safety and accuracy of, 303
  timing of, 297–298
  ultrasonography for, 298, *298*
Amniotic fluid, 297
Amplicon, 345
Amplification
  definition of, 341
  oncogene activation due to, 254, *254*

by polymerase chain reaction, 73, 76, 77
Anaphase, *19*
Anemia
  Cooley's, 108, *108*, 112–113, *113*
  Fanconi, 177, 264
  glucose-6-phosphate dehydrogenase deficiency and, 117, 121
  sickle cell, 91, 96–102, *97–101* (*See also* Sickle cell anemia)
  thalassemias, 104–113,127
Anencephaly, 292
Aneuploidy
  definition of, 162, 341
  in Klinefelter syndrome, 185
Angelman syndrome (AS), 174
  clinical features of, 174
  molecular basis for, 174, *176*
  paternal uniparental disomy for chromosome 15 in, 175, *176*
Animal models, 58, 227–228, 238, 238t, 324
Ankylosing spondylitis, 50, 211
Antenatal diagnosis. *See* Prenatal diagnosis
Anticipation, 30–33
  definition of, 341
  in myotonic dystrophy, 30–32
Anticodon, 15
Antisense DNA, 322, 341
α_1-Antitrypsin
  definition of, 341
  gene for, 125, 126
    mutations of, 126
    Pi genotypes, 125, 125t
α_1-Antitrypsin deficiency, 124–127
  as ecogenetic disorder, 127
  inheritance pattern of, 127
  liver disease and, 125–126
  prenatal diagnosis of, 304
  prenatal DNA diagnosis of, 126, 127, *127*
  smoking, emphysema and, 117, 125, *126*, 307
  treatment of, 126–127
    gene therapy, 126–127
    intravenous α_1-antitrypsin, 307–308, *308*
    lung transplantation, 126
    purified human inhibitor therapy, 126
Aortic aneurysm, 150
APC gene
  colon cancer and, 262t, 266–268, *267*, 275, *336*
  screening for mutations of, 270
Apolipoprotein E gene, 58
Apoptosis, 256, 263, 341
AS. *See* Angelman syndrome
Ascertainment, 341
Ashkenazi Jews
  BRCA gene-related breast cancer in, 270–271, 295, 304–305
  cystic fibrosis in, 296
  familial hypercholesterolemia in, 130

395